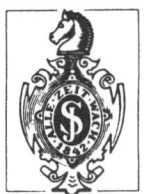

Angiocardiography
Current Status and Future Developments

Edited by
H. Just   P. H. Heintzen

With 323 Figures and 34 Tables

With Contributions by
H. E. Aldrige, J. S. Alpert, I. Amende, K. Bachmann,
R. Balcon, R. Brennecke, J. H. Bürsch, Ch. Chen, H. T. Dodge,
P. A. Doriot, G. Fredzell, H. Freudenberg, U. Gleichmann,
P. Heintzen, G. Hellige, F. W. Hofmann, T. E. H. Hooghoudt,
J. Jehle, H. Just, P. E. Lange, J. P. LeChevallier, P. Marhoff,
J. Meyer, K. L. Neuhaus, Y. Pochon, W. Rafflenbeul,
J. H. C. Reiber, W. Rogers, F. K. Schmiel, P. W. Serruys,
C. J. Slager, U. Sigwart, R. Simon, J. F. Spann, P. Spiller,
T. v. Volkmann, H. Woelke, E. Zeitler

Springer-Verlag
Berlin Heidelberg New York
London Paris Tokyo

Prof. Dr. H. Just
Med. Universitätsklinik
Abt. Innere Medizin
– Kardiologie –
Hugstetter Straße 55
7800 Freiburg i. Br.

Prof. Dr. P. H. Heintzen
Klinikum der Universität Kiel
Abt. Kinderkardiologie und Biomedizinische Technik
Kinderklinik
Schwanenweg 20
2300 Kiel 1

ISBN 978-3-662-00822-5   ISBN 978-3-662-00820-1 (eBook)
DOI 10.1007/978-3-662-00820-1

© Springer-Verlag Berlin Heidelberg 1986
Softcover reprint of the hardcover 1st edition 1986

2119/3140-543210

Preface

Angiocardiography has undergone tremendous development. It currently represents the imaging system offering the highest resolution and greatest detail information.

A widely applicable, complex technique able to meet high standards was required by the increasing number of coronary bypass interventions as well as by the advent of interventional catheter techniques, such as transluminal percutaneous catheter balloon dilatation, recanalization techniques, and intracoronary thrombolytic procedures. At the same time, improved image resolution began to furnish information on intracoronary flow dynamics and anatomy, thereby opening a new avenue of acquiring prognostically and therapeutically important pathophysiologic information. In spite of rapid improvements in the equipment, there are still demands for improved resolution, image quality, and methods of image processing.

In this situation, the need was felt to describe the current status of equipment, angiocardiographic systems, image intensifiers, photographic materials, and processing techniques. Furthermore, the attempt was made to describe evaluation techniques using manual or computer-assisted semi- or fully automated procedures to estimate left ventricular volumes, ventricular mass, cardiac function, anatomy, and flow dynamics of the coronary arterial system. This book assembles original work presented at a symposium held by the European Society of Cardiology, the *Deutsche Gesellschaft für Herz- und Kreislaufforschung,* and the *Deutsche Gesellschaft für Biomedizinische Technik.* It was the aim of the symposium to outline the current state of the art and to define a process for further improvement.

It is our hope that the material assembled in this book gives an overview of what is currently available and what can be done with angiocardiography. In spite of the advent of newer, noninvasive imaging techniques, such as echocardiography, computer tomography, and magnetic resonance imaging, angiocardiography has remained the gold standard for the delineation and quantification of anatomical detail and the analysis of heart function. In addition the experience gained with digital angiocardiography will in all probability improve imaging techniques as far as the presentation of detail and quantification is concerned.

We are grateful to the Bayer Pharmaceutical Company, Leverkusen, and especially for the help and understanding of Dr. Günther Albus, whose continued support has made the symposium and the publication possible.

P. Heintzen, Kiel   *H. Just,* Freiburg

Table of Contents

Equipment for Angiocardiography

G. FREDZELL

Research and Development (Röntgen), Siemens-Elema AB, Solna, Sweden

When Forssmann, in 1929 in Berlin, introduced a catheter into his own right auricle via a cubital vein, he performed the first heart catheterization. He failed, however, to visualize the chambers of the heart when in 1931 he injected an iodide solution. The first researchers who managed to outline the right heart (in children) were Castellanos et al. in Havana, in 1937.

Robb and Steinberg (in New York) successfully visualized the right and left heart as well as parts of the great vessels in man. They used 35 cc 70% diodrast injected for 2 s in the basilic or cephalic vein of the arm. The patient was seated with arms raised. Two films were taken in different projections as single shots. For different circulatory phases the injection had to be repeated. Their method which was described in detail in 1939, became the standard one until the late 1940s.

Timing of the exposures was a problem, and the need for rapid series of films was obvious.

Film Changers

Several pioneers in different countries tried the indirect technique by filming a fluoroscopic screen. However, due to poor image quality, this method was abandoned. Instead, more or less homemade vertical and horizontal cassette tunnels and cassette changers with rotating wheels and drums were used during the 1940s.

A changer for a maximum of twelve 10 × 12 in. cassettes originally designed for cerebral angiography by Sanchez-Perez (1943) became commercially available and was extensively used in the USA.

In 1948 Scott (in St. Louis) and Dotter et al. (in New York) (1949) used a Fairchild serial camera converted for 9½ in. X-ray film. This unit was similar to a roll film changer designed by Gidlund (Stockholm) (1949).

In Sweden angiography was emphasized from the very beginning. The first commercial cassette changer appeared in 1946. It was manufactured by Georg Schönander AB according to the requirements established by Axén and Lind (1948, 1950) and later by Jönsson et al. (1951). It operated with two piles of ten standard 30 × 40 cm cassettes perpendicular to each other up to a maximum

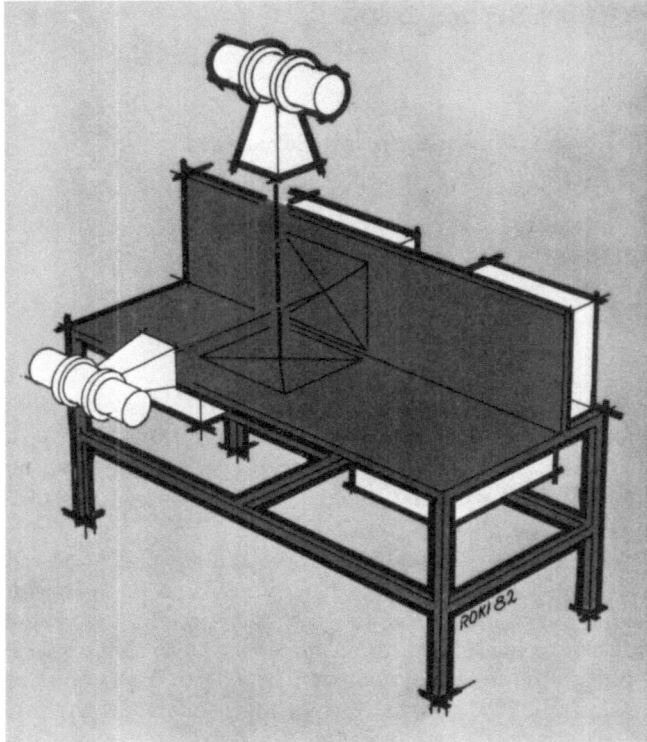

Fig. 1a

Fig. 1a,b. Axén-Lind cassette changer

speed of 1.5 cassettes per s (Fig. 1a,b). Soon enough, the need for higher speeds was experienced.

A big step in this direction was taken in 1949 with the Wegelius/Lind changer designed for children (Lind et al. 1949; Fredzell et al. 1950). Here again piles of cassettes were used, but now up to 50 in each plane. The 18 × 24 cm cassettes were of a special light-weight design using cardboard envelopes with metal reinforcement of their corners (Fig. 2a,b). The actual changing mechanism was two rotating circular disks with a radial slit, very much like the sausage-cutting machines of today. The uppermost cassette of each pile was cut off and placed on top of the disk during exposure. The disk itself protected the rest of the pile from radiation. After exposure the cassette was thrown out in a bag, while simultaneously the subsequent cassette was cut off the pile. This changer had two rather remarkable features. When it worked – in other words, when the knife cut between the cassettes and not through them – the maximum speed was 12.5 films per s. The exposure angle, i.e., the portion of the cycle allowed for exposure, was 270°. Even today this record is unbeaten.

The Gidlund roll film changer of 1949 rapidly developed to the Elema biplane roll film changer (Fig. 3a,b) (Magni 1954). The Film width was 30 cm. By 1971

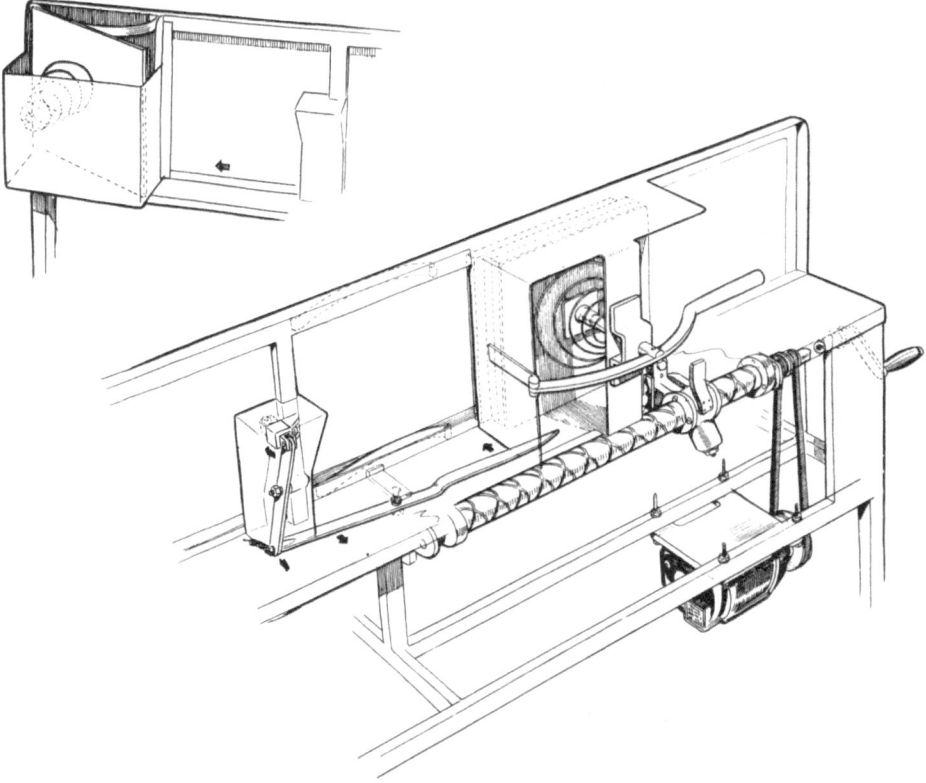

Fig. 1 b

several hundred of this model had been manufactured. Maximum speed was 12 frames/s. The high exposure rates of both the Wegelius/Lind and the Gidlund changers necessitated the design of new high power generators with electronic exposure switches (Fredzell et al. 1950, Grim 1962).

Parallel with the roll film innovations, development of cut film changers went on. The initial changers of standard cassettes, via special cassettes, became the cassetteless cut film changer AOT (Sjögren and Fredzell 1953). The three letters stand for AngiO-Table and, as seen in Fig. 4a, b, the first biplane design included the examination table. The maximum speed was, and still is, six per s. By the end of 1981, 14 300 AOTs had been delivered.

There is no doubt the Gidlund roll film changer and the AOT cut film changer have played a notable role in the development of angiographic techniques over many years.

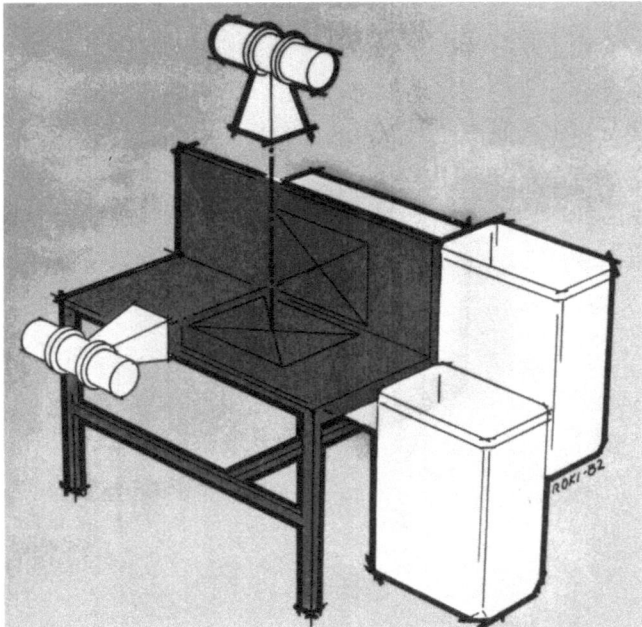

Fig. 2 a

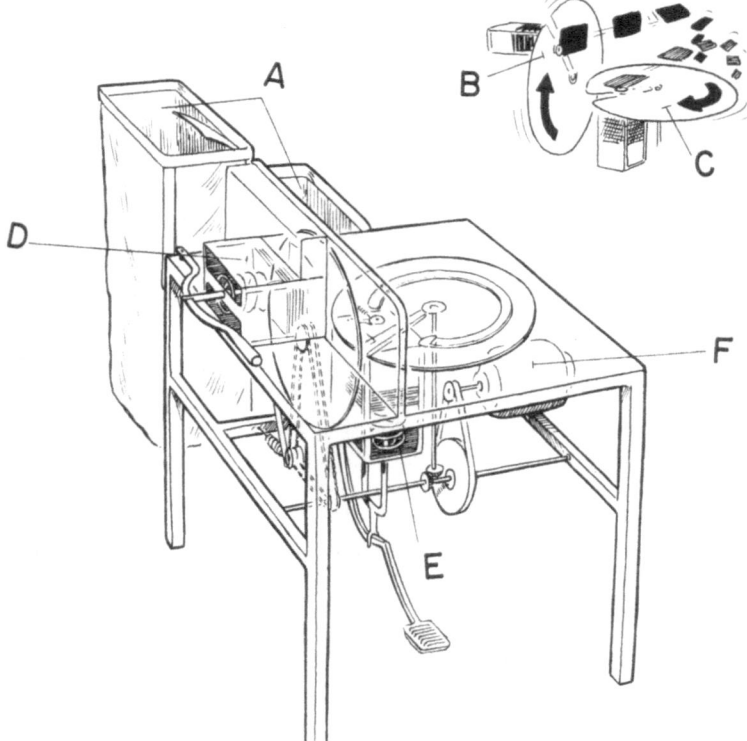

Fig. 2 b

Fig. 2a, b. Wegelius/Lind changer 12 cassettes per s

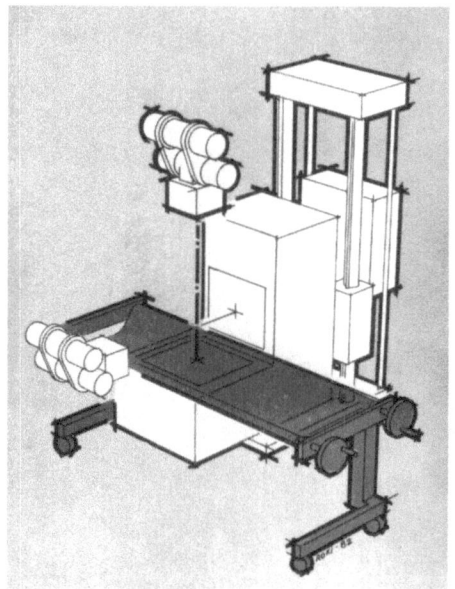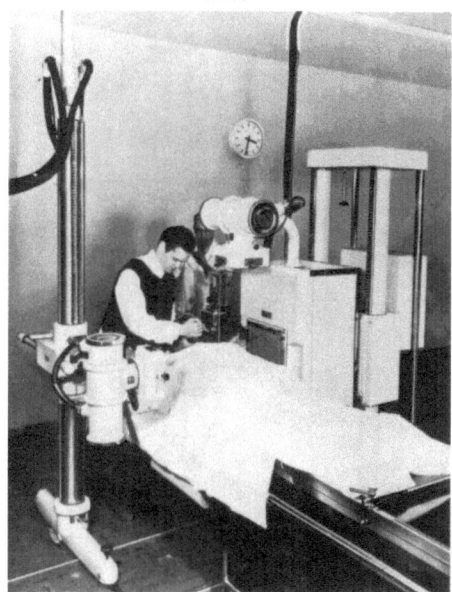

a   b

Fig. 3a,b. Gidlund roll film changer

Examination Systems

Fluoroscopy was a great problem in the early days. Sometimes it had to be performed using screens and mirrors (Fig. 4a,b). When the image intensifier appeared, therefore, it was immediately incorporated into the angiographic systems. Cine cameras attached to the image intensifier tube were also tried early on in order to increase the speed. However, image quality was not good enough until the end of the 1960s. Various examination systems around the film changers were developed. In Fig. 5a,b, the intensifier is below the table. As catheter material and manipulation technique improved, more selective injections took place. Access to the patient and protection against radiation for the staff members became matters of consideration. The X-ray tube was located under the table, where it has remained (Fig. 6a,b).

Until the early 1970s only straight vertical and horizontal ray directions could be used. For oblique projections the patient had to be turned. At this time coronary arteriography was becoming increasingly frequent and the importance of adequately selected oblique projections was recognized, so a cradle was added to the existing patient tables (Fig. 7a,b).

The image intensifier as well as cine cameras had reached such a degree of perfection that the cine films became an alternative to the film changers. Interesting research had been conducted to determine the clinically adequate number of frames per s. Cameras taking several hundred frames per s were tried

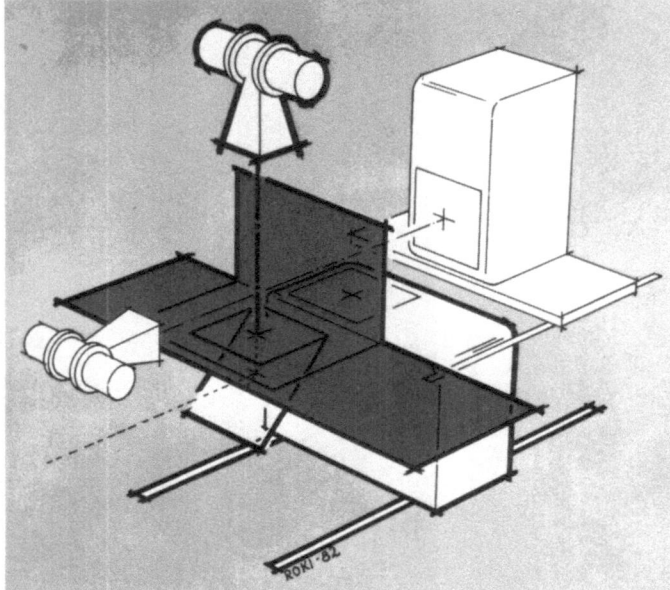

Fig. 4 a

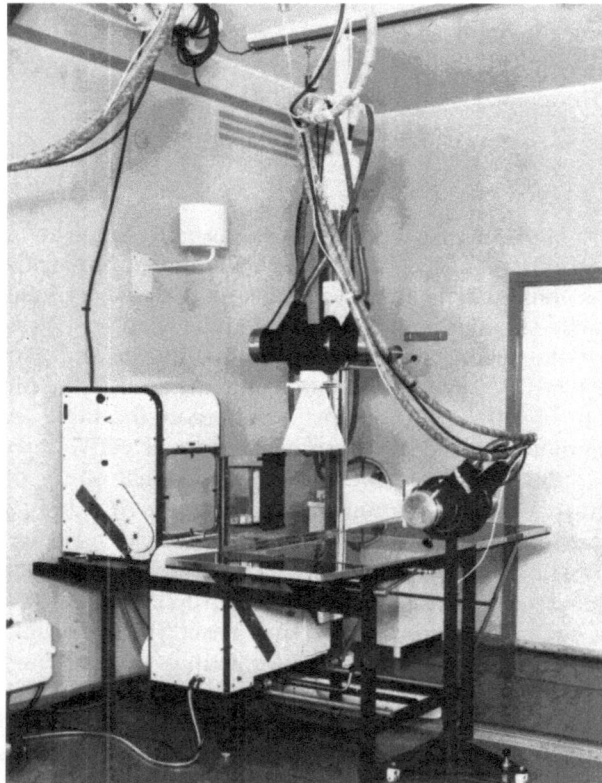

Fig. 4 b

Fig. 4a,b. Early design of AOT cut film changer; note fluoroscopic image seen via mirror

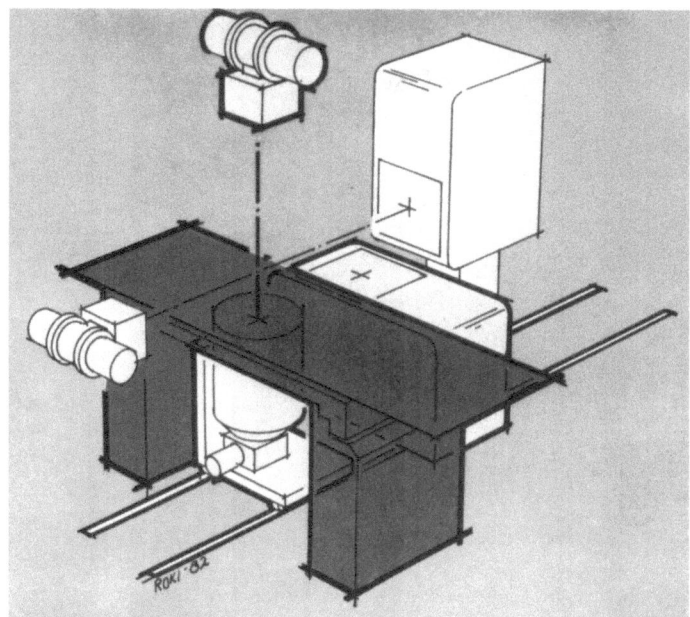

Fig. 5 a

Fig. 5 b

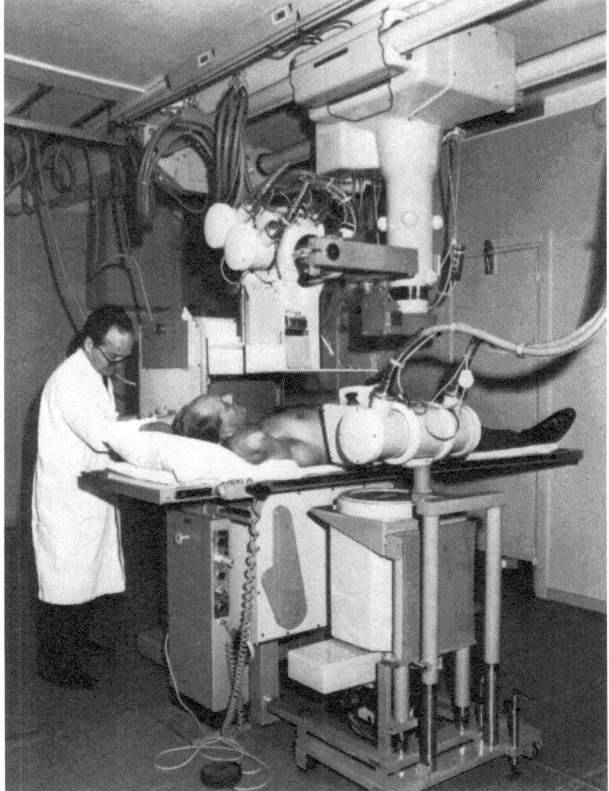

Fig. 5 a, b. Tunnel unit for rapid exchange of under-table image intensifier and film changer

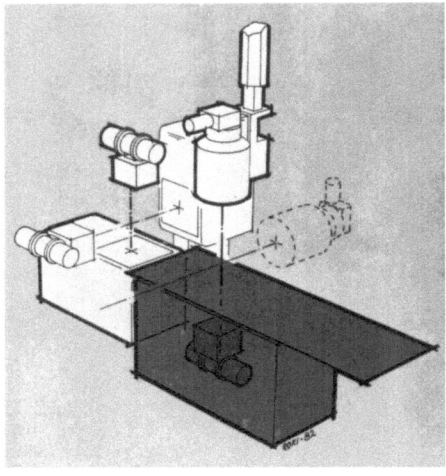

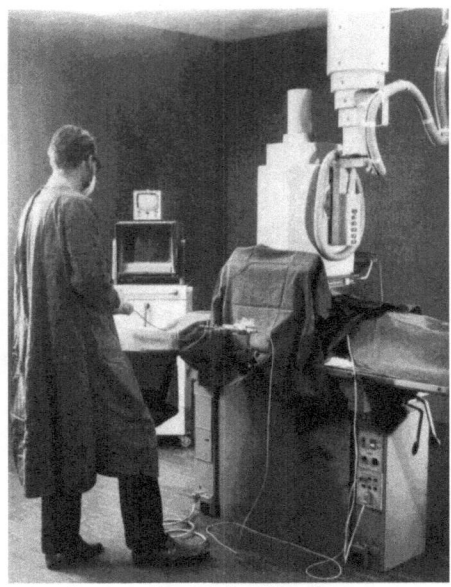

a

b

Fig. 6a, b. Over-table fluoroscopy. Table-top longitudinally adjusted for film changer operation

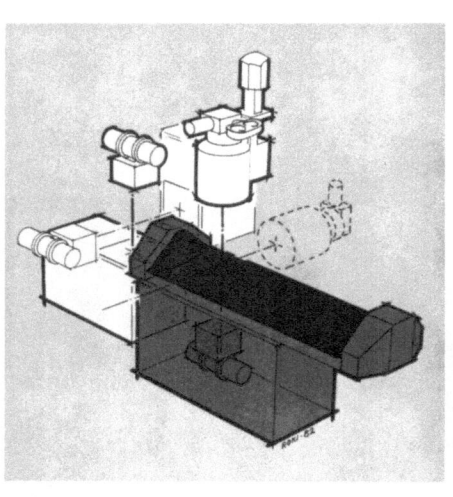

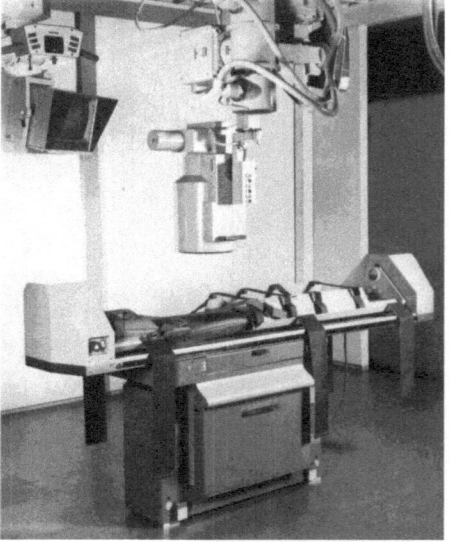

a   b

Fig. 7a, b. Patient cradle for oblique projections

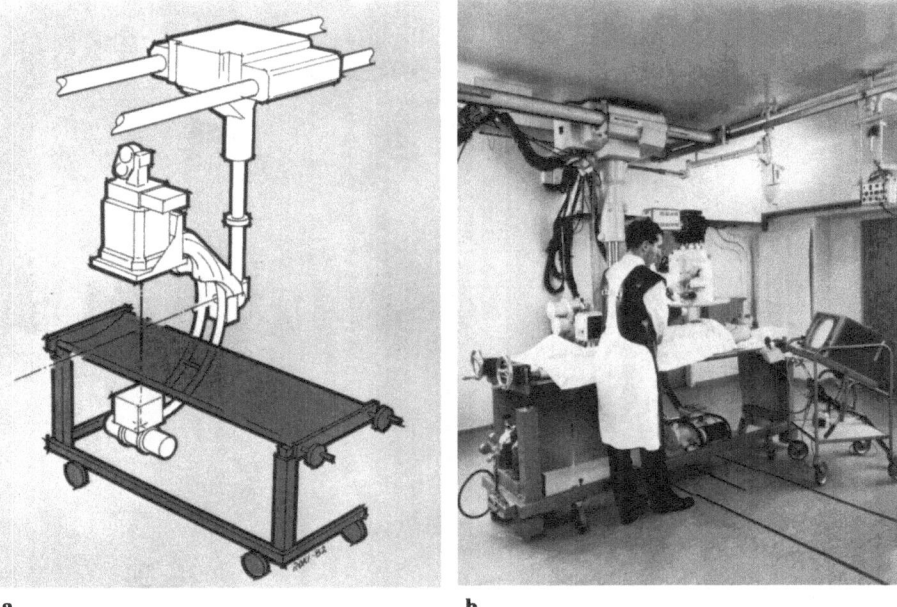

a   b

Fig. 8a, b. Ceiling suspended C-arm unit combined with "roll-cloth" patient support; Norden-ström 1960

until the present speed of 50 was established. The importance of craniocaudal oblique projection especially during coronary examinations had been noticed early on. For that purpose the unit in Fig. 8a, b was introduced by Nordenström in 1960 (Nordenström and Magni 1966).

With the number of coronary arteriographic examinations rapidly increasing, a simplified single plane U-arm unit was designed by Mason Sones in 1970. Since these units are only adjustable in a vertical plane around the patient, craniocaudal tilts are achieved by rotation of the patient table around a pivot in the floor (Fig. 9a, b).

We have now arrived at today's equipment. The next logical step was to keep the patient stationary in a supine position and move the unit around him. This can be achieved either by turning the X-ray unit instead of the patient table, or by replacing the U-arm with a parallelogram or – as shown in Fig. 10a, b – by replacing the U-arm with an arc (Fredzell and Borggren 1977).

In order to fully utilize a multidirectional isocentric unit of this kind, the patient support must not contain any metal framing which might be superimposed on the object. A table-top made of carbon fibre-reinforced plastic eliminates the need of framing and in addition offers less absorption than materials used previously. When a patient table-top of this kind is suspended from the ceiling there are no restrictions on the movements of the patient, and the floor is kept free from interfering objects (Fig. 11a, b).

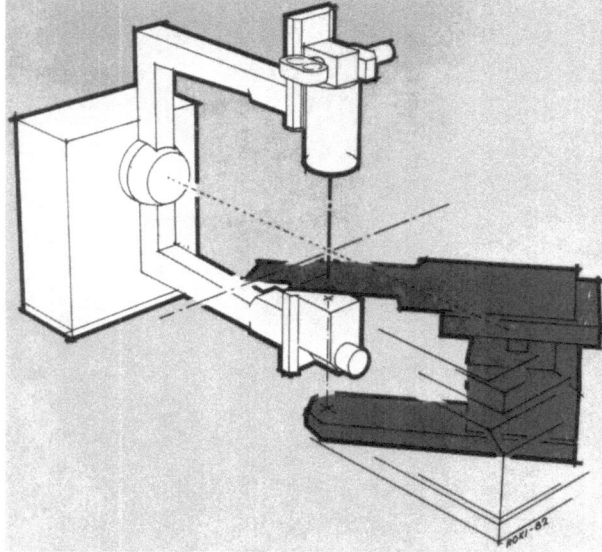

Fig. 9 a

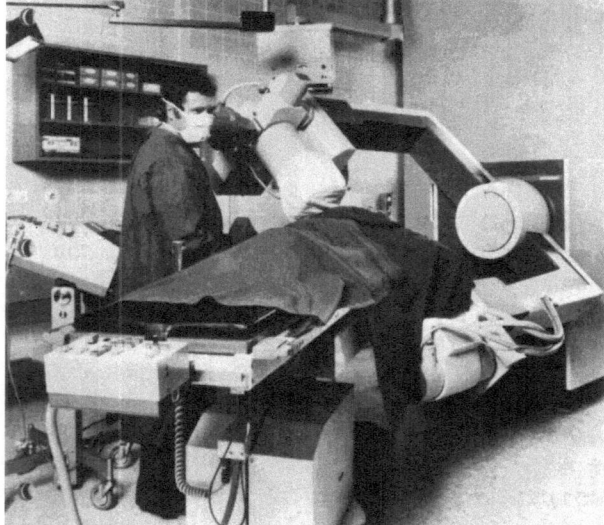

Fig. 9 b

Fig. 9 a, b. Isocentric U-arm unit. Craniocaudal tilts by rotation of table

Before the introduction of the simplified U-arm units, all angiocardiographic units were biplane. Since investigation of the dynamics of the heart chambers has not decreased in importance, it is not surprising that the tendency today is in the direction of biplane multidirectional systems (Nordenström and Holmström 1980).

Besides the obvious arguments in favour of biplane simultaneous operations, such as requiring less contrast medium, minimizing the amount of time the

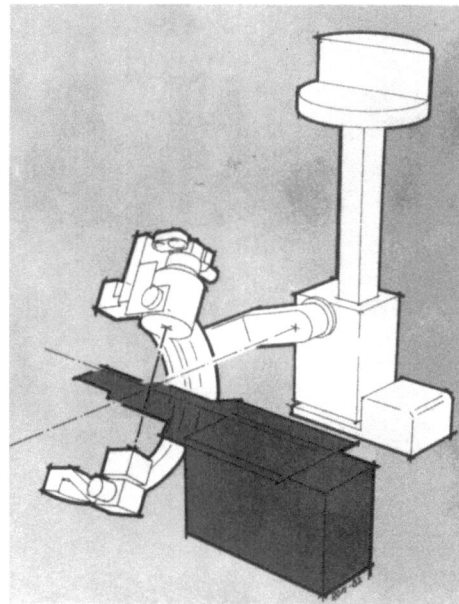

Fig. 10 a

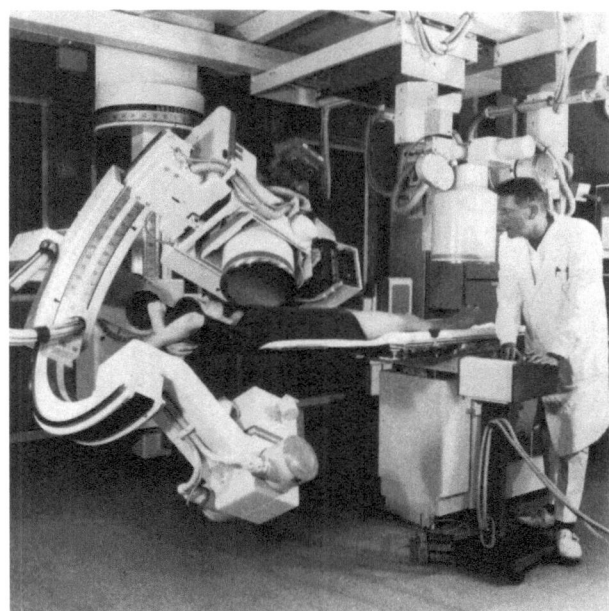

Fig. 10 b

Fig. 10 a, b. Isocentric multidirectional C- + L-arm unit

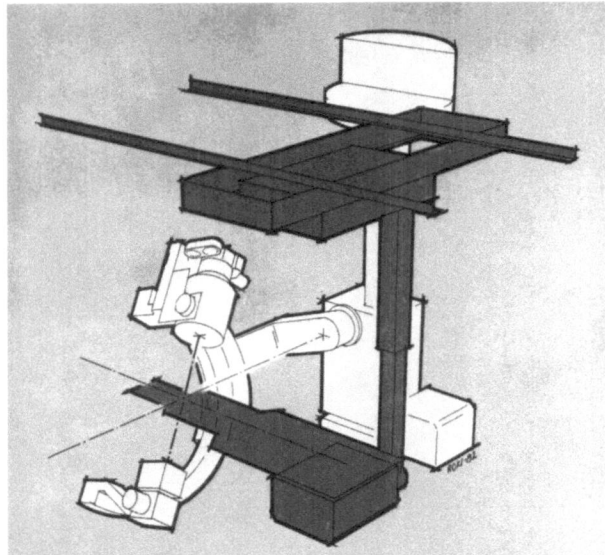

Fig. 11 a

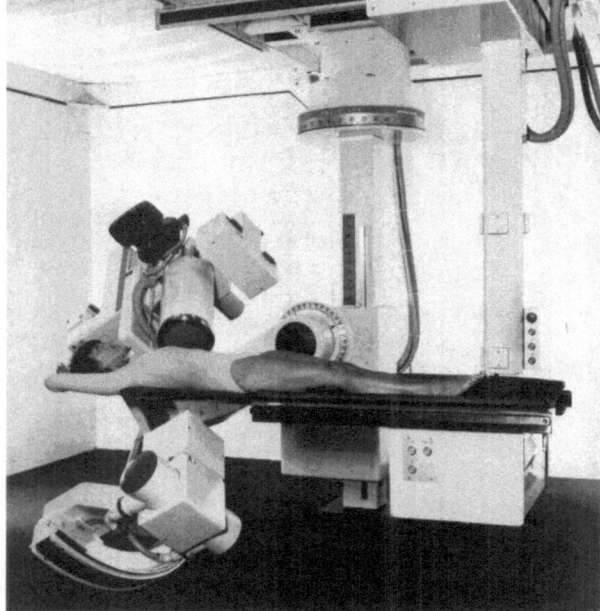

Fig. 11 b

Fig. 11 a, b. Carbon fibre ceiling suspended patient table

catheter tip must be in a critical location, and making volumetric calculations possible, the biplane systems are most valuable in interventional procedures like angioplasty. Their main drawback is the impairment of access to the patient when he is surrounded by double sets of tube and receptor units. Present biplane systems (Fig. 12a, b) (Crochet et al. 1980) therefore combine both

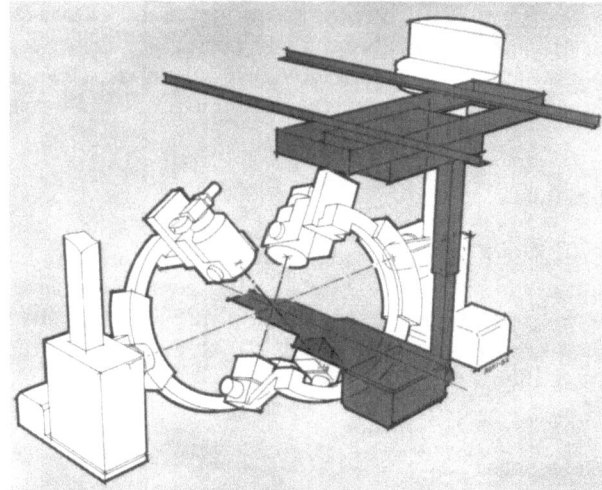

Fig. 12 a

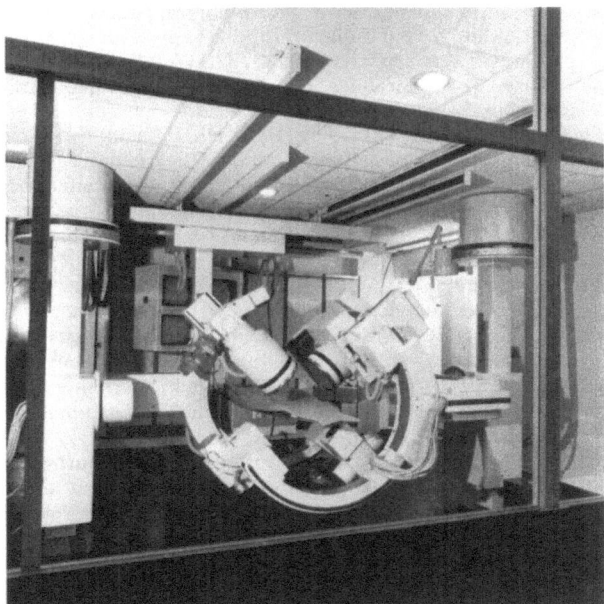

Fig. 12 b

Fig. 12a, b. Biplane isocentric multidirectional unit

single-plane and bi-plane modes of operation in such a way that one plane can be swung or moved aside when not needed.

Angiography has considerably influenced the development of conventional radiological systems. It is the most demanding technique with regard to short, rapidly repeated powerful exposures, alternative ways of documentation, and image quality.

As the present biplane multidirectional examination stands reach maximum usefulness, the next steps will be further improvements to the image-forming parts of the system. Improved X-ray tubes, films, screens and imaging intensifiers resulting in higher resolution of individual images could then be expected.

Summary

Equipment systems for angiocardiographic examinations have now existed for more than 30 years. Their development could serve as a model for a logical step by step procedure, each step alternatively taken by members of the medical and technical professions. In this paper the most characteristic technical steps have been identified and illustrated.

References

Axén O, Lind J (1948) Om angiocardiografi på späda barn Nord Med 38:1143–1144

Axén O, Lind J (1950) Table for routine angiocardiography; synchronous serial roentgenography in two planes at right angles. JAMA 143:540–542

Castellanos A, Pereiras R, Garcia A (1937) La angio-cardiografia radio-opaca. Arch Estud Clin Habana, Sept–Oct 1937

Crochet D, Först H, Petitier H (1980) Die Bedeutung der Zweiebenen-Angioskop-Technik in der Kard- und Koronarangiographie. Electromedica 4:110–117

Dotter C, Steinberg I, Temple H (1949) Automatic roentgenray roll-film magazine for angiocardiography and cerebral arteriography. Am J Roentgenol 62/3:355–358

Forssmann W (1929) Die Sondierung des rechten Herzens. Klin Wochenschr 8:2085–2087, addendum 8:2287

Fredzell G, Borggren A (1977) The angioscope – a new multidirectional examination unit for advanced radiological examinations. Electromedica 3/4:137–141

Fredzell G, Lind J, Ohlson E, Wegelius C (1950) Direct serial roentgenography in two planes simultaneously at 0.08 second intervals. Am J Roentgenol 63:548–558

Gidlund Å (1949) New apparatus for direct cineroentgenography. Acta Radiol 32:81–88

Grim S (1962) Röntgenapparate für Schnellserienaufnahmen und Kinematographie. Radiologe 11:420–425

Jönsson G, Brodén B, Karnell J (1951) Thoracic aortography with special references to its value in patent ductus arteriosus and coarctation of the aorta. Acta Radiol [Suppl] 89

Lind J, Wegelius C, Fredzell G, Wasser E (1949) Direct angiocardiography; experiencies with 10 exposures per second. J Fac Radiol 1:87–97

Magni G-A (1954) Technical problems in rapid serial radiography. Acta Radiol [Suppl] 116:638–648

Nordenström B, Holmström L (1980) Versatile single and biplane systems for radiologic procedures. In: Anacker H et al. (eds) Percutaneous biopsy and therapeutic vascular occlusion. Thieme, Stuttgart, pp 90–96

Nordenström B, Magni G-A (1966) Catheterization unit for fluoroscopy and roentgenography. Radiologe 6:419–421

Robb GP, Steinberg I (1939) Visualization of chambers of heart, pulmonary circulation, and great blood vessels in man. Am J Roentgenol 41:1–17

Sanchez-Perez J (1943) The cranial seriograph and its utility in neurologic radiology for cerebral angiography. Surgery 13:661–666

Sjögren S-E, Fredzell G (1953) Apparatus for serial angiography. Acta Radiol 40:361–368

Image Intensifiers

F. W. HOFMANN

Siemens AG, UB Med, Henkestraße 127, 8520 Erlangen, FRG

For many radiologists the image intensifier is only a black box whose input is an X-ray beam and whose output is a small, bright visible image. It may therefore be worth our while to start by reviewing the working principles of the X-ray image intensifier.

An image intensifier is a vacuum tube enclosing a large volume. Its wall material is glass or metal. Figure 1 shows a cross-sectional view. The X-ray beam, modulated by the patient, enters through an input window and falls on an input screen where it is transformed into a visible image, just as in a fluoroscopic screen. On the surface of the input screen an extremely thin semiconductor layer is vapour-deposited. It consists of caesium and antimony. It absorbs the light emitted by the input screen and transforms it into a corresponding flux of electrons which are emitted into the open volume of the tube.

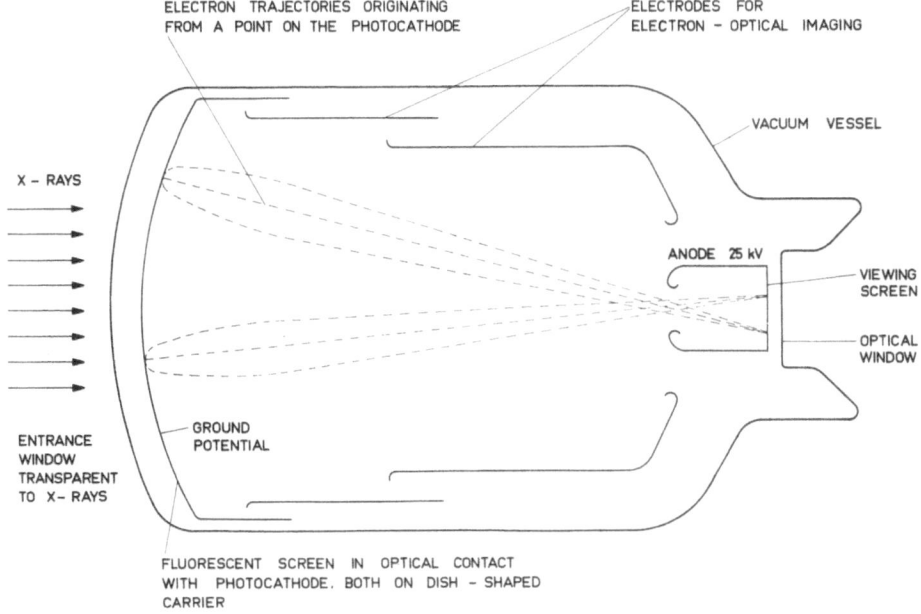

Fig. 1. X-ray image intensifier, schematic

The next step is the focusing of these "photo"-electrons on a second screen, much smaller than the first, the output screen. This is achieved by an appropriately shaped electric field, a so-called electron lens. In contrast to an optical lens, which can gather only a small fraction of the light coming from the object even at high aperture, the electron-optical focusing has the remarkable property of collecting *all* electrons emitted by the photocathode surface, regardless of their initial direction. The electric focusing field accelerates the photoelectrons from a practically negligible initial energy to between 25 and 35 keV at the output screen, sufficient energy for each electron to generate at least 1000 light quanta in the output screen.

The efficiencies of the three information-converting layers, namely the input screen, the photocathode and the output screen, and in addition the final energy of the photoelectrons, determine the amplification of the total light flux, or the "gain". Usually, however, the luminance, i.e. the light flux per unit area of the output screen, is of greater interest. The "conversion factor" is the luminance at the output screen per unit exposure rate at the input. The conversion factor also depends on the demagnification ratio of the electron optics. The more the flux of the photoelectrons emitted from the large photocathode surface is concentrated, the higher is the luminance at the output screen. When the image is electronically "zoomed", the focusing electric field is changed in such a way that only a concentric inner part of the photocathode is focused on the full output screen. In other words, the demagnification is thereby reduced, and so is the conversion factor.

We have seen that the primary "detection", i.e. the conversion into light of the X-ray quanta incident on the image intensifier input, occurs in the input screen. In order to be an efficient converter, the input screen has to have the following properties: it has to attenuate the X-ray beam greatly, and the interaction has to result in the emission of light with a high yield. However, since we also want a high resolving power for our X-ray image, the input screen should be a thin layer, which apparently contradicts the requirement of high attenuation for X-rays.

Modern X-ray image intensifiers contain input screens consisting of an evaporated layer of caesium iodide, activated by a small admixture of sodium (Fig. 2). This screen material is exceedingly suitable with regard to the necessary trade-off between the requirements of adequate spatial resolution – or modulation transfer function (MTF) – and high yield of the conversion of X-ray quanta, since it consists entirely of heavy elements, and since the evaporated layer can be made to grow as small crystals oriented perpendicular to the substrate surface. The spatial resolving power of such a screen is higher than one might expect from its thickness. This is due to the formation of minute cracks between groups of CsI crystals. The cracks impede the spreading of the light from the scintillations in the crystals. Thus the scintillation light is preferentially conducted in the direction perpendicular to the screen surface; that is, towards the photocathode.

It goes almost without saying that a high quantum yield is desirable for a detector of diagnostic X-rays. The rapidly developing technique of digital radiography with its exciting possibilities for image enhancement has intensified

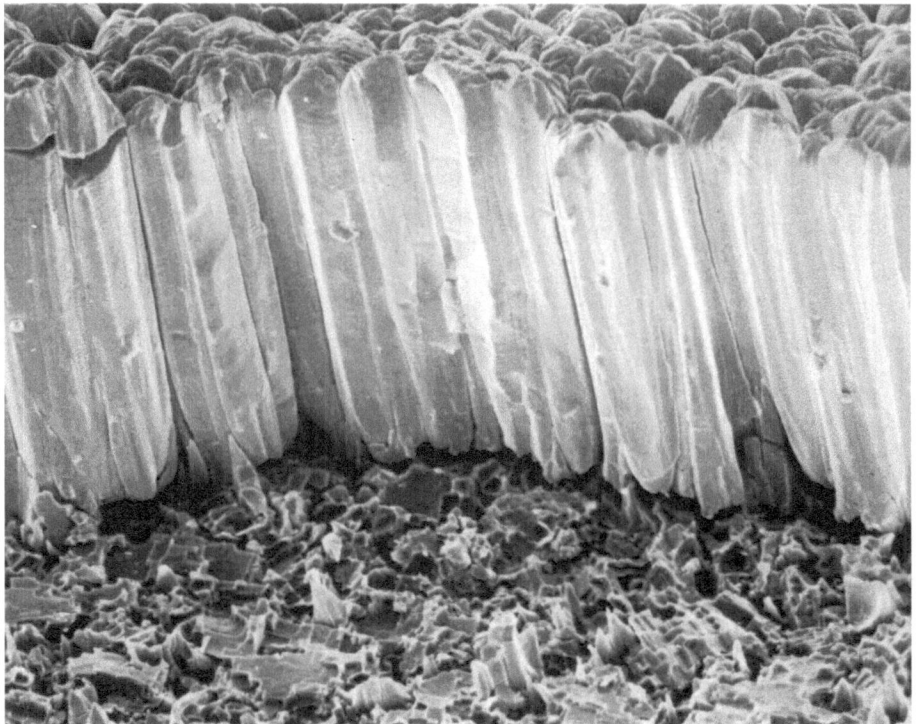

Fig. 2. Broken-off edge of a caesium iodide X-ray screen on a rough aluminium substrate (scanning electron micrograph)

the quest for a high detective quantum efficiency (DQE). Digital radiography usually starts out from individually stored X-ray television "frames", each exposed with only a few μR in the detector plane. Particularly in subtracted images, where we try to detect very small contrasts, the quantum noise is often the factor which limits the perceptibility of the diagnostically relevant features. A high DQE may therefore be even more important than high spatial resolution. The DQE depends strongly on the X-ray spectrum, i.e. on the kilovoltage of the generating tube. It is therefore customary to state the DQE at a standardized ICRU[1] radiation quality, characterized by a half-value layer of 7 mm aluminium. At this "ICRU radiation", the DQEs of contemporary image intensifiers are between 40% and 70%. Current developments aim at maximizing the MTF at a high value of the DQE.

Besides the input screen, several other image intensifier components contribute to the MTF: the output screen (which should be as fine-grained as possible), the electron-optical imaging, and also less obvious components such as

---

[1] International Commission on Radiological Units and Measurements

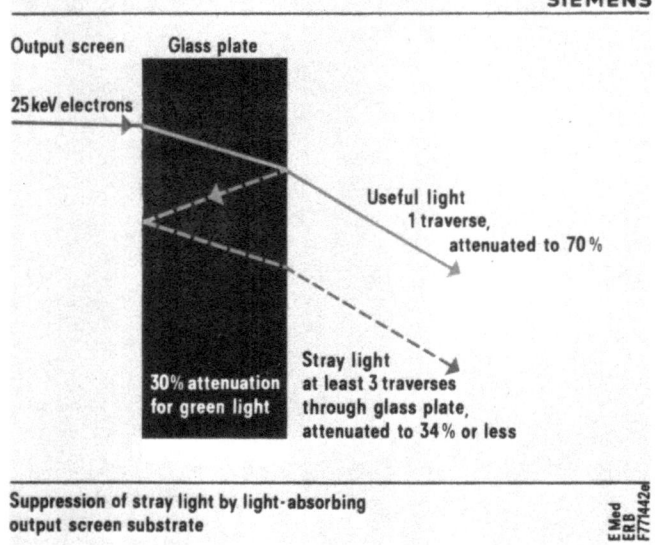

SIEMENS

Output screen   Glass plate

25 keV electrons

Useful light
1 traverse,
attenuated to 70 %

30% attenuation   Stray light
for green light   at least 3 traverses
through glass plate,
attenuated to 34 % or less

Suppression of stray light by light-absorbing
output screen substrate

Fig. 3. Contrast enhancement of a phosphor screen deposited on *tinted* glass

the input window and the substrate of the output screen. Until a few years ago, the entrance window of an X-ray image intensifier was made of glass, as was the entire vacuum envelope of the tube.

Replacing glass by metal, i.e. a thin sheet of aluminium or titanium, reduces the scattering of the X-rays and thereby increases contrast. The improvement is particularly noticeable in large-format image intensifiers.

Another major source of contrast loss is the conduction of light, by internal reflexions, in the glass plate which carries the output screen. The contrast can be markedly increased – although at some expense of gain – by using a tinted glass which transmits about 70% of the useful light, but a much smaller fraction of the parasitic light whose average path in the glass is longer (Fig. 3). Another very effective way to increase the contrast of the output screen is to deposit it on a fibre optic plate which prevents lateral light conduction.

The quality of any televised image has an obvious limitation on account of the fixed number of TV lines available for a given picture height. There is a similar limitation in the horizontal direction which is set by the band width of the TV signal transmission. This means that a given TV system transmits a certain number of picture elements, regardless of the size of the object field. Spatial resolution can therefore be increased by transmitting only a reduced object field, a procedure known as "zooming".

In a movie camera, the image is zoomed by changing the effective focal length of the objective lens. In an image intensifier to television chain, the lens train which transmits the image from the image intensifier output to the light-sensitive layer of the TV pickup tube is left unchanged, and the zooming is done in the electron-optical imaging system of the image intensifier. The total accelerating voltage between the photocathode and the output screen, however, is held constant. The fact that the photoelectron flux from an area smaller than the full input field is imaged on the full output screen means that a smaller conversion factor is obtained when the image is zoomed. The conversion factor decreases proportionally with the photocathode area which is imaged, i.e. with the square of the input field diameter.

In order to achieve high spatial resolving power in televised X-ray images, particularly in those which are stored and processed digitally, it is desirable to have large zoom factors available, such as from a full field diameter of 27 cm down to 8 or 10 cm, i.e. a factor of about 3.

Since the TV pickup tube requires a roughly constant amount of light per frame, the reduced conversion factor, during zoomed operation, has to be compensated by either increasing the aperture of the optics or the radiation exposure, or a combination of these measures. One should not be misled into believing that zooming irresponsibly increases the patient's radiation hazard. When the image is zoomed, the X-ray beam has to be coned down by the same factor by which the dose rate increases, so that the product of dose and exposed area remains constant. It can even decrease when the aperture of the optical system is opened.

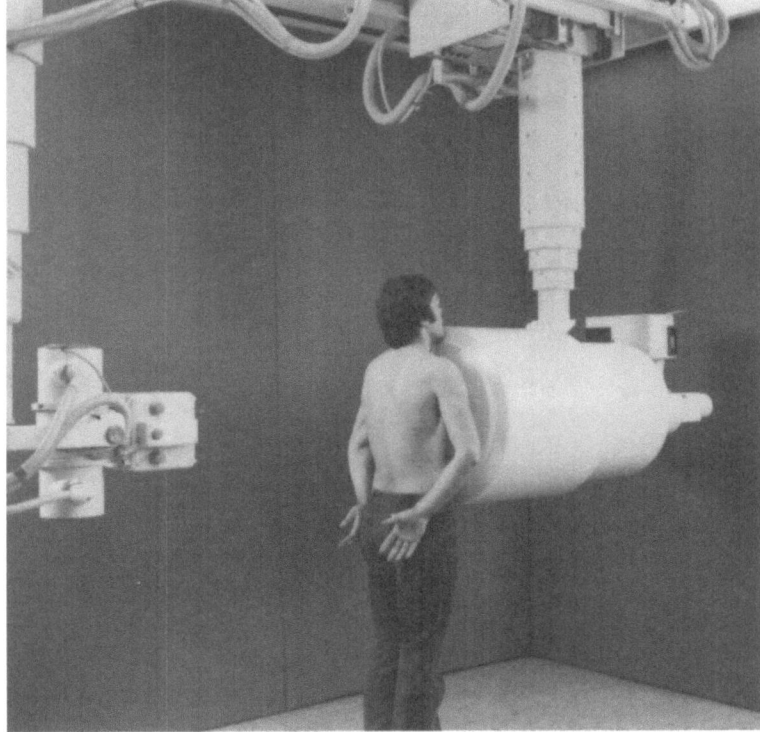

Fig. 4. Taking a chest radiograph through a 57-cm X-ray image intensifier with a 100-mm sheet film camera

I would like to end this paper with some remarks on image intensifier field sizes. Until now, commercially available X-ray image intensifiers have had input field diameters of between 15 cm and 35 cm. The emerging trend toward indirect and digitized radiography may require larger fields. There is no principal technical impediment against building larger image intensifiers; it is only a question of cost and of increased demands on mechanical tolerances. To prove this, we have built a few experimental image intensifiers for taking indirect chest films on 100-mm film (Fig. 4). The input field diameter is 57 cm; it accommodates an inscribed 40 cm by 40 cm square, which is the usual chest film size. Clinical testing has shown that the image quality is sufficient for routine chest examinations and it is certainly far better than in photofluorographic chest films. We may therefore expect that the range of field sizes of commercial X-ray image intensifiers will be extended in the near future. Indirect radiography and current developments involving digitized images should benefit from such larger image intensifiers with commensurate extension of the pixel matrix.

New Developments in Video Systems: Camera Tubes and Storage Devices

P. Marhoff

Siemens AG, Bereich Medizinische Technik, Henkestraße 127, D-8520 Erlangen, FRG

Angiocardiographic X-ray examination demands high-grade technical equipment which frequently includes a biplane operation, making better spatial orientation possible. While the stereo technique also appears to be very suitable, so far it has only been applied in individual cases [1]. Instead of the cut film changer with its frame speed limitation, nowadays, without exception, the image intensifier cine technique is used for documentation. Only in this way can the high demands regarding image quality and dynamic resolution be satisfactorily met. For routine work, extremely high frame speeds (up to many hundreds per s) are unneccessary [2]; the emphasis is more on the range of 50–100 per s [3].

Cine film is used in routine operation, primarily for visual evaluation and morphological interpretation. The extensive literature on the topic [e.g., 4–7] shows the necessity of quantifying the examination results, not only in order to objectify them but also in order to derive additional information. If extensive introduction of this into the daily routine has still, so far, not taken place, this is due to several reasons, one of which may be the relatively complicated procedure, as illustrated in Fig. 1. The normal image production and evaluation process involves a number of stages in the image intensifier cine technique. The information-carrying X-ray beam is absorbed in the X-ray image intensifier and transformed into an output image which is led via a light distributor to the cine camera where the film is exposed. Here, first of all, the chemical process of film development must take place before visual evaluation is possible using a film viewer or projector.

At this point it is possible, using an electrooptical converter, to transform the fully processed cine film into an electrically, analogically, or digitally evaluable signal via a film projection or scanning device.

In general practice it is usual that, parallel to the exposure of the cine film, a proportion of the available light is deflected to the TV camera, so that direct observation is possible simultaneously with the cine scene. It is an obvious step to use the video signal directly for quantitative evaluation, or to record it in parallel, so that this electronic recording (usually on magnetic tape) can be used subsequently for further observation and/or repeated processing.

If, therefore, the video technique provides significant advantages compared with the cine technique in being a simpler procedure and offering more rapid availability of processed data, then the question must be asked: Why has it not

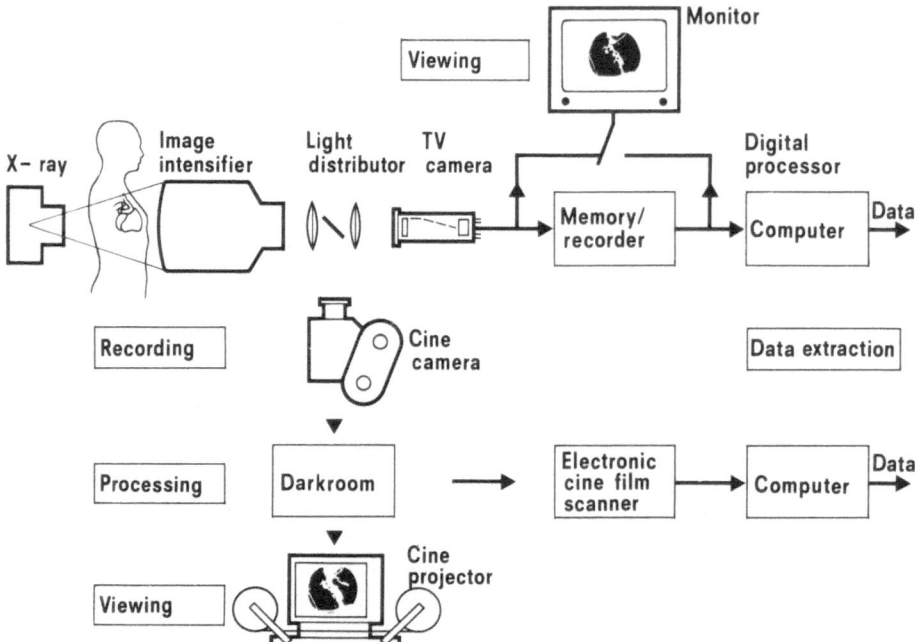

Fig. 1. Angiocardiographic equipment for cine and video imaging, recording, and computerized data extraction

been applied more for documentation and processing? The reasons are, in the first place, the reduced image quality of the standard TV system as opposed to the cine film, and the additional loss in quality due to the analog recording principle of the available videotape recorders. With regard to quantitative evaluation, there are additional problems caused by the analog signal processing technique which is typical for standard videometry [8, 9].

Concerning image quality, however, important advances have been made in recent years as a result of the development of high-resolution, high line-rate TV systems. The digital video technique whose application to digital video subtraction angiography [10] has been so successful, and which has led to particular optimism, has now also initiated development in X-ray image storage and processing which sets new standards. It is thus to be expected that the video technique and digital signal processing will prove the best options for application in angiocardiography, not only to increasingly replace the cine film, but especially to introduce quantitative analysis on a routine basis.

In the following, these new developments are presented with special regard to the requirements of angiocardiography. Digital video technique, together with its possible consequences for signal storage, is briefly discussed.

High-Resolution Video Systems: Camera Tubes and Video Recorders

State-of-the-art high-resolution X-ray television has already been discussed [11]. Here, we will examine in detail the characteristic features of the camera tube, the decisive element in the production of the video signal: for the properties of the camera tube dictate the quality it is possible to achieve in all other components of the transmission channel. Today, the 1-in. vidicon is used almost exclusively, and other tube types [12, 13] no longer have practical significance in X-ray TV.

As material for the photosensitive layer, antimony trisulfide and lead oxide (e.g., Plumbicon) are the preferred materials today; no other materials have yet become standard in X-ray application. Silicon diode array tubes, for example, showed great promise for industrial and broadcasting applications, but did not come up to expectations. New materials have also been adopted in Pasecon tubes that seem well suited for special X-ray purposes [14]. Similarly, this may prove to be the case for the Saticon tube, but this has not been sufficiently tested so far. Both Saticon and Pasecon use selenium-based photoconductive layers and will be dealt with later on. For many years now, work has been proceeding on the development of solid-state image sensors [15]. Compared to camera tubes, their small volume and low energy consumption represent advantages. However, it is not expected that solid-state components will be competitive in price and capacity to high-resolution camera tubes in the foreseeable future.

Figure 2 shows the modulation transfer of three different camera tubes. Line pairs per picture height have been selected as a standard of spatial frequency, so that a direct comparison is possible despite various image sizes at the photosensitive layer. It can be clearly seen that with the high-resolution TV system, it is important to have the largest possible image diameter. This has been realized by the Hivicon (image diameter 16 mm) shown here. In the standard equipment,

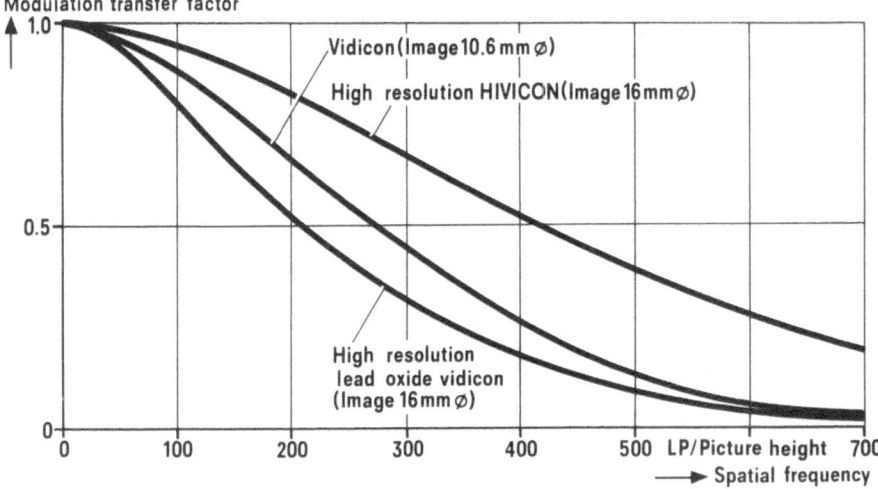

Fig. 2. Spatial modulation transfer functions of TV camera tubes

Modulation transfer factor

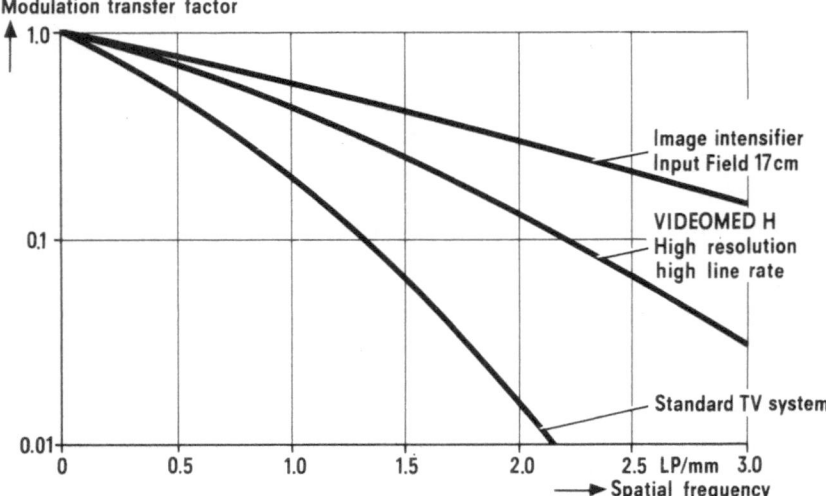

Fig. 3. Modulation transfer function of an image intensifier Sirecon Optilux 27-17 HN coupled to a standard 625-line TV system and to a high-resolution, high line-rate Videomed H TV system

the image diameter is 13 mm or less, so that the transfer characteristics are correspondingly poorer. However, the selection of the image size is not entirely a matter of free choice, but is subject to an optimizing process between a number of conflicting criteria, such as uniformity over the surface including modulation transfer, freedom from blemishes, and cost. In the lead oxide vidicon, which is frequently used in equipment for cardioangiography because of its good reproduction of moving objects, the modulation transfer is decidedly poorer. Even if the input diameter is exploited to the maximum, the quality of the standard vidicon is not quite achieved. Lead oxide tubes with a larger diameter have indeed been specially developed [16]; however, these tubes are only produced in small numbers and are therefore not yet suitable for wider application.

Let us now consider the modulation transfer function (MTF). The MTF achieved by a high-resolution image intensifier in conjunction with a high-resolution, high line-rate X-ray TV installation, gives the curve shown in Fig. 3 and marked Videomed H. For comparison, the transfer function of the standard installation is also shown, as well as that of the image intensifier tube alone. With regard to "imaging faithfulness", which requires the best possible modulation transfer, the high-resolution system is significantly superior to the standard system. Figure 4 shows on the left an optical pattern transmitted by a standard TV installation and on the right the transmission by a high-resolution, high line-rate installation.

In Fig. 5, the X-ray image intensifier is also included in the transmission and the "grainy" background structure corresponds to the X-ray quantum noise for a normal fluoroscopic dose rate. Here, again, the standard installation is shown on the left and the high-resolution unit on the right.

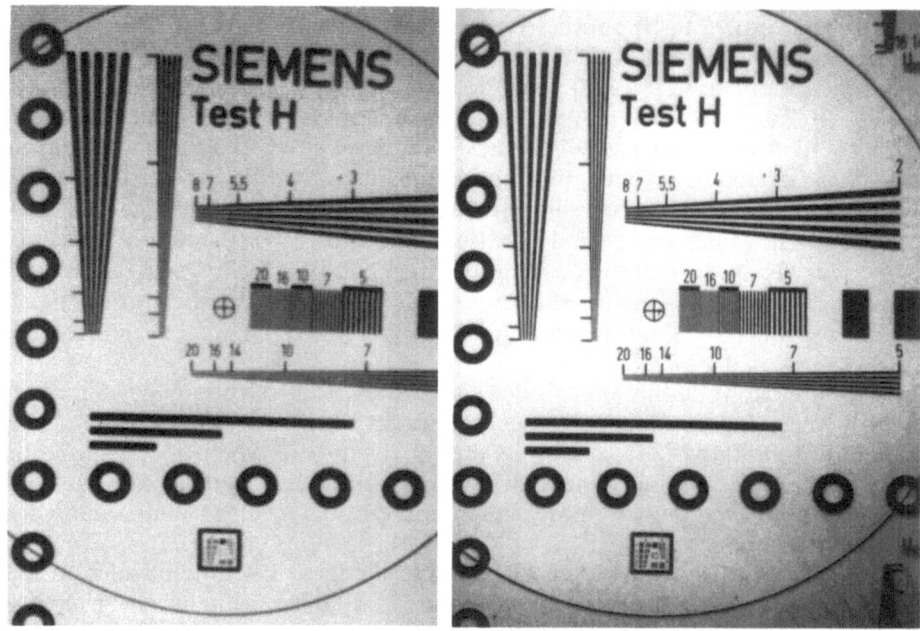

Fig. 4. Comparison of standard (*left*) and high-resolution (*right*) TV systems

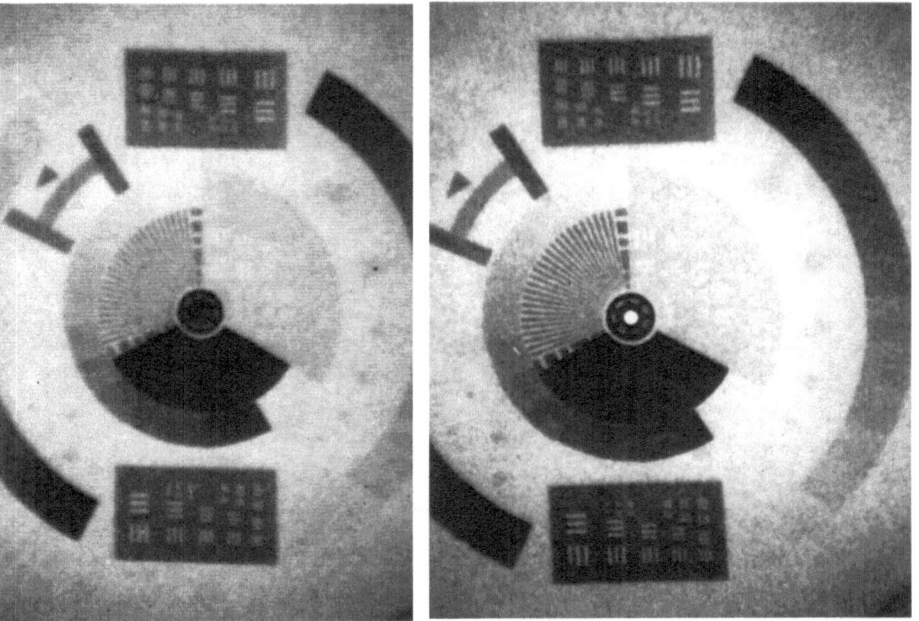

Fig. 5. Comparison of fluoroscopic images obtained with standard (*left*) and high-resolution (*right*) TV systems

A further aspect to be considered in image quality is the capability of transmitting dynamic processes. For this, the temporal transmission characteristic of the TV camera tube [17, 18], commonly designated as "lag" in the case of broadcast TV, is decisive. Even the established rate of 50 fields per s constitutes a substantial limitation which becomes even more severe when the interlacing process is taken into account, since it normally takes two fields to constitute one frame. According to the sampling theorem of communication theory, at least two sampling values per period of a sine wave must be provided for transmission. This "Nyquist limit" is 25 Hz in the case of 50 TV fields (equivalent to 50 sampling values) per s and is shown in Fig. 6 as a dashed vertical line. Higher signal frequencies will not be transmitted properly and will lead to interference effects.

A useful feature of this effect is derived by the use of a stroboscope, since very rapidly recurring moving processes appear to be greatly slowed down. The generally well-known effect seen in the movie theatre when, for example, in spite of the obviously high speed of a vehicle, the wheels appear to be turning only slowly or even in the opposite direction, is also a result of contravening the sampling theorem.

In Fig. 6, a transfer function is allocated to the ideal TV system which results from the fact that over an imaging period, i.e., 20 ms, summation or storage takes place. Naturally, the remaining transfer functions which are shown also contain this component which arises from the effective exposure time of 20 ms per image. This component can be considerably reduced, in that the exposure is not continuous, but pulsed, as is usual in the case of X-ray cine operation. With a pulse duration of, for example, 2 ms, the curve for the ideal TV system runs

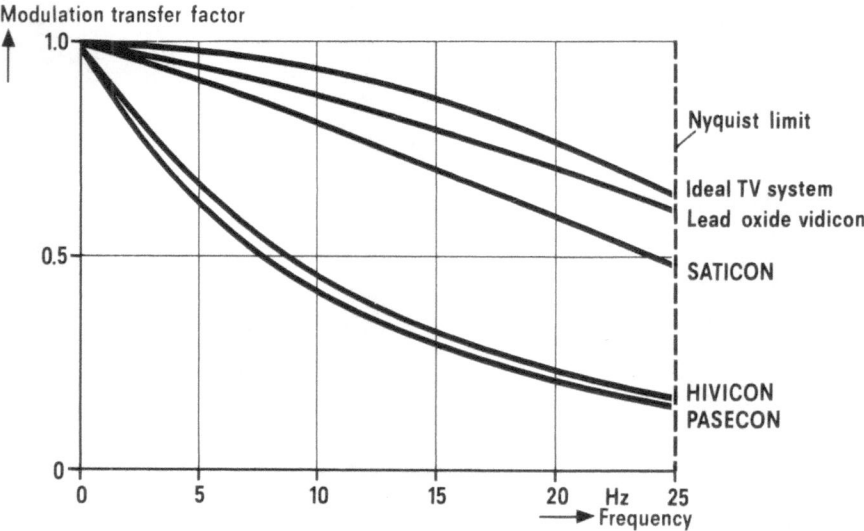

Fig. 6. Temporal modulation transfer function of TV camera tubes measured with a sinusoidally varying illumination. The minimum and maximum values of the illumination have been set so as to give a signal current of 120 and 180 nA respectively, at a frequency of 0.3 Hz. Measurements of the signal current at higher frequencies are referred to this value

practically horizontally, and all the remaining curves are improved by a corresponding amount in the case of pulsed exposure.

The lead oxide vidicon is undisputedly superior to all other tubes for the reproduction of movement. However, one of the newly developed tubes already mentioned, the Saticon, possesses a lag characteristic similar to the lead oxide vidicon and, in addition, has a very high spatial resolution. Because of this favorable combination of characteristics, this tube could in the future acquire significance for angiocardiographic application.

The smallest possible lag is not always desirable, since although lag causes rapid dynamic processes to be blurred (that is, reproduced with less contrast), the intensity of the interfering quantum noise also becomes less. The optimum lag is thus a compromise between two opposing effects, desirable noise reduction and disadvantageous loss of contrast in the case of movement.

Both the Hivicon, which is a high-resolution vidicon with an antimony trisulfide photolayer, and the Pasecon have considerable lag and are therefore very useful in producing low quantum noise fluoroscopic images.

Although lag can be classified by objective characteristic data, experience shows that subjective assessments of lag do not always conform with these data. This is a general problem of the subjective assessment of image quality, and of attainable diagnostic information, which is partly due to the fact that it is not always possible to change parameters independently; but it is also due to such nonquantifiable factors as familiarity, experience, and additional knowledge of the situation under assessment.

The storage of the X-ray TV signal is of especial importance in angiocardiography, for the rapidly moving processes involved demand the possibility of repetition as desired, without further exposure to radiation or application of contrast medium. Whereas the vertical resolution which is determined by the number of lines (shown dashed in Fig. 7) is not influenced by the recording and reproduction via the video tape recorder, the limited bandwidth of 5 or 10 MHz means a significantly steep drop in modulation transfer in the horizontal direction at spatial frequencies corresponding to this electrical frequency.

With a recorder having a bandwidth of 5 MHz, there is a balanced relationship between horizontal and vertical resolution for the standard installation. In the case of high-resolution, high line-rate installations, the bandwidth of 10 MHz means that the horizontal resolution does not maintain the same relationship because of the high number of lines (1249). Here, further improvement would be desirable. At the present time, the technological possibilities are so far exhausted that within the basic concept prescribed, no appreciable further increase of the bandwidth is possible. Video tape recorders with the usual, analog recording principle influence not only the transfer quality by the limited electrical bandwidth, but also the signal-to-noise ratio (SNR), since they produce an additional noise component. If in the case of X-ray TV, the usual high-grade recorders using 1-in. magnetic tape are assumed, then under normal circumstances the additional noise is less than the corresponding quantum noise already contained in the noise proportion of the signal to be recorded, so that no visible deterioration arises. A perceptible quality bottleneck in recording with a video recorder could occur if, in future applications of digital video signal

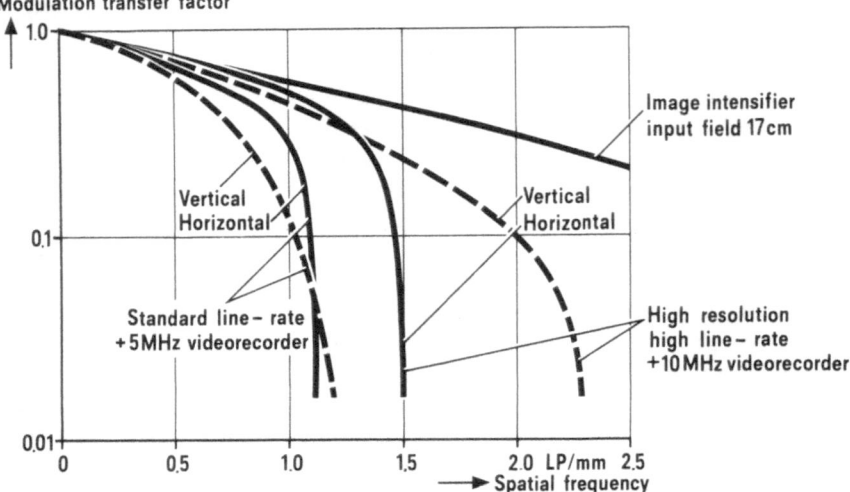

Fig. 7. Modulation transfer function of Sirecon Optilux 27-17 HN image intensifier with standard 625-line TV system and high-resolution Videomed H TV system and video tape recorder. *Vertical* modulation transfer differs from the curves shown in Fig. 3 only by taking into account the effect of sampling done by the line-scanning format of the TV system. *Horizontally* the limited bandwidth of the video tape recorders Sirecord X (5 MHz) and Sirecord XH (10 MHz) determines the shape of the transfer function as compared with Fig. 3

processing, appreciably higher dose rate values are required than is usual at present.

Digital Video Technique: Image Storage

On the basis of the recording principle used at present there appears to be no possibility of an appreciable improvement in quality, so that only a digital recording procedure can fulfill the appropriate quality requirements. Because of the necessary throughput and quantity of data, there is today, still no economically justifiable solution to the problem of storing angiocardiographic scenes in real time.

Digital storage of individual images in image memories built up from semiconductor components, in which writing and reading can be performed in real time (e.g., 20 ms per image), is starting to be introduced into X-ray TV techniques [14]. Referring to Fig. 8, some fundamental concepts of digital storage are touched upon. First of all, the analog video signal must be converted into digital information. For this purpose, the analog-to-digital converter is used, and this is characterized by the conversion rate R and the number of amplitude levels Q which are coded with "el" ld Q bit. With 256 amplitude levels this is 8 bit, for $2^8 = 256$. The so-called quantizing error, that is, the exactness with which

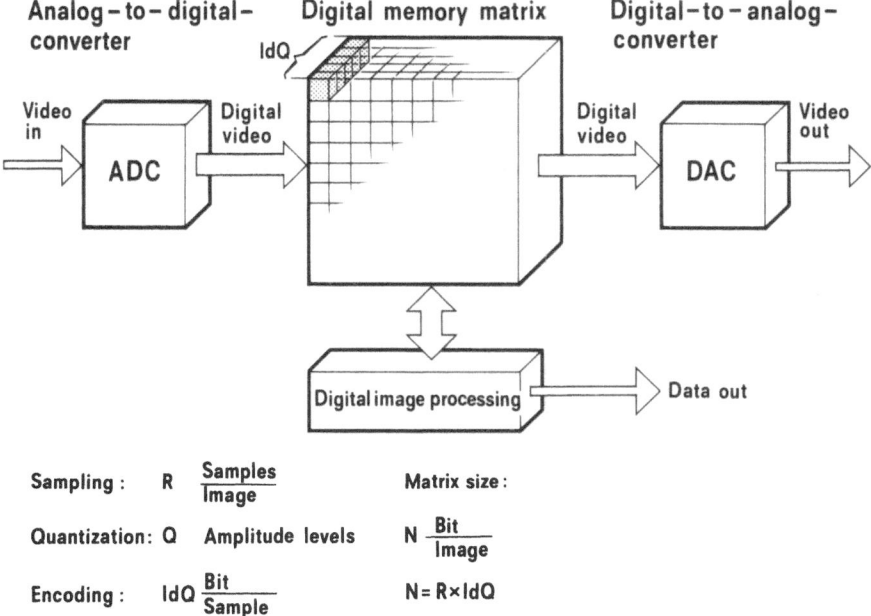

Fig. 8. Basic concept of digital video system

a specific amplitude value can be recalled after digitization, amounts to $\pm \frac{1}{2}$ which, in the example given, is 1/512, or 0.2%. The necessary conversion speed is obtained from the number of picture elements or pixels desired per image; in the case of X-ray TV, because of the round image-intensifier field, these are expediently so selected that the image is divided into the same number of elements both horizontally and vertically. With a total of N pixels a square matrix of $\sqrt{N} \cdot \sqrt{N}$ pixels results. The number of bits which have to be stored is obtained from the multiplication of the number of pixels N and the bit depth ld Q. The digital image memory itself can be appropriately visualized as being organized into rows and columns corresponding to the matrix, in which every pixel is allocated a number of ld Q memory cells. Signal processing demands access to the content of the memory matrix. The stored signal can be converted into a standard video signal again by means of a digital-to-analog converter and observed on a monitor.

Digital Video Technique: Signal Processing

Because of their inherent exactness and reproducibility, digital techniques are particularly suitable when cardioangiographic examinations have to be quantitatively evaluated. Figure 9 shows a systematic summary of the many possible processes.

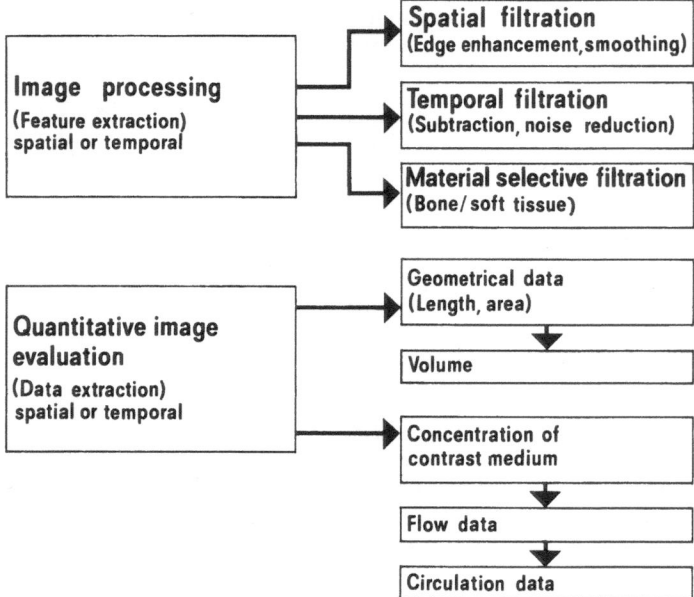

Fig. 9. General classification of digital image processing

In the following papers, the processes designated as quantitative image evaluation or data extraction, or the extracted results, will be examined more closely. However, digital techniques also show themselves to be advantageous in general image processing, as indicated in Fig. 9, as feature extraction. This type of image processing is not only significant for visual image evaluation – in order to make the morphological information more conspicuous [19] – but can also be a preliminary stage for subsequent quantitative evaluation, as in the case of temporal or material-selective filtering [20].

References

1. Kunnen M, DePinte (1972) Stereokino und Stereofernsehdurchleuchtung in der 2-Ebenen-Angiokardiographie. Vortrag Angiographiekongreß Salzburg 1972
2. Gimenez JL, Stewart GH, Lynch PR (1968) High speed (540 frames per second) biplane cineradiography. Invest Radiol 3:51–55
3. Bove AA, Ziskin MC, Freeman E, Gimenez JL, Lynch PR (1970) Selection of optimum cine-radiographic frame rate. Invest Radiol 5:329–335
4. Rutishauser W (1969) Kreislaufanalyse mittels Röntgendensitometrie. Huber, Bern
5. Heintzen P (ed) (1971) Roentgen-, Cine- and Videodensitometry. Fundamentals and applications for blood flow and heart volume determination. Thieme, Stuttgart
6. Snellen, HA et al. (eds) (1972) Quantitation in cardiology. University Press, Leiden
7. Vanselow K, Heuck F (1975) Neue Grundlagen und Theorien zur Verbesserung der Angio-Cine-Densitometrie. Fortschr Röntgenstr 122:453–456, 123:268–273, 358–363, 468–475, 567–570

8. Silverman NR (1970) Television fluorodensitometry. Invest Radiol 5:35–45
9. Wood EH, Sturm RE, Sanders JJ (1964) Data processing in cardiovascular physiology with particular reference to roentgen videodensitometry. Mayo Clin Proc 39:849–865
10. Mistretta CA, Crummy AB, Strother CM (1981) Digital angiography: a perspective. Radiology 139:273–276
11. Haendle J (1979) Der Entwicklungsstand des Röntgenfernsehens. Radiol Diagn 20:554–569
12. Gebauer A, Lissner J, Schott O (1974) Das Röntgenfernsehen. Thieme, Stuttgart, p 74
13. Heimann B, Heimann W (1978) Fernsehkameraröhren – Eigenschaften und Anwendungen. Fernseh Kino Tech 32 (9/10):1–13
14. Haendle J, Hohmann D, Maaß W (1981) Das elektronische Röntgenbild in der peroperativen Röntgendiagnostik. Electromedica 49:74–79
15. Reimers K (1981) Halbleiter kontra Röhre. Funkschau 53:71–74
16. Franken A (1981) Eine neue hochauflösende Plumbiconröhre. Rundfunktechn Mitt 25:49–53
17. Marhoff P (1967) Übertragung von Bewegungsvorgängen beim Röntgenfernsehen. Deutscher Röntgenkongreß 1966. Thieme, Stuttgart, pp 190–193
18. Pfeiler M, Jooß B (1969) Zum Zeitverhalten eines Bildübertragungssystems am Beispiel des Röntgenfernsehens. NTZ 22:88–92
19. Schott O (1967) Elektronische Informationsaufbereitung in der Röntgendiagnostik. Elektromedizin 12:204–215
20. Riederer SJ, Kruger RA, Mistretta CA (1981) Three-beam K-edge imaging of iodine using differences between fluoroscopic video images: theoretical considerations. Med Phys 8:471–479

Digital Acquisition and Processing of Video Angiocardiograms *

R. BRENNECKE[1] and P. H. HEINTZEN

Department of Pediatric Cardiology and Biomedical Engineering, University of Kiel, Kiel, FRG
[1] Present address: II. Medizinische Klinik und Poliklinik der Universität Mainz, FRG

Introduction

Angiocardiographic diagnosis is still mainly based on the visual assessment of radiographic projection images recorded on photographic film. Considerable amounts of contrast material have to be selectively injected into the circulation in order to make the regions of diagnostic relevance visible in the superposition of the shadows of tissue and bone structures displayed in these transmission images. In addition, selective angiocardiography requires exact positioning of the catheter, a time-consuming procedure which is not without risk. The processing of the angiographic films obtained is difficult to maintain at a constant high quality level, and this introduces an disadvantageous delay between image recording and diagnostic evaluation. Electronic techniques of image recording and processing based on analog devices have not been able to replace film as the primary image storage medium in angiocardiography. However, the rapid development of digital microelectronic technology promises to offer the technical prerequisites for both high quality, flexible electronic image recording and reproducible image evaluation. The need for image processing, in addition to recording, results from two general requirements:

1. A wider demand for less invasive diagnostic procedures. The high sensitivity of the selective contrast material display offered by certain digital image processing techniques results in reduced patient load or makes possible an increased number of examinations at constant load, needed for follow-up studies, screening, or intervention angiocardiography.
2. The need for extraction of quantitative parameters characterizing functions such as regional blood flow or ejection fraction. The quantification of these parameters can help to support diagnostic decisions and to evaluate the success of a therapy. Analog videodensitometry and videometry can be applied to extract these data, but their application in a clinical environment has been limited by the need to interface the additional equipment necessary and its relatively complicated operation.

Thus, digital video techniques presently being evaluated and developed can offer a solution for some of the most severe technical and diagnostic problems discussed above. We shall review here the principles of digital acquisition and

* This work was supported by the Deutsche Forschungsgemeinschaft

processing of video angiocardiograms. The framework for the discussion of the many achievements and problems of this rapidly developing new branch of radiology will be taken from concepts of signal and image processing (Schüssler 1973; Peled and Liu 1976; Pratt 1978). We hope in this way not only to provide a description of already existing methods, but also to stimulate the wider use of tools developed in other fields of information processing.

Digital Radiographic Imaging Modalities

Radiographic imaging of tissue structures is limited by the central problem that only transmission images can be generated. In these images, the shadows of all transradiated structures are shown superimposed. An early systematic overview of radiologic transmission imaging methods has been given by Mistretta (1974). Since 1972, when computer tomography (CT) was introduced, a number of digital imaging modalities have been developed to separate radiologic details from background. All of these techniques generally still require the injection of contrast material into the circulation if used for cardiac imaging. The most important of these methods have been collected in Fig. 1. By their digital electronic implementation, they all differ from conventional film techniques. However, there are also fundamental differences between these techniques in regard to methods of data acquisition and digital signal processing.

The fan beam systems shown in the upper part of Fig. 1 offer the advantage of direct digital data acquisition and good contrast resolution due to the high

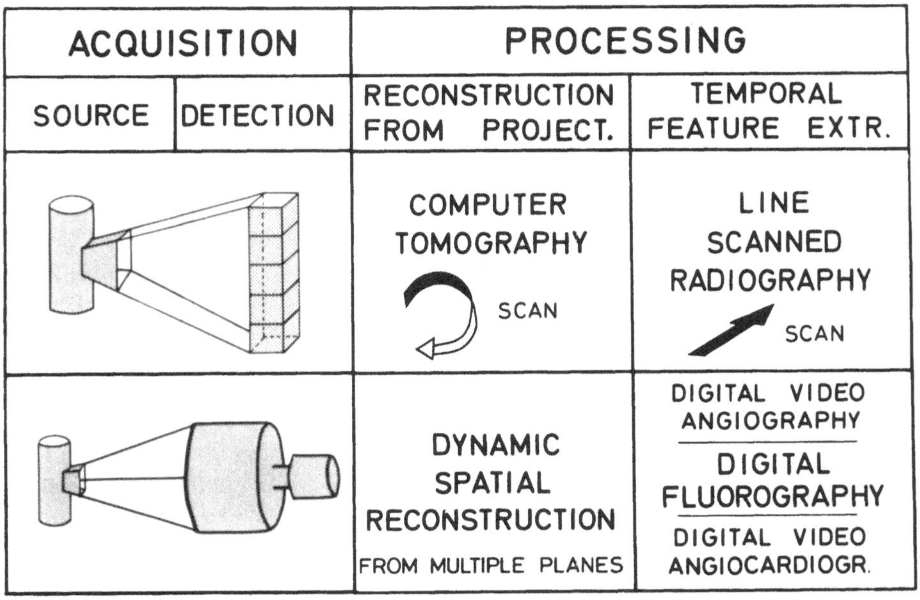

ACQUISITION		PROCESSING	
SOURCE	DETECTION	RECONSTRUCTION FROM PROJECT.	TEMPORAL FEATURE EXTR.
		COMPUTER TOMOGRAPHY ↺ SCAN	LINE SCANNED RADIOGRAPHY ↗ SCAN
		DYNAMIC SPATIAL RECONSTRUCTION FROM MULTIPLE PLANES	DIGITAL VIDEO ANGIOGRAPHY ––––– DIGITAL FLUOROGRAPHY DIGITAL VIDEO ANGIOCARDIOGR.

Fig. 1. Modalities of digital radiographic imaging systems. These systems are compared with regard to the image acquisition mode used and the class of image processing methods typically applied

signal-to-noise ratio of the detectors used and the low amount of scattering components. However, both CT (rotating imaging system, cross-sectional reconstruction algorithms) and line scanned radiography (linear movement of imaging system, temporal feature extraction algorithms; Brody 1981) are limited in their temporal resolution. Only area beam systems seem to be capable at present of providing the high radiographic image data flow necessary for a detailed study of dynamic structures such as the heart. To obtain the high temporal resolution required and at the same time extract quantitative three-dimensional (spatial) absorption data is the aim of dynamic spatial reconstruction (DSR; Wood 1977). This complex system combines a number of complete X-ray systems with a high speed digital processor system. Pfeiler (1981) has discussed some basic problems of this approach which may limit its applicability.

Because of the reasons described above, only the techniques collectively named "digital fluorography" in Fig. 1 are left for routine angiocardiographic imaging. They are characterized by the following features:

1. Image acquisition using fluoroscopic system components (area beam radiation source, image intensifier, video camera). However, in some angiographic applications, the radiation exposure per image may be 10 to 100 times higher than in standard fluoroscopy. This dose is then concentrated in a few images.
2. Analog or digital recording of the video signal.
3. Digital processing of the video data, primarily based on the extraction of temporal parameters instead of cross-sectional or spatial reconstruction from projections.

A large number of names have been coined for this new field including digital video angiography, digital intravenous vascular imaging, computerized angiography, computerized fluoroscopy, digital subtraction angiography, and digital fluorography (DF). Since the term "cine fluorography" is already in use, we will use the term "digital fluorography". Most of the techniques employed are based on the concept of radiographic image subtraction going back to film subtraction work pioneered by Ziedses des Plantes (1961). After the advent of the digital computer, subtraction of digitized film images was repeatedly described (Selzer 1968; Chow et al. 1973). Quantitative video techniques for angiocardiography and their digital implementations were developed very early by groups at the Mayo Clinic and in the Kinderklinik in Kiel (Sturm and Wood 1971; Heintzen 1971a; Heintzen and Bürsch 1978). Hardware and software developed at Kiel in the years between 1972 and 1977 showed most of the features of current digital fluorography systems, including: a) real-time temporal subtraction imaging (Brennecke et al. 1977); b) real-time subtraction recording for enhanced image storage (Brennecke et al. 1976, 1977); c) postprocessing capabilities for video recorded images (Heintzen et al. 1975; Brennecke et al. 1976, 1977; using a conventional minicomputer software implementation); and d) application in intravenous (Brennecke et al. 1977) and selective (Brennecke et al. 1976, 1977) angiocardiography and angiography.

At Madison, Mistretta, Kruger, and coworkers developed a purely hardware-oriented architecture (Kruger et al. 1978a, b) while the group of Capp, Nudelman and coworkers at Tucson designed a primarily software-oriented system featuring direct digital storage of serial angiograms (Ovitt et al. 1978). Design of commercially available processors was based on these architectures. Since 1980, clinical evaluation of these techniques is in progress in many clinics. This is, however, a topic outside the scope of this report on the technical and physical conditions of digital angiocardiography. Published results from experience with digital angiocardiography include reports from Madison (Crummy et al. 1982), Utrecht (Engels and Ludwig 1982), Kiel (Brennecke et al. 1982; Bürsch et al. 1982), Cleveland (Meaney et al. 1980), and Los Angeles (Vas et al. 1981). Many other applications have been made in carotoid, intercranial, and peripheral angiographic imaging. In the following paragraphs, we will discuss the adaptation of fluoroscopic equipment to the digital storage/processing system and the main processing algorithms used at present. Some trends in the development of X-ray sources, camera tubes, and image intensifiers are described in other chapters in this book.

Digital Representation of Radiographic Video Image Sequences

Some shortcomings of angiographic imaging techniques and of transmission imaging in general have been outlined above. The high degree of freedom in handling and processing data provided by digital systems has led to a search for digital implementations of image storage and data extraction techniques. However, in this time of transition from the analog to the digital approach of image storage and processing, it may be useful to remember that many digital systems can be regarded as simulations of analog systems (Papoulis 1977). This allows in digital signal processing, too, the use of the well-known concepts of (analog) system theory and, more specifically, of filter theory (high pass and low pass filters, modulation transfer function). Figure 2 shows this correspondence in more detail. The digital system has a defined transfer function which often can

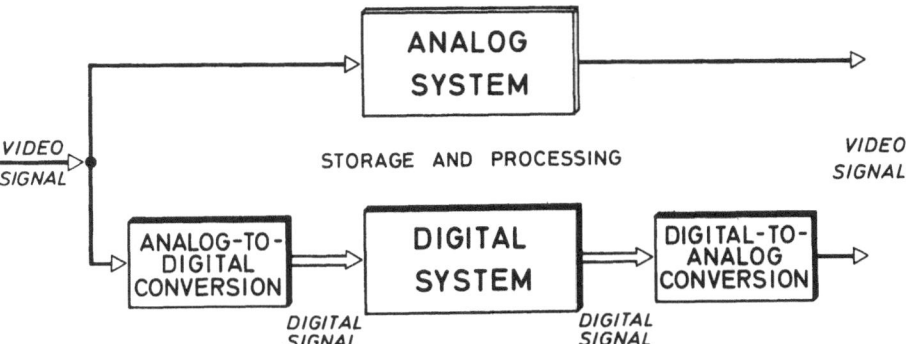

Fig. 2. Schematic comparison of analog and digital systems for storage and processing of radiographic video image sequences. The digital system can often be regarded as a simulation of an analog system. The conversion steps shown in Figs. 3 and 4 transform the video signal from the analog to the digital representation and vice versa

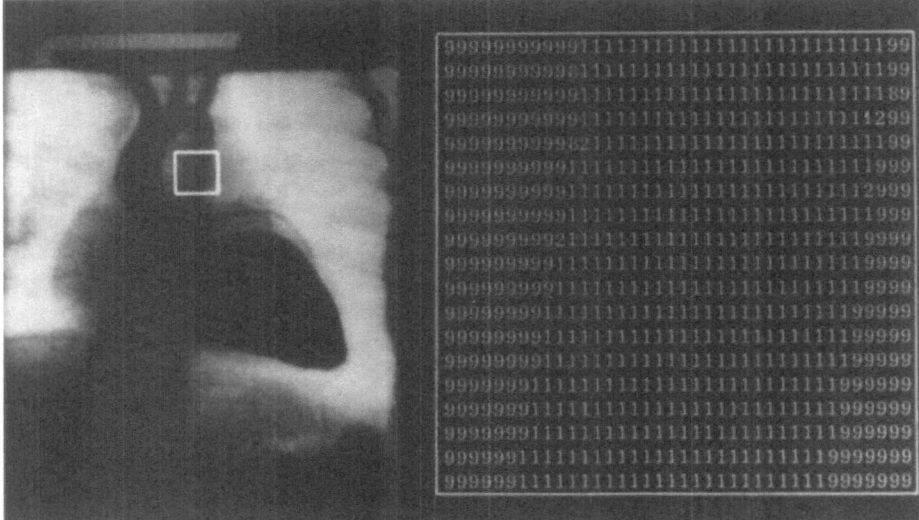

Fig. 3. Digitization of an angiocardiogram. A small region in the left image is converted into the digital subimage shown schematically at the right, i.e., an array of numbers describing the gray level values of the picture elements in the marked region

be chosen to simulate that of an equivalent analog system. Converters adapt the analog input signal to the digital system and transform the processed digital data back to an analog output signal. In many cases, the errors of the conversions can be made negligible.

The analog input signal is usually assumed to be continous with regard to time and amplitude. Specifically, radiographic images stored on photographic emulsion or on the target of a Plumbicon camera are often regarded as being recorded in continuous gradations of tone or charge across the two-dimensional surface of the medium. Digital systems, on the other hand, store and process image information in discrete numerical units. Figure 3 shows, on the left, an ordinary cardioangiographic image. On the right, the digital representation of a small region of this image is shown schematically. It consists of an array of integers. Image processing transforms these data into another array which is then converted back to a continuous image for viewing.

Image Data Sampling

The basic steps involved in the digitization of a one-dimensional, time-varying signal are shown in Fig. 4. This ist analyzed in more rigorous form in many textbooks (Peled and Liu 1976). In the first step, a conversion from continuous time to discrete time is performed by sampling the analog signal $y(t)$ at discrete time intervals τ:

$$t \rightarrow k\tau \tag{1}$$

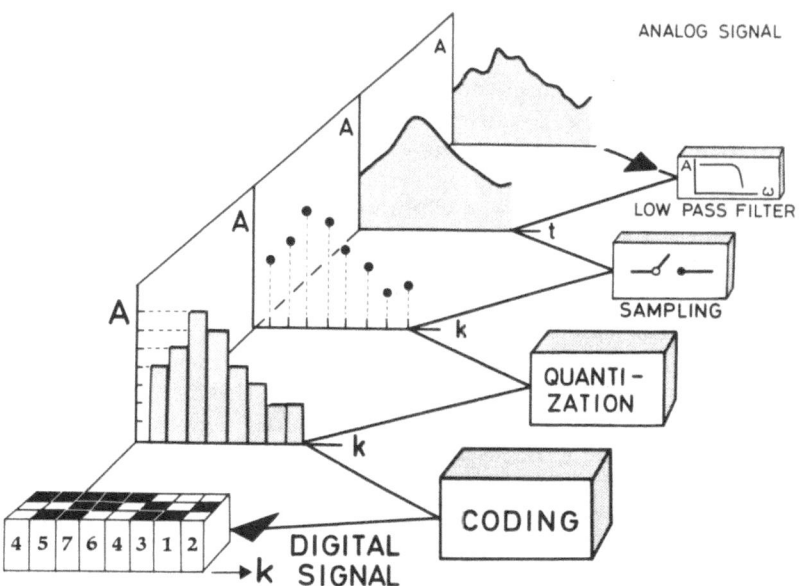

Fig. 4. General scheme for the digitization of an analog time-varying signal. A similar scheme is applied for the digitization of time-varying image sequences (Fig. 5)

The sampled signal is a function of discrete time k ($k = 0, 1, 2...$):

$$y(t) \rightarrow y(k) \tag{2}$$

This process is shown schematically in Fig. 3. In a second step, the discrete amplitude samples are quantized, i.e., they are approximated by a limited number P of different fixed amplitude values

$$y_1 < y_2 < ... < y_P \tag{3}$$

The true value of each time varying sample is represented by the fixed amplitude value with the smallest deviation from the value of the sample. Usually, the number P of discrete fixed amplitude values is given by a power N of 2 and the spacing Q between the discrete amplitudes is constant:

$$P = 2^N, \quad y_n - y_{n-1} = Q \tag{4}$$

Typically, for video signals 256 to 1024 different amplitude levels are used ($N = 8$ to $N = 10$). Due to this finite amplitude resolution, a statistical error is generated which is equivalent to a signal-independent (additive) noise amplitude. The useful dynamic range D of the analog-to-digital conversion is often approximated in decibel (dB) units to be at least:

$$D = 20 \log P = 6N \tag{5}$$

This value is than comparable with the contribution of other noise sources. The temporal sampling process preserves all information contained in the time-varying signal $y(t)$ if this continuous signal is appropriately band-limited by a low-pass filter as shown in Fig. 4. Under ideal conditions, the filtered analog signal may contain frequency components lower than half the sampling frequency. However, as discussed above, quantization of the amplitude samples is always an approximation process. As will be discussed below, it is usually technically feasible to make the error of this approximation so small that it can be neglected when compared with the unavoidable noise in the filtered continuous input signal.

The last step shown in Fig. 4 is signal coding. This transforms the quantized signal into a binary representation compatible with the organization of common digital storage elements and arithmetic functions; N bits (binary digits) are needed to code the P different amplitude levels defined in Eqs. 3 and 4 above.

The digitization of the information contained in the dynamic projection images from a moving object such as the heart is a much more complex process. Figure 5 shows the most relevant steps for a system applying video scanning of the radiographic images. Comparing this schematic with the digitization of a one-dimensional signal (Fig. 4), we notice that while quantization and coding appear to be similar, the sampling process is performed in several steps.

The first step in sampling a radiographic image sequence is the generation of discrete radiographic images by pulsed radiation of short duration and with a pulse rate matched to the fastest process to be imaged. Note that (with the exception of the small effect of the time lag of the camera tube) no band-limiting filter (Fig. 4) can be conceived in this case to avoid aliasing ("stroboscopic") effects due to a low sampling rate. Thus, the image generation rate is usually determined by the fastest moving structures of interest (Freeman et al. 1970; Ritman 1977) and the signals of the usually much larger static or slowly moving

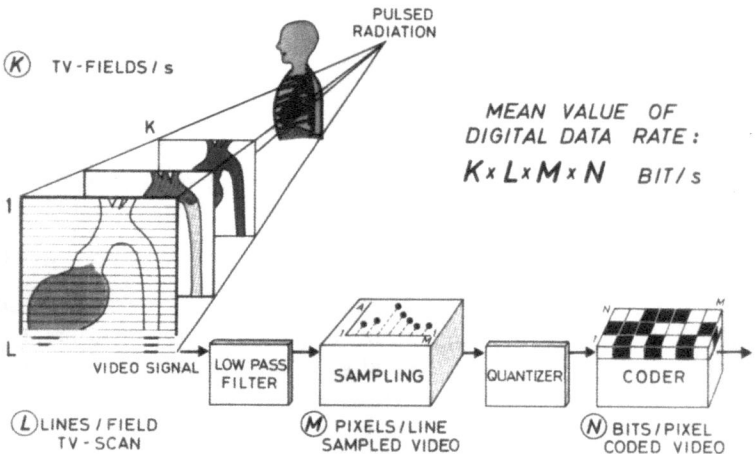

Fig. 5. Acquisition of digital image data describing a radiographic projection of the heart. The sampling of the video signal (*right*) is performed as shown in Fig. 4. The total digitization process for this dynamic information involves, however, two additional sampling steps (pulsed image generation and line sampling) as shown schematically in the *left* part of the diagram

image regions are over-sampled. This generates a high mean data rate and large amounts of data and requires a large radiation dose (Martin et al. 1981; Waldman et al. 1981). These problems may in future be solved by digital implementations of image data acquisition and processing. The data rate and capacity may be decreased in the coding process and both these parameters, and in addition the radiation dose, might in certain applications be reduced by noise reducers or temporal low-pass filters. These topics are discussed in the following paragraphs.

Presently, the typical imaging rate is 50/s or 60/s in video angiocardiography and the radiation pulse (aperture time) should not be wider than 2 ms to avoid motion blurring and a widening of the X-ray spectrum (Heintzen 1971 b; Haendle 1979). Lower pulse rates should increasingly be evaluated. In some applications, the generation of heart phase triggered images from end diastole and end systole should be sufficient (Wittmaack et al. 1980). This way of image data rate reduction is free from aliasing even though the mean sampling rate is low. One should also be conscious of the very high dose sometimes applied during catheter positioning. Digital storage of images can replace analog media in applications such as pathfinder techniques and low pulse rate fluoroscopy (Grolman et al. 1972; Wittmaack et al. 1980).

In a video system, the next partial step of the sampling procedure is the line scanning of the target of the Plumbicon camera (Fig. 5). The spatial frequency content ist limited to some extent by the finite focal spot size of the X-ray tube and the modulation transfer function of image intensifier and optics. Again, no sharp cutoff of the modulation transfer function can be provided to avoid (spatial) stroboscopic effects, but the width of the scanning beam introduces some blurring of horizontal edge information. Typical line sampling rate is about 500–600 lines per TV frame (33 or 40 ms). Interlaced scanning of TV lines in even and odd fields is commonly used to increase the perceived spatial resolution in static images without an increase of data rate requirements. This format is, however, not usable in low pulse rate applications, due to slow image buildup on the target of a video camera tube. Moreover, in any kind of stop action viewing it loses its spatial resolution advantage over repeat field (noninterlaced) systems, since in dynamic regions the two (312½-line) fileds comprising a (625-line) frame contain different information, so that only one field should be shown at a time. In subtraction imaging, the differencing of even and odd fields results in artifacts at vertical edge structures, if interlacing is used. Therefore, we expect that repeat field techniques (no interlacing of TV lines) using, e.g., 312 lines/50 Hz or 624 lines/25 Hz will increasingly be used in radiologic video systems in the future. The equivalent numbers for the US standard are 256 lines/60 Hz or 512 lines/30 Hz. A digital system can easily provide the scan conversion needed to display the recorded repeat field images on a standard interlaced monitor.

The last simpling step in a radiographic video system is the continuous to discrete conversion of the video signal resulting from line sampling (Fig. 5). This is the only sampling step used in a digital system in addition to those provided by an analog video chain. In a 512- or 624-line system, the sampling frequency has to be around 10 MHz to provide 512 samples per line (visible part of each line about 50 µs). These samples are called picture elements or pixels. Stroboscopic effects due to vertical edge information with high frequency components and the effect of high frequency noise can be reduced by a conventional electronic filter shown in Fig. 5. A passband of about 5 MHz is allowed by the sampling frequency of more than 10 MHz. The nonlinear phase characteristics of a sharply band-limiting analog filter may, however, introduce some "ringing" which turns up as a decorrelation of nearest neighbors on a TV line in the performance of certain types of quantitative analysis.

The quality of the digitization and image analysis process is, in addition to the above-mentioned considerations, determined by the degree of the temporal reproducibility of the three sampling processes. Specifically, any time base error in the video sampling process (pixel sampling) is translated into subtraction noise originating at vertical edge structures of the background. The tolerable amount of relative shift of pixel positions in the images to be subtracted is of the order of only 10–20 ns (less than ¼ of pixel time interval), depending on the contrast of the background and the signal-to-noise ratio of the original images. This stability is required for some seconds. The time base jitter is also a severe problem in recording video images on video tape or disc recorders before digitization.

Image Data Quantization and Digital Real-Time Storage

Following the sampling processes described, the resulting time discrete signal is quantized. From Eq. 5, we can derive that it is easy to make quantization-induced errors small compared with the noise level of standard radiographic TV systems (about 43 dB or 140:1) which is limited by the mainly additive noise of the video amplifier. A conversion with $N = 8$ bits (signal-to-noise ratio of more than 48 dB) is sufficient in this case. Other considerations apply if a high signal-to-noise ratio (e.g., 300:1) is obtained for the camera so that the multiplicative quantum noise becomes determining. The amplitude of quantum noise becomes low in dark regions of the image so that the quantization noise of the conversion process may become limiting. Some digital fluoroscopy systems therefore apply a logarithmic amplifier before digitization to expand small signal levels so that they cover more of the quantization steps than in linear quantization. However, logarithmic video amplifiers exhibit a complex signal-dependent frequency response. Thus, it seems to be more appropriate to use a quantizer with nonuniform sampling steps. It is, however, more common to apply standard 9- or 10-bit converters and perform a logarithmic conversion by a digital look-up table after analog-to-digital conversion.

The coder (Fig. 5) transforms the quantized signal into a digital code. The video (pixel) sampling in combination with the quantization and coding process is usually called "analog to digital conversion." The total information capacity, as determined by the three sampling steps and the quantization process, is given by the equation derived in Fig. 5 ($\times T$):

$$C = K \times L \times M \times N \times T \tag{6}$$

where T is the duration of the scene (in seconds). For $K = 25/s$, $L = 512$ lines/ frame, $M = 512$ pixels/line, $N = 8$ bits/pixel and $T = 10$ s, we obtain a data capacity of 50 Mbytes.

Different tradeoffs are possible between temporal resolution (K) and spatial resolution ($L*M$). The same amount of data is produced at high spatial and low temporal resolution as is generated at a high frame rate combined with a lower geometrical resolution. The meaningful choice of these parameters is determined not only by the cost and complexity of the digital storage necessitated, but also by the radiation dose required to provide a sufficient signal-to-noise ratio at the level of the picture elements at a given frame rate and geometrical resolution.

The present resolution limit of X-ray TV systems (1024*1024 pixels at a 40 ms frame period; Haendle 1979) is still lower than that provided by the cine film. This may be a limitation in applications such as coronary angiocardiography.

The amount of data generated in digital angiocardiography and their rate are large even when considering the high state of the art of computer peripherals such as digital disc and tape recorders. The mean data rate is larger than 50 Mbit/s and the required data capacity around 400 Mbit (50 Mbyte) per scene. For comparison, standard disc technology delivers mean data rates around 7 Mbit/s. Discs which store at rates up to about 30 MHz and offer a capacity of about 500 Mbytes will probably soon become available (Hedberg 1982). Even then, several channels have to be used in parallel for the continuous storage of video image sequences. The higher error rate of these devices should be tolerable for image recording. This makes possible an increase in storage density and, correspondingly, in data rate, given a certain state of disc technology. Development along this line will certainly soon lead to cost-effective solutions of the storage problem even for the high data rates encountered in digital angiocardiography.

An alternative way to solve the digital storage problem is to apply techniques for data reduction. In the transmission and storage of quantitative data, the goal of data reduction is to transmit only information that cannot be derived from data which have been sent earlier. Thus, redundancy is reduced. We were able to reduce by a factor of ½ the data rate and data capacity for the storage of radiographic images (256*256 pixels) by an intraframe information-preserving predictive coder (Brennecke et al. 1978a). This relative gain should be even greater at higher spatial resolution and when more advanced adaptive coding schemes are applied (Musmann 1979). The storage problem will also be discussed in the context of image processing in the next section.

Future Developments of Digital Radiographic Image Acquisition

We expect that future radiographic video systems will depart more and more from commercial TV standards. These standards were optimized on the basis of subjective display criteria. Digital technology helps to optimize separately the image formation and coding processes (based on quantitative requirements such as signal-to-noise ratio, entropy and sampling rate) and the image display

process (psychovisual requirements). The fidelity of the digitization process is mainly limited by two sources of error:
1. Quantization errors
2. Time base errors in the sampling processes

By careful design, these errors can be held sufficiently low. More subtle error sources may originate from the nonideal band-limiting characteristics of the filters preceding the various sampling processes. The extremely high mean data rates typical for angiocardiographic image sequences require an approach to digital data transmission and storage that deviates from the methods used for program and data handling in general purpose computer systems.

Digital Processing of Angiocardiograms

The main medical motivations for handling radiographic image data by digital techniques result from the need for more flexible handling of stored images (compared with film), from the necessity to obtain quantitative morphological and functional information, and/or from the requirement to reduce patient load. Here we describe the processing techniques available for the large amount of image data generated at an extremely high rate using the digitization process.

Electronic Storage of Angiocardiograms in Digital Fluorography Systems

Image storage has to be provided for the primary image sequence and this sequence has to be accessible for further processing. The solution chosen for image storage in a digital fluorography system has far-reaching consequences for the architecture of the whole processing system and for its overall performance. In fact the three main system architectures found today in digital fluorography can be discriminated by the implementation of their image data storage.

Figure 6 gives an overview of the most frequently applied architectures. The conceptually simplest configuration (A) is a system performing both storage and processing by digital devices. However, because of the present excessive cost of digital real-time video storage (see above) angiocardiographic systems apply hybrid architectures combining (analog) video storage devices and digital processing devices. In the configuration B shown in Fig. 6, the angiographic image sequence is recorded on high quality video tape (¾ or 1 in.) or a video disc recorder. The image sequence can then be replayed from tape or disc and various digital processing techniques applied in real time while viewing the results. In addition, the images can be digitized in a stroboscopic mode (Brennecke et al. 1977) and transferred to a digital disc for flexible processing using a standard computer. In an optimized design this takes typically 4 min for 10 s of input data. The principal disadvantage of this approach is that the signal-to-noise ratio is limited by the recording process (magnetic and electronic noise, time-base jitter), at least in applications where quantum noise is low and where the background possesses a high contrast. For these cases we developed a scheme for subtraction recording (Brennecke et al. 1976, 1977) which is now also found in some commercial systems. As shown in Fig. 6c, during recording the digital processor is used to extract by background subtraction the relatively small contrast-material signal. The remaining specific signal is multiplied by an integer factor (typical contrast enhancement factor: 2–4) and this expanded signal is stored on video tape or disc after digital to analog conversion. Thus, the specific contrast material signal is amplified with respect to storage media and electronic noise. Wie also described a technique to reconstruct the full image information (including background) with low noise from the video tape recording. The limitation of this technique of subtraction recording results from motion of background structures, which may produce signals overloading the dynamic range of the system even at conservative contrast enhancement factors. This clipping destroys irreversibly the image information in the moving region. Large enhancement factors of 8 or 16 sometimes found in the literature increase this risk. Certainly, less critical techniques for reduction of tape noise can be developed.

We expect that the evolution of future systems integrating the image processing steps (e.g., real-time processing and postprocessing) will lead to an increased development of exclusively digital systems (Fig. 6a). The image processor ISAAC (Image Acquisition and Analysis Computer) developed by our group represents an approach to integrate image data acquisition (including digital control of the X-ray generator, the storage of physiological data, and image processing) in a programmable digital system (Brennecke et al. 1980).

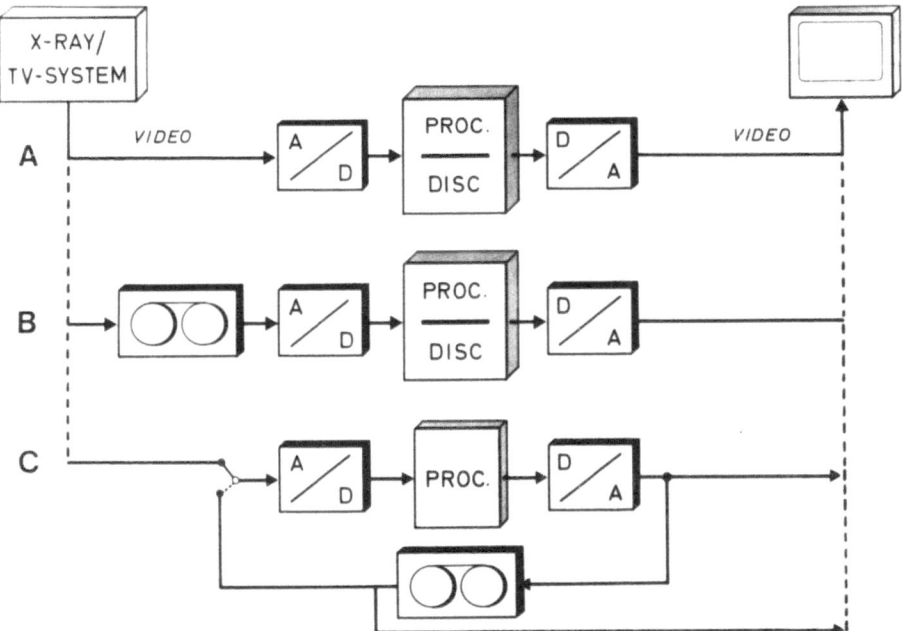

Fig. 6. Principal architectures of image acquisition and processing systems for digital fluorography. The three system designs vary primarily with respect to the method chosen for image sequence storage. Digital (*A*), analog (*B*), and hybrid (*C*) storage concepts are shown

However, hybrid systems will for quite a while have the advantage of lower cost and higher mobility, especially when applied in intensive care units and similar applications and when only a limited degree of flexibility is needed. Moreover, at present the video tape seems to be the only electronic medium applicable for clinical archival storage of image sequences, considering the fact that one angiocardiographic scene is typically equivalent to 25–50 Mbytes of digital data. The integrity of this storage is, however, only guaranteed for a few years. Although technical systems for archival storage are not yet ready for general application, work is in progress to solve the problem of managing the image data archiving and communication tasks in a digital imaging system (Meyer-Ebrecht 1980; Meyer-Ebrecht et al. 1982; Cox et al. 1982).

Digital Image Processing Techniques for Radiographic Detail Extraction

The basic goal of the image-processing techniques presently evaluated on a broad scale in angiocardiography is the selective display of regions of the circulation opacified by contrast material. By eliminating superimposed shadows of bone and tissue structures, the details of interest are selectively displayed. In this process, the contrast of these structures is usually expanded. The prerequisite of this selectivity is the injection of contrast material into the circulation. It is the temporal change in X-ray absorption provided by the passage of this bolus which is evaluated by the image-processing techniques commonly applied in digital fluorography.

It has been known for decades (Ziedses des Plantes 1961) that a sensitive selective display of opacified regions can be obtained by using image subtraction techniques. A mask image (without dye) is subtracted from an opacified image to make visible the regions containing contrast material. In recent years, the flexible, reproducible, and efficient operation of digital implementations of these techniques have led to their wider use. In addition, other modalities of the subtraction scheme were evaluated and subtraction was combined with preprocessing and postprocessing techniques. The need for the automatic processing of whole image sequences and for the flexible reduction of subtraction artifacts was one of the driving forces for this development, the requirement to extract quantitative parameters the other. Because of this rapid development, it seems worthwhile to seek a systematic framework for description and differentiation. This framework is offered by the terminology of electronic signal processing and digital image processing.

The basic operators for processing a digital image sequence are the following:
1. Point operators: linear and nonlinear mapping of the gray levels of each pixel
2. "Spatial" (planar) filters applied to a neighborhood of each pixel in a single image
3. Temporal filters applied to a temporal sequence of brightness values, taken pixelwise over the image sequences. If, e.g., the spatial resolution of each image in a sequence is equivalent to 64 000 pixels, the temporal filtering of this sequence is equivalent to the processing of 64 000 one-dimensional time-

varying signals, each describing the temporal brightness variations at a given pixel location over time. More complex operators can be obtained by linear or nonlinear combinations of the three basic steps. In digital fluorography, the main gain has been obtained by application of temporal filters while image processing is otherwise usually associated with spatial filtering. These temporal filters are implemented in the time domain, but realizations using Fourier techniques will certainly follow.

Temporal Subtraction and Filtering Methods

The main temporal detail extraction techniques presently being evaluated are shown in Fig. 7. Subtraction is the basic method applied. In angiocardiography, the optimum matching of the mask image is obtained by ECG-gated subtraction (Fig. 7, left). In its simplest implementation, from each contrast image a single background image (mask) recorded at the same heart phase is subtracted after logarithmic conversion of the brightness values. The exact reference to the heart phase may not always be necessary. Kruger et al. (1979) generated mask images by integrating pixelwise a complete heart cycle before opacification (Fig. 7, right). This reduces random noise in the subtraction image by a factor of about 1.4 (3 dB) as compared with the subtraction of an image pair.

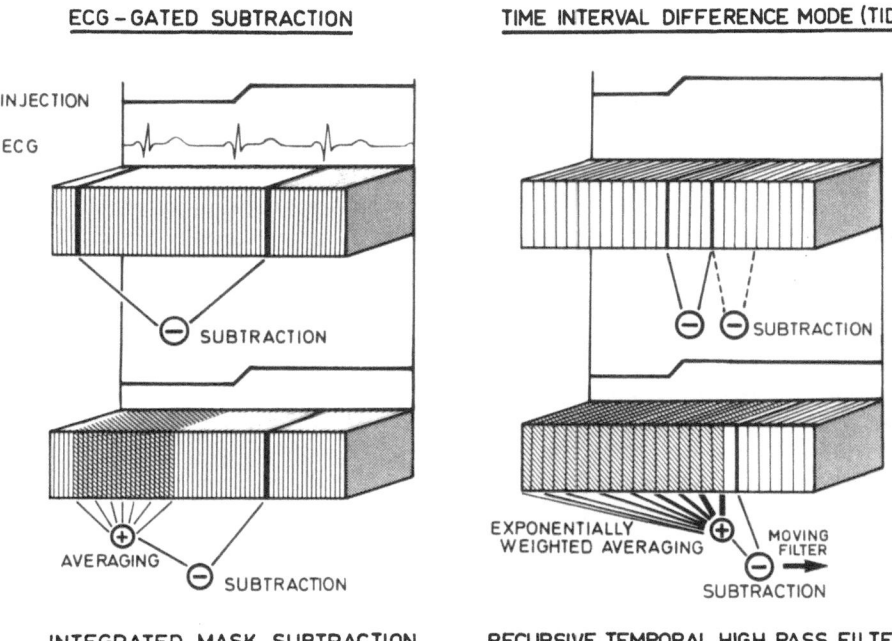

Fig. 7. Principal algorithms for radiographic feature extraction used in current generation systems for digital angiocardiography. The schemes shown on the *left* are based on temporal image subtraction, the schemes on the *right* on temporal high-pass filtering of image sequence data

Table 1. Temporal Feature Extraction

Image subtraction/registration
  cancelling of
  interferring background
  (structured noise)
Image integration
  reduction of
  random noise
Parametric imaging

Image Enhancement

Gray level mapping
  contrast expansion

While the techniques described above extract opacified regions from the unspecific background, it seems sometimes more interesting to look at phasic changes of the area of the opacification. Detail motion extraction is performed by the techniques shown in Fig. 7 (left and right, bottom). Time interval differencing (TID) as implemented in the processor of the Wisconsin group (Kruger et al. 1979) subtracts each TV field from the field taken N periods earlier. Typically, $N = 4$, thus making the time interval equal to 67 ms (US standard) or 80 ms (European standard). This difference image is shown for another N-1 field periods until a new subtraction is performed. This scheme is simple to implement, but the effective imaging rate is reduced by a factor of 4 and aliasing may occur. The (recursive) high-pass filter (Pfeiler 1969; Brennecke et al. 1978a; Kruger 1981) shown in Fig. 7 (right, bottom) performs the same task of detail motion extraction. Here, however, continuous operation is obtained (50 or 60 new fields/s). Each opacified image is subtracted from an image calculated by temporal low-pass filtering of the previous image sequence.

The performance of the temporal filters described is not without severe limitations. The subtraction techniques (Fig. 7, right and left, top) require the suspension of respiration. Otherwise, the alignment of the images to be subtracted may be imperfect resulting in subtraction artifacts especially at high-contrast background structures in the images being subtracted. The process of alignment is called registration.

When respiration cannot be suspended for the duration of the angiocardiographic recording, good results can often still be obtained by respiration-gated subtraction. In the scheme shown in Fig. 8, a number of mask images taken from a respiration cycle are stored in a large random-access memory. The optimum mask is found from this background sequence by spatial cross correlation (similarity detection) of a region of interest in the opacified image with the same region in all of the mask images (Brennecke et al. 1978a). The motion extraction techniques shown in Fig. 7 (right top, left bottom) are less susceptible to motion artifacts than ECG-gated subtraction, but they usually possess a much lower contrast sensitivity and they do not show radiographic details but short-

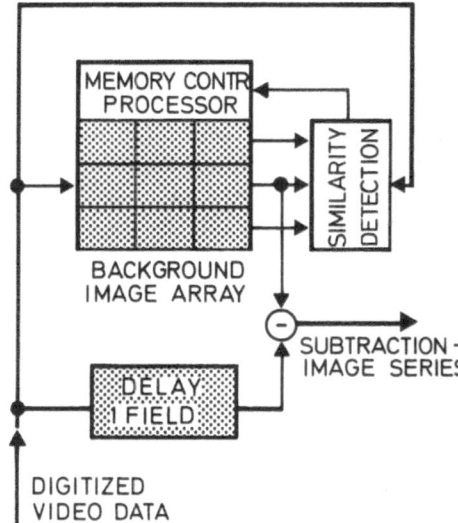

Fig. 8. Schematic diagram of a system for respiration gated subtraction

term changes in the projection area or in the thickness of details (Brennecke et al. 1978a, 1982). Modifications such as the subtraction of end diastolic and end systolic frames may provide some functional information (Kruger et al. 1979), but this can also be obtained by dynamic viewing of normal subtraction images obtained at these cardiac phases.

Remaining imperfections in the registration of background structures of the subtracted images are the main source of subtraction artifacts. The simple shifting of one of the images before subtraction by interactively determined amounts may reduce these artifacts in many cases. More automatic techniques of image registration are known from the image processing literature in the field of reconnaissance (Rosenfeld 1961; Lillestrand 1972), but they are computationally costly and still seem to apply to simpler situations. Thus, the avoidance of misregistration during the recording of the scene must remain of primary importance. Much experimental work has been done to obtain iodine contrast material signal extraction by combination of images recorded at different X-ray energies (Kelcz and Mistretta 1977; Macovski 1978). Dual-energy imaging (Brody 1981; Keyes et al. 1982), possibly in combination with temporal feature extraction, may in the future be used to create mask images which are updated when the patient moves.

Temporal Image Sequence Averaging

By (ideal) subtraction of background structures, the relatively small detail signals are extracted and thus their dynamic range can be expanded by simple multiplication of the density differences found at each pixel in the subtraction image. However, random noise components in the original images are not cancelled in the subtraction process. Statistically, the noise amplitude (measured as the noise in a region of constant gray level) will even be increased in the subtraction process by a factor of 1.4 (3 dB) if the noise is random with zero mean value.

The primary random noise component is caused by fluctuations in the number of photons received at the image intensifier entrance in the area equivalent to a given pixel. Additive noise is superimposed which is especially critical in the input stage of the video amplifier and – if analog storage of the image data is used – in the magnetic tape (disc) recording process. Since the quantum noise decreases in proportion to the square root of the mean number of received photons, while the video noise is much less signal dependent, the video noise becomes limiting especially when small amounts of contrast material are imaged which pass over dark areas of the background. The video noise sources also limit the contrast material sensitivity obtainable by using a higher radiation dose per image.

Random noise can be reduced by averaging N image frames pixel by pixel (see, e.g., Fig. 7, right bottom). In static imagery and linear averaging the noise is decreased by the factor $1/\sqrt{N}$. However, moving structures will be blurred in this process. ECG-gated averaging (Brennecke et al. 1977) helps to keep blurring effects small. It has to be decided from application to application if at a given total radiation exposure it is to be preferred to record image data at a relatively low pulse rate (high radiation per image, low random quantum noise) or at a high pulse rate (higher quantum noise) and then reduce the random noise by temporal averaging. Advantages of the latter technique are the possibility to use standard X-ray generators, tubes, and relatively noisy video amplifiers and recorders (Kruger 1981), and the possibility to reduce stroboscopic effects by the careful design of the digital filters used off line. In some cases it will also be advantageous to be able to decide at the time of image processing (and not at the moment of image recording) at which specific time the feature of interest is best observed. On the other hand, the data rate to be stored is higher in this scheme. Performing the temporal filtering in real time solves this storage problem, but in this process an irreversible information loss is encountered. More specifically, the image averaging approach to noise reduction can produce motion blurring of dynamic structures. Noise reducers (Rossi 1978) originally developed for commercial broadcasting applications can adapt the frequency response of the filtering process to the rate of brightness change estimated separately for each pixel and can, in principle, avoid the blurring effect. It remains to be seen if this technology can be adapted for use in diagnostic imaging.

The preceding discussion is one example of the unified view of image generation and image processing conditions (Kruger 1982) necessary for the optimization of radiography imaging. Digital control of imaging parameters combined with digital image processing provide the degrees of freedom for this optimization process.

Image Contrast and Density Correction

The detail extraction provided by image subtraction and temporal filtering is usually preceded by the conversion of image brightness values to logarithmic (density) values. This point operator corrects for the exponential law of X-ray absorption (Lambert-Beer Law). Due to this effect, even after ideal subtraction of a mask image from an opacified image, the background signal would be visible by "cross-talk" in the contrast material regions if (linear) brightness values were subtracted. It has to be taken into account, however, that even after logarithmic conversion some of this cross-talk is still present due to light scattered into the region of interest from neighboring areas (Brennecke et al. 1978b). Correction of this type of interference is one of the most important goals of the future both in qualitative and quantitative image evaluation.

Another point operation is used for the rescaling of subtracted images before displaying the image on a monitor for visual assessment. Depending on the many parameters of image operation and processing, the useful contrast of the subtraction images may vary widely. Although optimization of the display by multiplying the subtraction signal by a fixed factor and manipulating the controls of the display monitor is sometimes thought to be sufficient, some more reproducible techniques can be found in the literature (Brennecke et al. 1976; Christenson et al. 1980). In our experience, automatic analysis of the amplitude histograms of the subtraction images leads to reproducible results.

Discussion of Image Processing Techniques

The basic goal achieved by the digital processing techniques described is the extraction of radiographic details from background structures interfering with their intelligibility. When we define as the signal the transient change in X-ray absorption produced by the contrast material, we can regard the methods described above as filters extracting this signal from random or deterministic interference or noise. The generation of random noise is unavoidable in the image formation process (quantum noise) and electronic noise is added in the detection process. Similarly, the superposition of shadows of background structures upon the shadows of opacified regions can be regarded as deterministic interference or structured noise. The processing of image sequences by the subtraction operators described above can then be regarded as a modality of (deterministic) noise cancelling. After noise cancelling, the signal may still be hidden in random noise, which may be reduced by temporal (or spatial) averaging.

To define the subtraction operators in terms of extraction from interference seems to be more general than the definition "increase of conspicuity" which is sometimes found in the radiologic literature to describe the effect of subtraction. The use of the latter term stresses the subjective effects of these signal-processing techniques, although most of the methods described above also form the basis for automatic analysis techniques. Moreover, the description of detail extraction in terms of noise reduction is a reminder of the fact that the reduction of structured noise is a common problem which has found solutions in radar and communication systems (Widrow et al. 1971). Dual energy imaging instead of temporal mask subtraction (or their combination) may be one way to create the reference signal needed in classical schemes of structured noise cancelling.

Based on the extracted signal, a number of image analysis techniques can be used to provide quantitative data (Heintzen et al. 1978). The interactive measurement of the ejection fraction from subtraction images (Vas et al. 1981) seems to be the first example of a systematic evaluation of such a technique in digital angiocardiography. Parametric or functional imaging first developed in scintigraphy and for radiographic images of the abdominal circulation (Höhne et al. 1978; Böhm and Höhne 1981; Bürsch et al. 1981) will be applied to the analysis of the function of the heart chambers and the vessels (Brennecke et al. 1979).

The following list gives an overview on the modalities of the image processing techniques discussed:
1. Temporal feature extraction:
   a) image subtraction/registration, cancelling of interfering background (structured noise);
   b) image integration, reduction of random noise; and
   c) parametric imaging
2. Image enhancement: gray level mapping, contrast expansion

In addition, a large number of methods of feature extraction from image sequences have been developed in other fields of application; Nagel (1981) has recently given an overview and stressed certain trends of this development. We expect that a much wider spectrum of methods will develop as soon as digital systems for software-controlled processing of angiocardiograms will be more common than they are today.

Clinical Applications

In this report on the development of digital image processing we cannot go into details of the clinical applications in angiocardiography. Some early reports on specific clinical applications have already been cited. More generally, the appearance of digital techniques of image processing have made us more conscious of hidden degrees of freedom in the diagnostic procedures applied in angiocardiography. Advantages offered by this progress in imaging should be optimized by also making use of some of the following developments:
a) optimization of projections (Bogren et al. 1981); for example, C-arm mounting of the source/detector combination facilitates this choice; and
b) improved nonionic contrast materials which may, for instance, reduce the problem of pulmonary passage of the contrast material.
In addition, the selection of catheter positions and the parameters of bolus injection will have to be carefully optimized.

The many conditions of acquisition and processing of angiocardiograms mentioned in this report can only be chosen on the basis of careful clinical evaluation. From early experience with some of the developments described in this article, we expect that digital fluorography will have the following clinical advantages:

1. Immediate availability of high quality X-ray images
2. Flexible interactive access to image data and the corresponding physiological data stored in a common data file
3. Flexibility to provide image data possessing either high temporal resolution, high spatial resolution, or an extremely high signal-to-noise ratio
4. Reduction of contrast material and X-ray dose obtainable in ventriculography can be used to reduce the load to the patient or to increase the number of examinations performed at constant dose
5. Feasibility of less-invasive diagnostic procedures
6. Storage of X-ray images in a format immediately applicable to digital image restoration, quantitative analysis (such as volumetric and densitometric measurements), and a digital archival system

References

Böhm M, Höhne KH (1981) The processing and analysis of radiographic image sequences. In: Höhne KH (ed) Digital image processing in medicine. Springer, Berlin Heidelberg New York, pp 42–92

Bogren HG, Bürsch JH, Brennecke R, Radtke W, Heintzen PH (1981) Intravenous angiocardiography using digital image processing: experience with axial projections in normal pigs and in pigs with experimentally generated left-to-right shunts. Proc SPIE 314:287–293, Bellingham, USA

Brody WR, Enzmann DR, Deutsch LS, Hall A, Pelc N (1981) Intravenous carotid arteriography using line-scanned digital radiography. Radiology 139:297–300

Brennecke R, Brown TK, Bürsch JH, Heintzen PH (1976) Digital processing of videoangiographic image series using a minicomputer. Proc Comp Cardiol, IEEE Computer Society, Long Beach, pp 255–260

Brennecke R, Brown TK, Bürsch JH, Heintzen PH (1977) Computerized video-image preprocessing with applications to cardio-angiographic roentgen-image series. In: Nagel HH (ed) Digitale Bildverarbeitung. Springer, Berlin Heidelberg New York, pp 244–262

Brennecke R, Hahne JH, Moldenhauer K, Bürsch JH, Heintzen PH (1978a) Improved digital real-time processing and storage techniques with applications to intravenous contrast angiography. Proc Comp Cardiol, IEEE Computer Society, Long Beach, pp 191–194

Brennecke R, Bürsch JH, Heintzen PH (1978b) Improvements in videodensitometric measurement techniques. In: Heintzen PH, Bürsch JH (eds) Roentgen-Video-Techniques. Thieme, Stuttgart, pp 15–22

Brennecke R, Hahne HJ, Moldenhauer K, Bürsch JH, Heintzen PH (1979) A special purpose processor for digital angiocardiography. Design and applications. Proc Comp Cardiol, IEEE Computer Society, Long Beach, pp 343–346

Brennecke R, Hahne HJ, Heintzen PH (1980) A multiprocessor-system for the acquisition and analysis of video image sequences. In: Pöppl SJ, Platzer H (eds) Erzeugung und Analyse von Bildern und Strukturen. Springer, Berlin Heidelberg New York, pp 113–122

Brennecke R, Bürsch JH, Bogren HG, Heintzen PH (1982) Digital intravenous imaging techniques in pediatric cardiology. In: Mistretta CA, Crummy AB, Strother CM, Sackett JF (eds) Digital subtraction arteriography: an application of computerized fluoroscopy. Year Book Medical Publishers, Chicago, pp 133–141

Bürsch JH, Hahne JH, Brennecke R, Grönemeier D, Heintzen PH (1981) Assessment of arterial blood flow measurements by digital angiography. Radiology, 141:39–47

Bürsch JH, Bogren HG, Radtke W, Brennecke R, Heintzen PH (1982) Cardiac imaging by digitized intravenous angiocardiography. Proc Comp Cardiol, IEEE Computer Society, Long Beach

Chow CK, Hilal SK, Niebuhr KE (1973) X-ray image subtraction by digital means. IBM J Res Dev 17:296–218

52   R. Brennecke and P. H. Heintzen

Christenson PC, Ovitt TW, Fisher HD, Frost MM, Nudelman S, Roehrig H (1980) Intravenous angiography using digital video subtraction: intravenous cervicocerebrovascular angiography. AJR 135:1145–1152

Cox JR, Blaine GH, Hill RL, Jost RG (1982) Study of a distributed picture archiving and communication system for radiology. Proc SPIE 318:133–142

Crummy AB (1982) Digital subtraction arteriography of the thoracic vasculature. In: Mistretta CA, Crummy AB, Strother CM, Sackett JF (eds) Digital subtraction arteriography: an application of computerized fluoroscopy. Year Book Medical Publishers, Chicago, pp 58–64

Engels PHC, Ludwig JW (1982) Digital subtraction arteriography of the left ventricle using time interval difference mode. In: Mistretta CA, Crummy AB, Strother CM, Sackett JF (eds) Digital subtraction arteriography: an application of computerized fluoroscopy. Year Book Medical Publishers, Chicago, pp 123–124

Freeman E, Ziskin MC, Bove AA, Gimenez JL, Lynch PR (1970) Cineradiographic frame rate selection for left ventricular volumetry. Radiology 96:587–591

Grolman JH, Klosterman H, Herman MW, Moler CL, Eber LM, MacAlpin RN (1972) Dose reduction low pulse-rate fluoroscopy. Radiology 105:293–298

Haendle J (1979) Der Entwicklungsstand des Röntgenfernsehens. Radiol Diagn 4:554–569

Hedberg DJ (1982) A real time digital video disc recorder for medical imaging. Proc SPIE 318:47–55

Heintzen PH (1971a) Roentgen-, Cine- and Videodensitometry. Fundamentals and applications for blood flow and heart volume determination. Thieme, Stuttgart

Heintzen PH (1971b) Videodensitometry with pulsed radiation. In: Heintzen PH (ed) Roentgen-, Cine- and Videodensitometry. Thieme, Stuttgart, pp 46–56

Heintzen PH, Bürsch JH (1978) Roentgen video techniques for dynamic studies of structure and function of the heart and circulation. Thieme, Stuttgart

Heintzen PH, Brennecke R, Bürsch JH, Lange P, Malerczyk V, Moldenhauer K, Onnasch D (1975) Automated video-angiocardiographic image analysis. Computer (IEEE) 8: 55–64

Heintzen PH, Brennecke R, Bürsch JH (1978) Computer quantitation of angiocardiographic images. Proc SPIE 167:17–21

Höhne KH, Böhm M, Erbe W, Nicolae GC, Pfeiffer G, Sonne B (1978) Computer angiography: a new tool for X-ray functional diagnostics. Med Progr Technol 6:23

Kelcz F, Mistretta CA (1977) Absorption edge fluoroscopy using a 3-spectrum technique. Med Phys 3:159–165

Keyes GS, Pelc NJ, Riederer SJ, Sieb LE and Enzmann DR (1982) Digital fluorography. General Electric Medical Systems Operations, Milwaukee

Kruger RA (1981) A method for time domain filtering using computerized fluoroscopy. Med Phys 8:466–470

Kruger RA (1982) Combined acquisition/processing for data reduction. Proc SPIE 318:256–260

Kruger RA, Mistretta CA, Houk TL, Riederer SJ, Shaw CG, Ergun DL, Carbone D, Kubal W, Crummy AB, Zwiebel W, Rowe G, Flemming D (1978a) Real-time computerized fluoroscopic cardiac imaging. Proc SPIE 167:77–82

Kruger RA, Mistretta CA, Lancaster J, Houk TL, Goodsitt M, Shaw CG, Riederer SJ, Hicks J, Sackett J, Crummy AB, Fleming D (1978b) A digital videoprocessor for real time X-ray subtraction imaging. Optic Eng 17:652–657

Kruger RA, Mistretta CA, Houk TL, Riederer SJ, Shaw CG (1979) Computerized fluoroscopy in real time for noninvasive visualization of the cardiovascular system. Radiology 130:49–57

Lillestrand RL (1972) Techniques for change detection. IEEE Trans Comp, 21:654–659

Macovski A (1978) Iodine imaging using spectral analysis. Proc SPIE 167:67–75

Martin EC, Olson AP, Steeg CN, Casarella WJ (1981) Radiation exposure to the pediatric patient during cardiac catheterization and angiocardiography. Circulation 64:153–158

Meaney TF, Weinstein MA, Buonocore E, Pavlicek W, Borkowski GP, Gallagher JE, Sufka B, MacIntyre WJ (1980) Digital subtraction angiography of the human cardiovascular system. AJR 135:1153–1160

Meyer-Ebrecht D (1980) The management and processing of medical pictures: an architecture for systems and processing devices. Proc Workshop Picture Data Description and Management, IEEE, pp 202–206

Meyer-Ebrecht D, Böhring D, Grewer R, Mönnich KJ, Schmidt J, Wendler T (1982) A hierarchical approach to distributed picture information systems. Proc SPIE 318:

Mistretta CA (1974) The use of a general description of the radiological transmission image for categorizing image enhancement procedures. Opt Eng 13:134–137

Musmann HG (1979) Predictive image coding. Advances in electronics and electron physics, Suppl 12, 73–112

Nagel HH (1981) Analysis of image sequences: What can we learn from applications? In: Huang TS (ed) Image sequence analysis. Springer, Berlin Heidelberg New York

Ovitt TW, Capp P, Fisher HD, Frost MM, Lebel JL, Nudelman S, Roehrig H (1978) The development of a digital video subtraction system for intravenous angiography. Proc SPIE 167:61–65

Ovitt TW, Christenson PC, Fisher HD, Frost MM, Nudelman S, Roehrig H, Seeley G (1980) Intravenous angiography using digital video subtraction: X-ray imaging system. AJR 135:1141–1144

Papoulis A (1977) Signal analysis. McGraw-Hill, New York

Peled A, Liu B (1976) Digital signal processing. Wiley, New York

Pfeiler M (1969) Image transmission and image processing in radiology. In: Grasselli A (ed) Automatic interpretation and classification of images. New York, pp 399–415

Pfeiler M (1981) CT techniques in medical imaging. Digital image processing in medicine (Höhne KH, ed.), Springer, Berlin Heidelberg New York, pp 42–92

Pratt WK (1978) Digital image processing. Wiley, New York

Ritman EL (1977) Quantitative transaxial imaging of the heart. Eur J Cardiol, 5:203–220

Rosenfeld A (1961) Automatic detection of changes in reconnaissance data. Proc 5th Convention Military Electronics, Los Angeles, 492–499

Rossi JP (1978) Digital techniques for reducing television noise. J SMPTE, 87:134–140

Schüssler HW (1973) Digitale Systeme zur Signalverarbeitung. Springer, Berlin Heidelberg New York

Selzer RH (1968) Digital computer processing of X-ray photographs. Proc. Rochester Conf. on Data Acquisition in Biology and Medicine, Vol. 5:309–325, Pergamon, Oxford

Sturm RE, Wood EH (1971) Roentgen image-intensifier, television, recording system for dynamic measurements of roentgen density for circulatory studies. In: Heintzen (ed) Roentgen-, Cine- and Videodensitometry. Thieme, Stuttgart, pp 23–44

Vas R, Diamond GA, Forrester JS, Whiting JS, Swan HJC (1981) Computer enhancement of direct and venous-injected left ventricular contrast angiography. Am Heart J 102:719–725

Waldman JD, Rummerfield PS, Gilpin EA, Kirkpatrick SE (1981) Radiation exposure to the child during cardiac catheterization. Circulation 64:158–163

Widrow B, Mantey P, Griffiths L, Goode B (1971) Adaptive filters. Aspects of network and system theory (Kalman R, DeClaris N, eds), Holt, Rinehart and Winston, New York, pp 563–587

Wittmaack W, Brennecke R, Heintzen PH (1980) Mikroprozessoreinsatz bei der Aufnahme von Videoangiokardiogrammen. Biomedizinische Technik, Ergänzungsband 25, pp 101–103

Wood EH (1977) New vistas for the study of structural and functional dynamics of the heart, lungs and the circulation by noninvasive numerical tomographic vivisection. Circulation 56:506–520

Ziedses des Plantes BG (1961) Subtraktion. Thieme, Stuttgart

Principles and Methods of Roentgen Densitometry for Circulatory Studies *

J. H. BÜRSCH

Department of Pediatric Cardiology and Bioengineering, University of Kiel, FRG

Densitometric studies in angiocardiography are basically performed by the recording of temporal changes in X-ray absorption induced by a contrast medium bolus injected selectively just upstream of or directly into the circulatory segment under study. The theory of indicator dilution applies very much to roentgen density measurements and actually provides the basis for the assessment of circulatory parameters. Consequently, most of the principles of the conventional dye techniques had been tested in angiographic contrast studies taking advantage of the noninvasive sampling procedure of radio-opaque dye. However, according to practical experience over almost two decades, certain limitations in roentgen densitometry evidently limited in turn the general application of indicator dilution principles, but otherwise indicated very specific advantages of this technique.

It is the purpose here
a) to survey those methods that have gained diagnostic relevance in clinical studies and
b) to outline some new developments made possible by the digital processing of roentgen images.

Methods

Practical Considerations

An early illustration from Heintzen et al. (1967) indicates three methods for the recording of densitometric curves; cine techniques, video techniques, and direct fluoroscopic densitometry (Fig. 1). The picture from the mid-1960s points to a question that is relevant even today: Which of the methods is the most adequate, versatile, and reliable? From the standpoint of practical application, video densitometry has the advantage of real-time data analysis which has always been found an important feature for clinical studies, because diagnostic information can be obtained immediately, even during the patient's examination. Video techniques, in addition, provide indicator sampling within large

* This investigation was supported by research grants from the Deutsche Forschungsgemeinschaft and the Bundesministerium für Forschung und Technologie

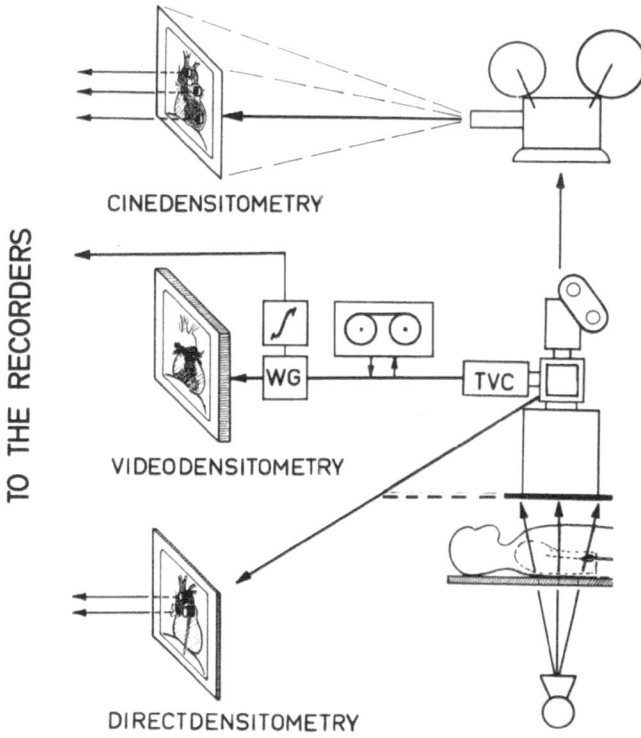

Fig. 1. Three methods for recording contrast dilution curves in angiocardiography. *TVC*, television camera; *WG*, window generator. (From Heintzen et al. 1967)

regions of interest (windows) of any desired shape; and, finally, they are most adequate for the digitization of image data. On the other hand, cine films certainly have a significantly higher spatial resolution and are most adequate for analyses with high temporal resolution because more than 100 frames/s can be obtained. Cine densitometry, initiated by Moros et al. (1953) for indicator dilution studies, therefore, is quite advantageous if extremely small structures (vessels) have to be analyzed and/or high speed flow studies are performed. Video densitometry, originally described by Wood et al. (1964), has the greatest versatility and applies mostly to the variety of densitometric principles, and therefore the latter technique will be discussed here, even though some methods apply equally to cine densitometry. Direct densitometry (Del Guercio et al. 1963) affords high radiation exposure particularly because detectors cannot be placed at the optimal sites of sampling and more than one contrast injection may be necessary. This procedure appears comparably less suitable for clinical studies.

Quantitative absorption measures are performed using fixed settings for X-ray tube voltage and current. Pulsed radiation or fluoroscopy conditions are adequate. In order to narrow the spectral distribution of X-rays, a copper filter (d > 0.2 mm) or aluminum is put in front of the X-ray tube. Angiocardiograms are usually recorded on videotape (or videodisc) for subsequent analysis using a video densitometer.

Assessment of circulatory volume and flow parameters, basically, relies upon quantitation of the amount of contrast medium. The mass of radio-opaque material transradiated is determined by measuring the difference in roentgen absorption with and without contrast medium from selected parts of the circulation. Measurement of roentgen absorption principally implies logarithmic data conversion of the regional intensity values, thereby providing, theoretically (Lambert-Beer law), a linear recording system. Unfortunately, the quality of linear data transmission in angiocardiography equipment is not ideal, owing mainly to scattering phenomena in the complex roentgen-optical system. Compensation for such effects is unavoidable if calibration of density signals (units of mass or concentration of indicator) is needed. However, procedures for both calibration and scatter correction afford additional radiation exposure and are somewhat difficult to practice as far as patient studies are concerned. Such difficulties have obviously prevented the establishment of clinical methods that require absolute measures of the amount or concentration of indicator (e.g., for cardiac output determination by the Stewart-Hamilton principle) even though a limited number of such studies have been performed (Cooley and Perry 1971; Bürsch and Heintzen 1973).

Consequently other methods were favored, utilizing comparative measurements only for the analysis of regional differences as well as temporal changes in angiocardiographic contrasts. For that purpose linearity of data recording was

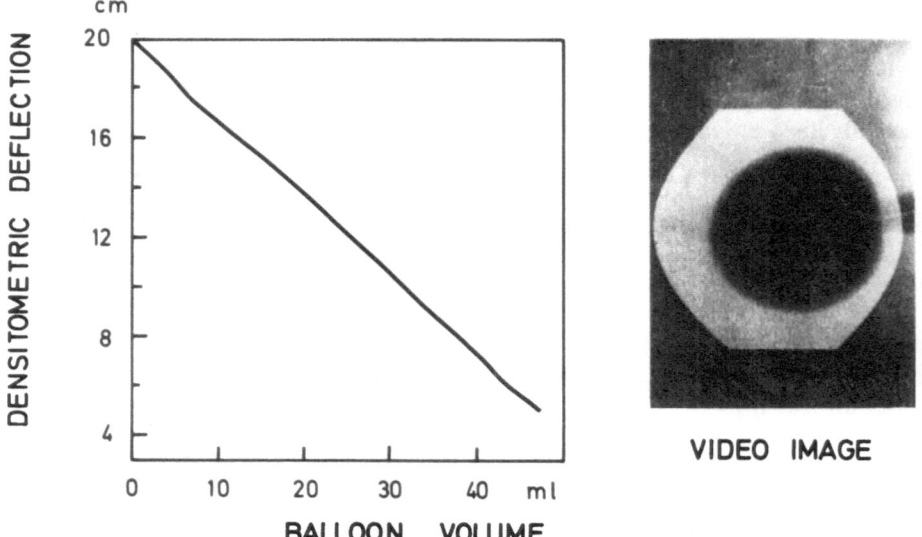

Fig. 2. Demonstration of linearity of densitometric recordings in an experimental study inflating a balloon with a Urografin solution with constant infusion rate. The bright area in the video image corresponds to the electronic sampling window

the precondition for adequate data recording and has been proven valid using video densitometry if absorption values by the contrast material did not exceed 30% of the total radiation intensity at the site of sampling (Fig. 2). The use of cine densitometry adds specific problems to straightforward processing of angiograms – in particular, uncertainties of linear data transmission (gradation of photographic material).

Special Applications

Video densitometry was found most appropriate for studies of ventricular ejection and filling characteristics using large sampling windows encompassing

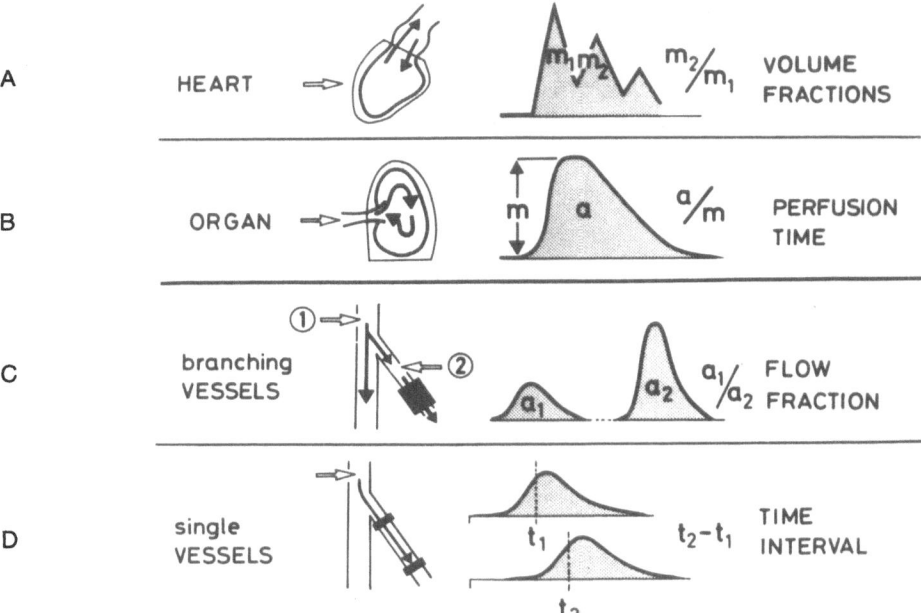

Fig. 3. Schematic drawing of the four basic principles for circulatory measurements by roentgen densitometry that are presently applied in clinical examinations. *a)* Aortic and pulmonic regurgitation measurements are calculated by relating the diastolic deflection (M_2) of the densogram to the according systolic deflection (m_1). The resulting regurgitant volume fraction value may be calculated from several cardiac cycles of the washout part of the curve. *b)* Perfusion-time measurements of the lungs or kidneys are determined by relating the area (a) of the curve to its peak deflection (m). *c)* Volume flow of an arterial branch is determined as a fraction of flow in the main artery by sampling two densograms from the branch following consecutive injections into the main artery ① and the daughter vessel ②. (The flow fraction is calculated by dividing curve area a_1 by curve area a_2.) *d)* Time interval measurements along nonbranched vessels are obtained by recording two densograms from one bolus injection and estimating the temporal delay of the downstream curve in relation to the upstream curve. Usually a representative time parameter is derived from each densogram and the time difference (t_2–t_1) is calculated

the end-diastolic contours of the left or right cardiac chambers (Bürsch 1973; Simon et al. 1973; Bürsch et al. 1974; Mennicken 1974; Simon 1981). Volume changes are derived from fractional changes of the amount of contrast medium; e.g., a diastolic increase of roentgen absorption over the ventricular chamber is indicative of valvular regurgitation of the contrast medium if the indicator was injected into the ventricle (Fig. 3a). By relating the magnitude of diastolic absorption changes to those of the according systoles, regurgitant fraction values are directly determined (Fig. 4).

A similar approach is used for ventricular ejection fraction measurements. If the change of absorption induced by systolic ejection of contrast medium from the ventricle is related to the degree of absorption at the termination of diastole, a measure of ventricular ejection is obtained. This method relies on homogeneous mixing and a uniform concentration of contrast medium in that chamber during the systolic phase. In order to partly overcome problems in cases of nonideal indicator mixing, a somewhat different principle of curve analysis has recently been applied (Falliner et al. 1981). Changes in amount of indicator from two consecutive cardiac phases were measured and related to each other for determination of the degree of indicator dilution, thereby yielding ventricular residual fraction. The methods described are based on the detection of

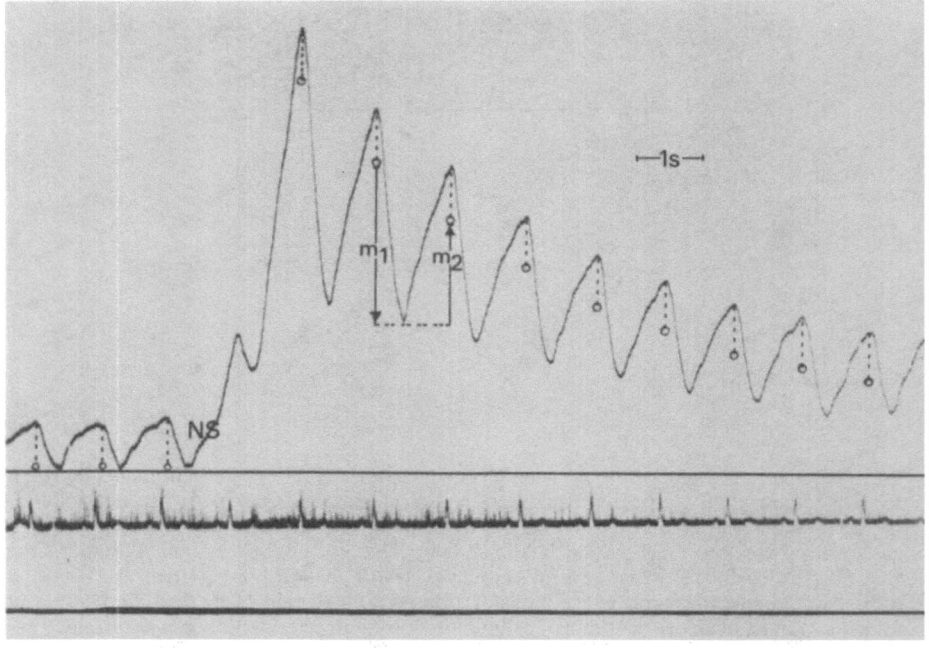

Fig. 4. Left ventricular densogram from a 16-year-old patient with significant aortic valve insufficiency; 15 ml Urografin 76% had been injected into the left ventricle by transarterial catheterization. Regurgitant volume as a fraction of total stroke volume was determined using the ratio of m_2/m_1. The maximum amplitude of nonspecific density variations (*NS*) is subtracted from the curve amplitudes at the termination of each end diastole. Regurgitant fraction 0.61 was calculated as the mean of fraction values from six cardiac cycles

ORIGINAL DENSOGRAM   CURVE ANALYSIS

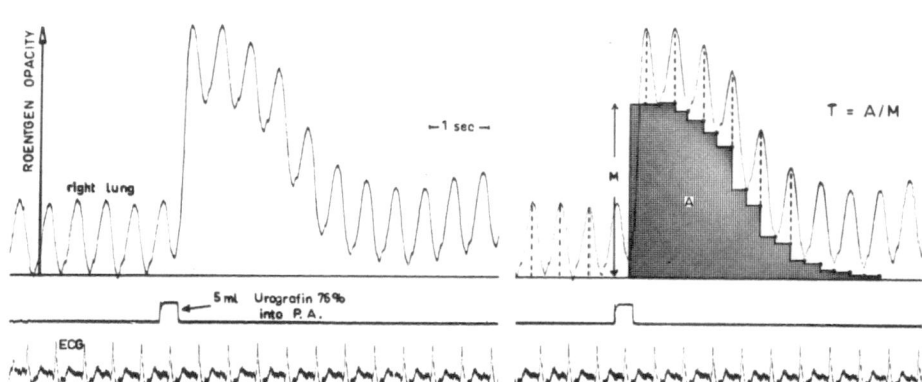

Fig. 5. Pulmonary densograms from a patient using a large sampling window that was contoured according to the external borders of the right lung field. Transit time (T) was determined by the ratio of the area (A) and the peak deflection (M) of the curve

changes of the total amount of indicator in the ventricle. For optimal windowing of the ventricular chambers, the video densitometer is equipped with a graphic tablet as a contour input device (Heintzen and Pilarczyk 1971).

Recording of contrast dilution curves using large sampling windows has been found appropriate for the determination of indicator transit times through organs such as the lungs (Bürsch and Heintzen 1978; Erikson et al. 1977). Recording of a mass-time curve from the entire organ is used to relate the area under the curve to its peak amplitude (Fig. 3b). The resulting measurement represents the magnitude of blood flow as determined by the total vascular volume perfused by the contrast medium (Fig. 5).

Video densitometry has been used to measure the total amount of contrast medium over arterial cross sections. The area under the mass-time curve is inversely proportional to the flow at the site of injection. If two injections are performed at different sites, e.g., the aorta and an arterial vessel, from which the densograms are recorded, the fraction of aortic blood flow in the artery under study is obtained (Fig. 3c). This technique has been established for clinical applications of flow fraction measurements in the various arterial vessels. It has also become of clinical importance for quantitating blood flow before and after pharmacologic or mechanical interventions. This last technique again emphasizes the potential value of roentgen densitometry for relative measures of roentgen absorption.

A completly different approach to roentgen densitometry aims at time interval measurements in arteries by sampling densograms from at least two sites of the vessel a certain distance apart from each other (Fig. 6). Linear recording of the mass of contrast medium is not essential in these studies for two reasons: firstly, the methods applied to determine a representative time value from a

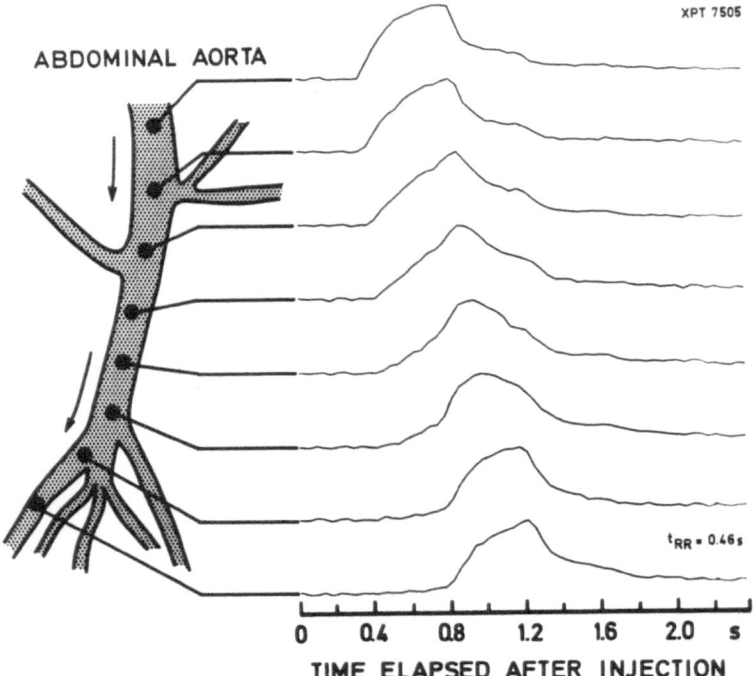

Fig. 6. Set of regional densograms from the abdominal aorta in a pig following bolus injection of contrast medium about 10 cm proximal from the renal arteries. The increasing delay of the appearance of the contrast dilution curves in flow direction is the basis for regional time interval measurements

single curve are not necessarily sensitive to nonlinear scaling of densitometric amplitudes, and secondly, the time intervals are derived from (two) curves of similar shape induced by an indicator bolus that will not have been significantly affected by dispersion along the short distance it has traveled.

These conditions are quite favorable to the use of cine densitometry as an alternative method to video densitometry for functional studies of blood flow, and, in fact, many of the studies published during recent years have used cine densitometry (Rutishauser 1969; Heintzen 1971; Heuck 1973). Regional flow measurements have to be performed at unbranched arterial segments by setting two windows in a fixed position over the vessel from which two densograms are recorded (Fig. 3d). This sampling technique has been modified by sophisticated procedures for compensation of changes in image background using additional windows adjacent to the vessels (Schmiel et al. 1979). This was useful specifically for coronary perfusion studies. Regional flow values are usually calculated from the volume of the vascular segment confined by the two windows (dimensional measures) and the time interval of bolus travel (densitometric measure).

Regarding time interval measurements by this method, two principal questions have repeatedly been raised. The one relates to optimal time parameter calculation from densograms and the other concerns effects of pulsatile blood flow on the shape of the indicator curve. Five time parameters were systematically tested in animal experiments for time interval measurements. These were: the gravity lines of curve areas, the appearance times, time of the half curve maximum, the mean of the times of the curve front, and a cross-correlation method (Rosen and Silverman 1973). The last two techniques mostly avoided errors associated with the physical effects inherent in contrast dilution methods, such as layering of contrast material, as well as effects of pulsatile flow on the shape of contrast density curves (distortion). The mathematical work entailed in such analyses, especially in cross-correlation techniques, indicates that computerized data analysis is extremely useful because calculations are performed with the highest possible speed and optimal reproducibility for parameter extraction. Involvement of digital computers has even become of vital importance for the latest advances in angiographic parameter extraction (Heintzen et al. 1975, 1978) because not only data analysis but even data acquisition can be established digitally (Brennecke et al. 1976, 1977, 1979).

Computerized image processing provides the technical solution for generating complete pictures of regional time parameters. According to the number of picture elements (256 × 256), up to 64 000 contrast absorption curves are obtained and used for automatic time parameter extraction. If the regional time parameters obtained from the perfused vessels are grouped (e.g., 40-ms time intervals) subsequently with the time elapsed after injection, a time-dependent

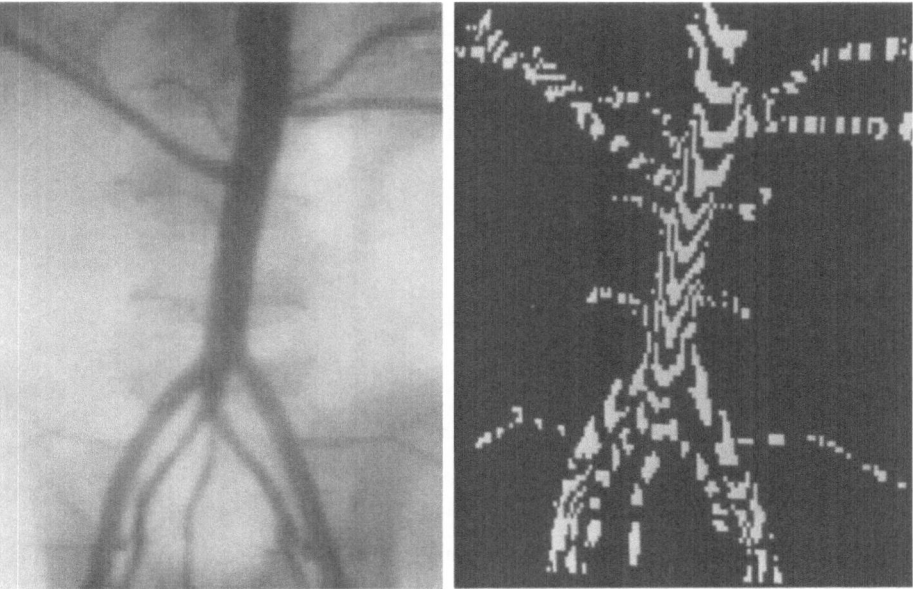

Fig. 7. Pictures of video monitor screen showing computer-processed images of the abdominal aorta. A bolus injection of 5 ml Urografin was performed in a 20-kg animal. *Left,* enhanced contrast image; *right,* segmentation of vessels by calculating time parameters with 40-ms time intervals (black/white)

segmentation of the vessels is achieved. Each segment indicates the distance of propagation within a (constant) time interval. Unlike cine and video densitometry, which perform time measurements along any arbitrarily chosen but fixed distance, digital densitometry enables one to use time as the determinant and thereby measure distances (Bürsch et al. 1979). One of the most appropriate examples is illustrated by short time interval segments that may have similar diagnostic qualities to flow velocity profiles (Fig. 7). In addition, quantitative measures of the mass of contrast material from larger segments (e.g., 80-ms time interval) can be derived. By this principle regional blood flow and flow distribution data are obtained and may be displayed as functional parameter images (Fig. 8).

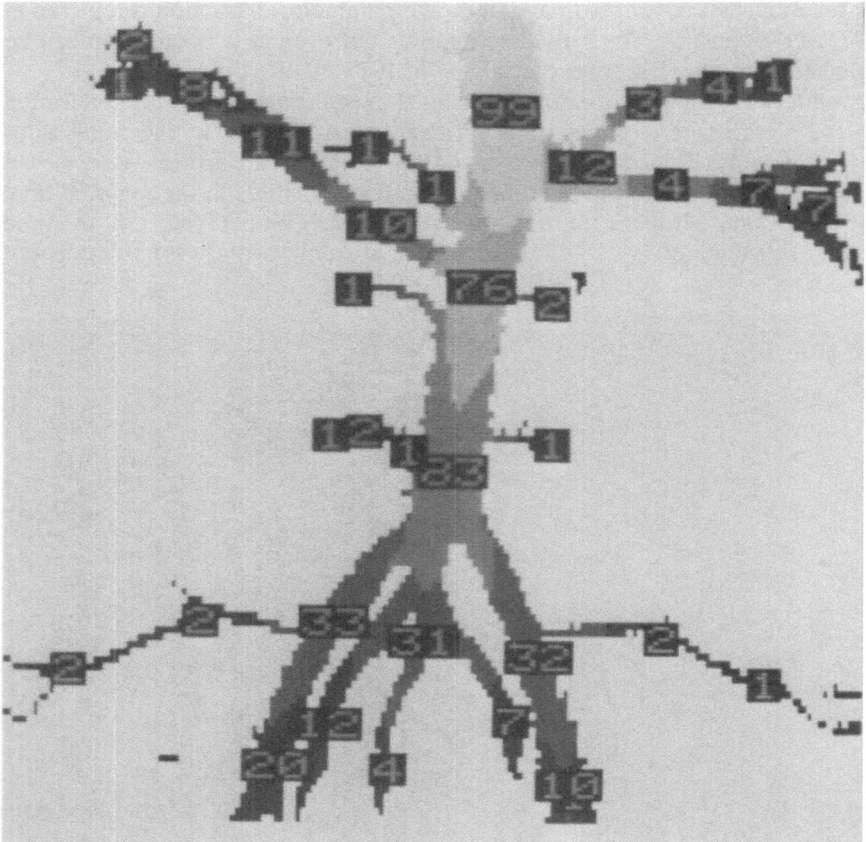

Fig. 8. Flow parameter image (video screen) from abdominal aorta indicating the propagation of the contrast bolus by increasing gray intensities as well as the rates of segmental volume flow that are expressed in percentage of the maximum flow rate (99 = 100%)

Validation of Methods

The accuracy of these techniques has been extensively studied during recent years by many investigators (e.g., Heintzen and Bürsch 1978). Some of the results may be presented as typical examples from these studies. Experimental pulmonary and aortic valve insufficiency demonstrated a high correlation between video densitometry and electromagnetic flowmeter data, with a correlation coefficient of at least $r = 0.94$ (Fig. 9). A similar correlation was found for

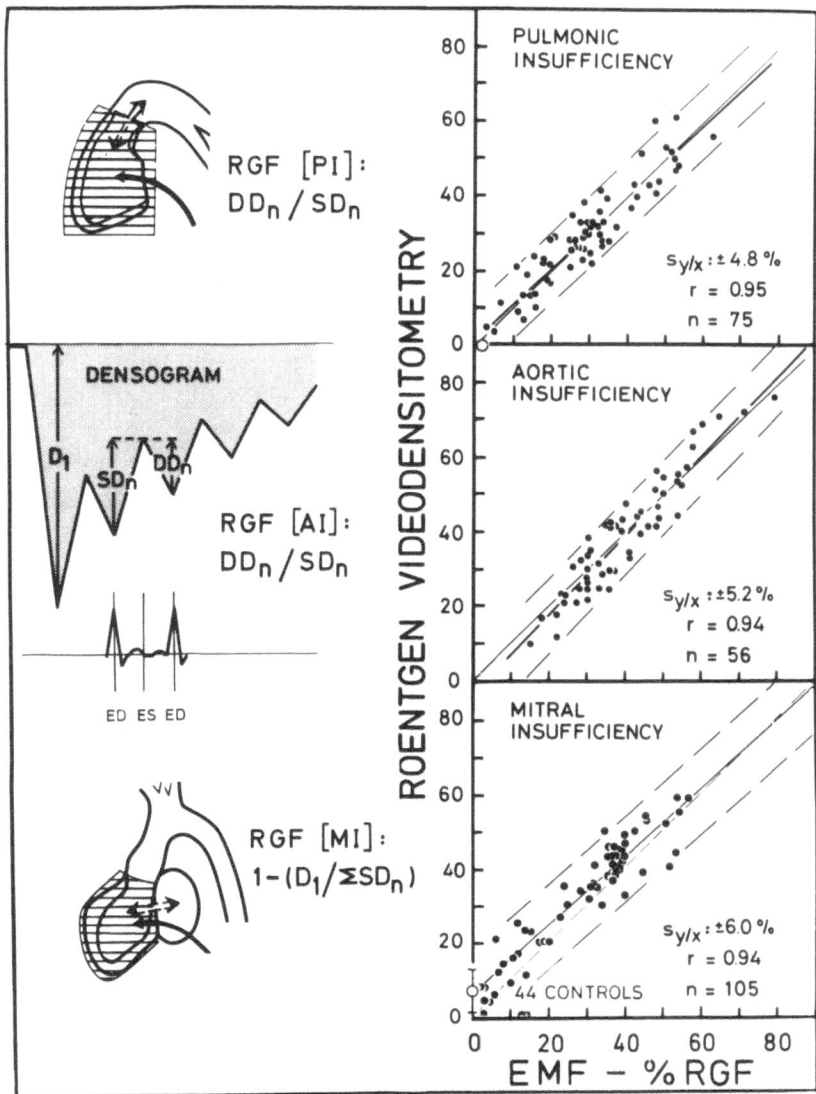

Fig. 9. Diagram depicting comparative measurements of experimental pulmonic, aortic, and mitral valve insufficiencies in animals using video densitometry and electromagnetic flowmetry. *RGF*, regurgitant fraction

experimental mitral valve incompetence. Routine application in our institution at present represents 350 patients with valvular insufficiency, indicating that this technique is highly suitable for clinical use.

Pulmonary transit time was studied experimentally for comparison with the cardiogreen dilution method. The correlation coefficient was found to be 0.94. A systematic difference was observed due to the higher distribution volume in the Cardio-Green method that involved left atrial sampling (Fig. 10). Clinical application was used to calculate pulmonary vascular volumes by the product of independently measured pulmonary flow and the transit time. A linear correlation was found between pulmonary volume and flow.

Regarding measurements of the flow fractions in branching arteries, we may refer to the data published by Lantz et al. (1980a, b) and Holcroft et al. (1980). Correlation coefficients using video densitometry and electromagnetic flowmeter data were found in the range of 0.91–0.98, depending on the circulatory region.

Coronary blood flow studies using by roentgen densitometry correlated well with independent methods as demonstrated by Rutishauser et al. (1970)

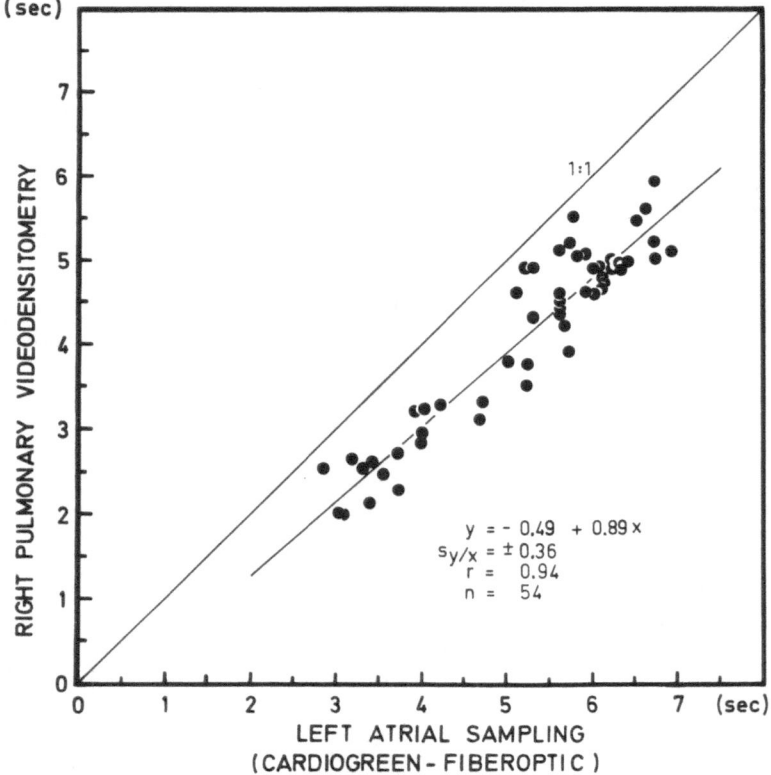

Fig. 10. Perfusion time measurements of the right lung using video densitometry and the Cardio-Green dye technique in an animal study

$(r = 0.93)$, H. Smith et al. (1971) $(r = 0.95)$, and Hackbarth et al. (1980) with intraoperative measurements $(r = 0.97)$. Our specific activities in this field were related to the optimization of data analysis on a more basic research level. Model and animal studies revealed correlation coefficients of about 0.95 between video densitometry and electromagnetic flowmeter data, but standard deviations varied significantly depending on the size of the vessel and the distance between sampling sites. Recent advances in digital angiography provided much more consistent data specifically for flow distribution and flow pattern analysis (Bürsch et al. 1981).

References

Brennecke R, Brown TK, Bürsch JH, Heintzen PH (1976) Digital processing of videoangiographic image series using a minicomputer. Proc Comp Cardiol, IEEE Computer Society, Long Beach, pp 255–260

Brennecke R, Brown TK, Bürsch JH, Heintzen PH (1977) Computerized video-image preprocessing with applications to cardio-angiographic roentgen-image series. In: Nagel HH (ed) Digitale Bildverarbeitung. Springer, Berlin Heidelberg New York, pp 244–262

Brennecke R, Hahne HJ, Moldenhauer K, Bürsch JH, Heintzen PH (1979) A special purpose processor for digital angiocardiography. Design and applications. Proc Comp Cardiol, IEEE Computer Society, Long Beach, pp 343–346

Bürsch JH (1973) Quantitative Videodensitometrie. Grundlagen und Ergebnisse einer röntgenologischen Indikatormethode. Dissertation, University of Kiel

Bürsch JH, Heintzen PH (1973) Methoden und Ergebnisse der Röntgendensitometrie in der Kardiologie. In: Heuck F (ed) Densitometrie in der Radiologie. Thieme, Stuttgart, pp 137–147

Bürsch JH, Heintzen PH (1978) Pulmonary perfusion measurements by videodensitometry. Methods and preliminary results. Ann Radiol 21:349–353

Bürsch JH, Heintzen PH, Simon R (1974) Videodensitometric studies by a new method of quantitating the amount of contrast medium. Europ J Cardiol 1:437–446

Bürsch JH, Hahne HJ, Brennecke R, Hetzer R, Heintzen PH (1979) Funktionsangiogramme als Ergebnis der densitometrischen Analyse digitalisierter Röntgenbildserien. Biomed Tech [Suppl] 24:189–190

Bürsch JH, Hahne HJ, Brennecke R, Grönemeier D, Heintzen PH (1981) Assessment of arterial blood flow measurements by digital angiography. Radiology 141:39–47

Cooley RN, Perry RR (1971) Angiographic determination. Invest Radiol 6:176–185

Del Guercio LRM, Goetz RH, Fawcett HN (1963) Roentgen densitometric dilution curves. Proceedings of conference on engineering in medicine and biology 5:56–57

Erikson U, Lindgren PG, Löfroth PO, Ruhn G, Wolgast M (1977) Measurements of total and regional renal blood flow by videodensitometry. Acta Radiol [Diagn] 18:225–234

Falliner A, Bürsch JH, Wessel A, Faltz HC, Heintzen PH (1981) Zuverlässigkeit der Röntgen-Videodensitometrie für Klappeninsuffizienzmessungen und für die Bestimmung der ventrikulären Auswurffraktion. Z Kardiol 70:754–760

Hackbarth W, Bircks W, Pölitz B, Körfer R, Schmiel FK, Spiller P (1980) Vergleich videodensitometrischer und elektromagnetischer Flußmessungen in aortokoronaren Bypassgefäßen. Fortschr Roentgenstr 132/5:554–560

Heintzen PH (ed) (1971) Roentgen-, cine and videodensitometry. Thieme, Stuttgart

Heintzen PH, Bürsch JH (eds), (1978) Roentgen-video-techniques for the analysis of structure and function of the heart and circulation. Thieme, Stuttgart

Heintzen PH, Pilarczyk J (1971) Videodensitometry with contoured and controlled windows. In: Heintzen PH (ed) Roentgen-, cine- and videodensitometry. Thieme, Stuttgart, pp 56–61

Heintzen PH, Bürsch JH, Osypka, P, Moldenhauer K (1967) Röntgenologische Kontrastmitteldichtemessungen zur Untersuchung der Herz- und Kreislauffunktionen. Elektromedizin 12:82–95

Heintzen PH, Brennecke R, Bürsch JH, Lange P, Malerczyk V, Moldenhauer K, Onnasch D (1975) Automated video-angiocardiographic image analysis. Computer (IEEE) 8:55–64

Heintzen PH, Brennecke R, Bürsch JH (1978) Computerized videoangiocardiography. In: Kaltenbach M, Lichtlen P (eds) Coronary heart disease. Thieme, Stuttgart, pp 116–121

Heuck F (ed) (1973) Densitometrie in der Radiologie. Thieme, Stuttgart

Holcroft JW, Lantz BMT, Foerster JM, Link DP (1980) Video dilution technique. An accurate measure of blood flow during routine arteriography. Arch Surg 115:1299–1303

Lantz BM, Link P, Foerster JM, Holcroft JW (1980a) Angiographic determination of splanchnic blood flow. Acta Radiol [Diagn] 21:3–10

Lantz BM, Foerster JM, Link DP, Holcroft JW (1980b) Angiographic determination of cerebral blood flow. Acta Radiol [Diagn] 21:147–153

Mennicken U (1974) Die Bestimmung der Herzkammervolumina und des Schlagvolumens des linken Ventrikels mit der videometrischen Dimensionsmessung, der videodensitometrischen Auswaschtechnik und der Pressure-Pulse-Methode im Tierexperiment. Dissertation, University of Cologne

Moros GG, Neri RJ, Villagordoa G (1953) Fluorodensography with radiopaque substance: a new method for hemodynamic investigation. Am Heart J 45:495–499

Rosen L, Silverman NR (1973) Videodensitometric measurements of blood flow using cross-correlation techniques. Radiology 109:305–310

Rutishauser W (1969) Kreislaufanalyse mittels Röntgendensitometrie, Huber, Bern

Rutishauser W, Bussmann WD, Noseda G, Meier W, Wellauer J (1970) Blood flow measurement through single coronary arteries by roentgen densitometry. I. A comparison of flow measured by a radiologic technique applicable in the intact organism and by electromagnetic flowmeter. Am J Roentgen 109:12–20

Schmiel FK, Hackbarth W, Politz B, Spiller P (1979) Simultane Hintergrundkorrektur zur videodensitometrischen Flußmessung am Koronargefäßsystem. Biomed Tech 24:158–159

Simon R (1981) Klinische Kontrastmittel-Densitometrie. Dissertation, University of Hannover

Simon R, Callesen C, Heintzen PH (1973) Videodensitometric determination of regurgitant fraction in pulmonic insufficiency by measuring the amount of indicator. Basic Res Cardiol 68:509–520

Smith HC, Frye RL, Donald DE, Davis GD, Pluth JR, Sturm RE, Wood EH (1971) Roentgen videositometric measure of coronary blood flow. Determination from simultaneous indicator-dilution curves at selected sites in the coronary circulation and in coronary artery-saphenous vein grafts. Mayo Clinic Proc 46:800–806

Wood EH, Sturm RE, Sanders JJ (1964) Data processing in cardiovascular physiology with particular reference to roentgen videodensitometry. Mayo Clinic Proc 39:849–865

Densitometry Using Polychromatic X-Ray Beams

Y. Pochon[1], P. A. Doriot[2], L. Rasoamanambelo[2], and W. Rutishauser[2]

[1] Institute of Applied Physics, EPFL, Lausanne, Switzerland
[2] Center of Cardiology, University Hospital Geneva, Switzerland

Introduction

The origin of our physical model for roentgen densitometry is the attempt to measure accurately the degree of stenosis in a coronary artery.

Densitometry has indeed the advantage of being independent of the noncircular shape of the stenotic cross section, which is an insurmountable obstacle to accuracy in any morphologic approach. However, densitometric methods have always been bound to the assumption of "sufficient monochromaticity" of the X-ray beam and to the restriction of using only small layer thicknesses of absorbing contrast medium (unless one uses a calibration wedge placed onto the patient [1]). These limitations cannot be respected in coronary angiography without considerable loss of image contrast. The model for densitometry using polychromatic X-ray beams and the derived correction procedure presented in this contribution removes these constraints.

Principle of Measurement

The principle of stenosis measurement consists in determining the quotient of the contrast medium volumes contained in two thin slices of the vessel, the first one taken in the stenotic segment, the second in the prestenotic section (cf. Doriot et al., this volume). These volumes are computed from the areas obtained by plotting the optical density of the cine film measured on scans across the vessel and subtracting the optical density of the background. However, the computed volumes are proportional to the areas only if the relationship between thickness × concentration of contrast medium and resulting optical density difference on the film is linear in each point (and if the constant of proportionality is constant over the region of interest). Unfortunately, this linearity cannot be assumed in coronary angiography.

Nonapplicability of the Lambert-Beer Absorption Law

The first attempt to establish theoretically the relationship between layer thickness of contrast medium and the resulting difference in optical density is to apply the Lambert-Beer absorption law for monochromatic radiation:

$$I = I_0 \exp(-\mu t) \tag{1}$$

where I_0 is the intensity of the incident monochromatic beam, I is the transmitted intensity, t is the thickness of the absorbing material, and μ is the absorption coefficient of the material.

By transformation of Ex. 1 we find:

$$t = \text{const.} \log(I/I_0) \tag{2}$$

which means there is proportionality between thickness of the absorbing layer and logarithm of the transmitted intensity.

However, X-ray sources used in diagnostic radiology are not monochromatic, so that Eq. 2 is only a rough approximation of the reality.

Bürsch et al. [2] have established the limits of applicability of this law for different concentrations of Urografin and various thicknesses of copper prefiltration of the beam. With fixed tube voltage, the additional filtration improved the monochromacy of the beam by absorbing the X-rays of low energy. But on modern X-ray machines which regulate the dose rate by varying the tube voltage, adding copper filtration leads automatically to higher voltage of the tube and a shift of the spectrum to higher energies without improvement of monochromaticity.

If we measure densitometrically the thickness of a wedge filled with Urografin 76%, we obtain the curve shown in Fig. 1. Bürsch et al. [2] have already found that such curves are sufficiently linear only in a very small thickness range (typically, less than 2 mm). A correction for this nonlinear effect is therefore necessary for accurate measurements of most vessels.

Model for Polychromatic X-Ray Beams

To design such a correction, we have developed a general model of the radiologic image formation [3], which will be presented in a simplified form in this section.

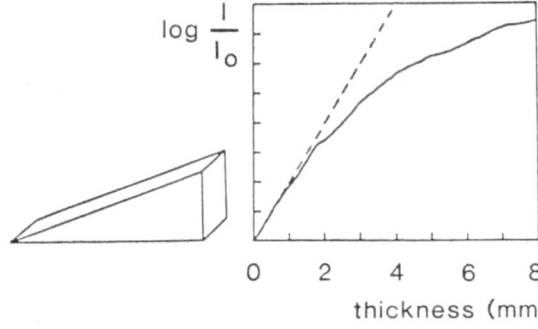

Fig. 1. Densitometric measurement of a wedge filled with Urografin 76% using 70 kV tube voltage

We consider the same point P on the vessel on two images. The first one is the image of the diseased area before injection of the contrast medium; the second one shows the passage of the contrast medium through the stenosis. We define the "luminescence contrast" $c(P)$ of the point P as

$$c(P) = \log L_2(P) - \log L_2^*(P) \tag{3}$$

where $L_2(P)$ and $L_2^*(P)$ are the light intensities incident onto the film in point P during the exposure of the first and the second image, respectively.

To express $L_2(P)$ [or $L_2^*(P)$], we take into account the polychromy of the X-ray beam, its absorption along the beam path P, and the spectral efficiency of the image intensifier input screen. This leads to

$$c(P) = \log \frac{\int_0^\infty [I_o(v) \exp(-\Sigma\mu_i t_i) + I_s(v)] R(v) dv}{\int_0^\infty [I_o(v) \exp(-\Sigma\mu_i^* t_i^*) + I_s(v)] R(v) dv} \tag{4}$$

where $I_o(v)$ is the spectrum of the X-ray source, $I_s(v)$ is the scattered spectrum reaching the input screen, $R(v)$ is the efficiency of the input screen, $\Sigma\mu_i t_i$ is the total absorption before injection of the contrast medium, and $\Sigma\mu_i^* t_i^*$ is the total absorption during the passage of the contrast medium.

It can be shown that this expression leads to a polynomial function for $c(P)$:

$$c(P) = A_1 t(P) + A_2 t(P) m(P) + A_3 t^2(P) + \ldots, \tag{5}$$

whereby the coefficients A_1, A_2, and A_3 depend upon the spectrum of the X-ray source, the scattered spectrum, the overall absorption of the beam, the absorption coefficient and concentration of the contrast medium, and the spectral efficiency of the image intensifier input screen.

The variable $m(P)$ represents the modulation of the contrast $c(P)$ on the opacified vessel due to the background nonhomogeneity.

On X-ray machines which regulate the dose rate by varying the tube voltage, overall absorption of the beam and spectrum of the source (or voltage of the tube) are related. The scattered spectrum is also related to the source spectrum and to the overall absorption; it is assumed to be homogeneous in the region of interest. So, for a given angiographic installation with preset pulse duration and tube current, the coefficients A_1, A_2, and A_3 depend in a first approximation only on the tube voltage.

Equation (5) is the expression of the nonlinear relationship between thickness and resulting contrast necessary to the description of the deviation from linearity observed in Fig. 1.

To verify the model and determine coefficients A_1 and A_3, we filmed the wedge in Fig. 1 filled with Urografin 76% first, and then after dilution of the Urografin 76% with water to a half, then a quarter of the initial concentration. The wedge was embedded in paraffin blocks (homogeneous background, $m = 0$) to simulate different patient absorptions, leading thus to different tube voltages.

The optical densities on the film (i.e., the densities on the wedge and on the adjacent background) were measured with the help of a microdensitometer.

The values obtained were then corrected for film nonlinearity with the help of a gray scale step wedge exposed on the same film, yielding new values proportional to the logarithmic exposure $\log L_2 \tau$ and $\log L_2^* \tau$. Finally, the differences between wedge values and background, i.e., the contrast $c = c(t)$ in arbitrary units, were computed.

The results are shown in Fig. 2. The curves labelled 1 were obtained with Urografin 76%, curve 2 with a half and curve 3 with a quarter of this concentration. In the left-hand panels the wedge was filmed without copper prefiltration, in the right-hand panels with a sheet of copper 0.2 mm thick.

A second order polynomial fit (smooth lines) of each experimental curve was performed according to the prediction of the model (Eq. 5). The deviation from

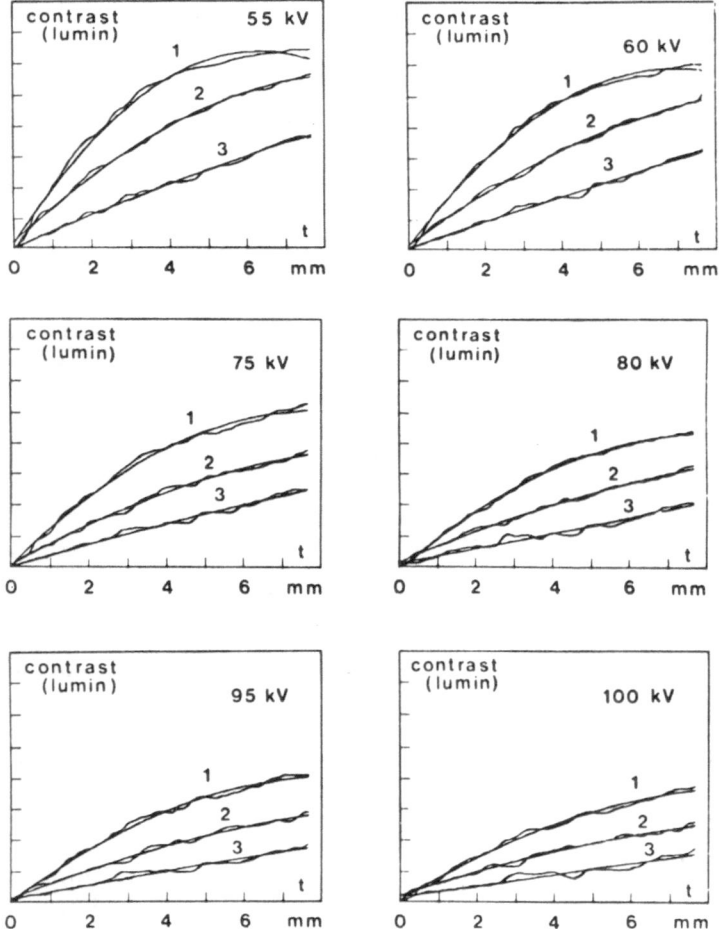

Fig. 2. Experimental curves and fitting functions obtained from measurements of a wedge filled with Urografin 76% (*1*), 38% (*2*), and 19% (*3*). *Left panels,* without copper prefiltration; *right panels,* with a sheet of copper 0.2 mm thick

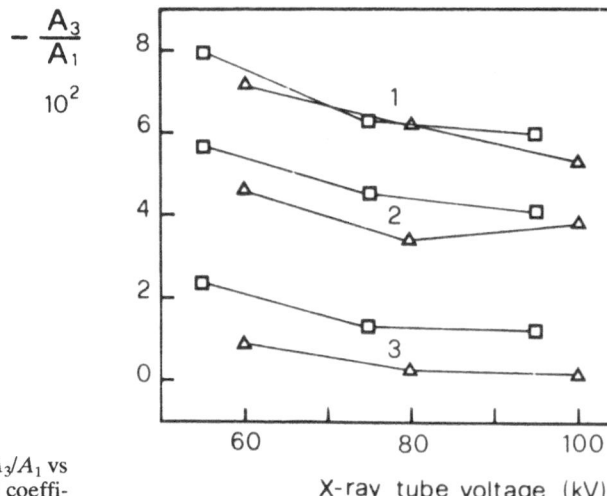

Fig. 3. Measure of linearity $-A_3/A_1$ vs tube voltage obtained from the coefficients A_1 and A_3 of the fitting functions of Fig. 2. The numbers *1, 2, 3* correspond to the concentrations of Urografin 76%, 38%, and 19%

△ .2 mm Cu filtration

▢ no filtration

linearity of each curve can be expressed by the ratio $-A_3/A_1$ of the fitting coefficients A_1 and A_3, which are also the coefficients of Eq. 5.

The values $-A_3/A_1$ obtained on our X-ray machine for different tube voltages are shown in Figure 3. The ordinate gives the deviation from linearity in percentages for a 1-mm thickness of contrast medium. For solution 1 (Urografin 76%) and 80 kV, for example, we find approximately 6% deviation. A 4-mm thick layer of Urografin would therefore produce 25% deviation. We also see that the additional copper filtration does not specifically improve the linearity for solution 1. The only effect of this additional filtration is to increase the tube voltage, as is done when studying corpulent patients. Note also the well-known fact that linearity is improved by using a lower contrast medium concentration. This may not, however, be advisable in many situations because of the resulting contrast degradation; because of decreasing signal-to-noise ratio it is also not advisable for accurate measurements.

Correction for the Polychromy of the Beam

For simplicity, the principle of the correction procedure for the nonmonochromaticity of the beam will be exposed under the assumption of homogeneous background ($m = 0$).

For a given tube voltage and a given contrast medium concentration, the nonlinear relationship between thickness and luminescence contrast is determined by the coefficients A_1 and A_3, as stated before.

$$c = A_1 t + A_3 t^2, \tag{6}$$

where t is the thickness we should integrate under the scanned areas mentioned previously to obtain the contrast medium volumes in the two slices. Since in this application of densitometry we need only proportional and not absolute values, we can for convenience define a new thickness variable A_1t, which is also the corrected contrast c_{corr} we want to obtain. Resolution of Eq. 6 yields:

$$A_1t = c_{corr} = \frac{-1 + \sqrt{1 + 4A_3c/A_1^2}}{2A_3/A_1^2} \tag{7}$$

By developing the square root we obtain a point by point (or pixel by pixel) correction of the actual luminescence contrast c, which allows computation of the corrected contrast:

$$c_{corr} = c\,(1 - A_3c/A_1^2 + 2(A_3c/A_1^2)^2 - 5(A_3c/A_1^2)^3 + - \dots) \tag{8}$$

The correction is a function of parameters A_1 and A_3. These can be determined once and for all by a wedge measurement for a given X-ray machine and a given X-ray tube (with unchanged pulse duration and tube current).

The complete correction procedure and its effects on a wedge of Urografin 76% are summarized in Fig. 4. First, the nonlinearity of the film is corrected.

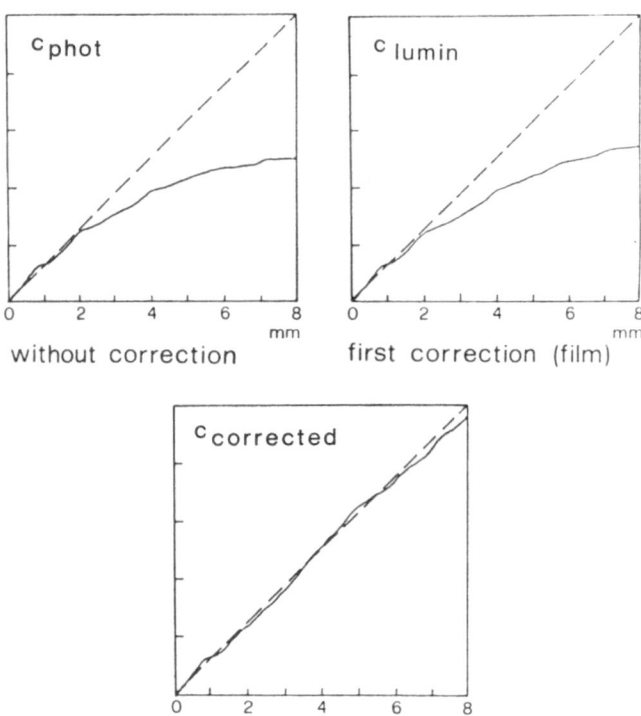

Fig. 4. Two-step correction procedure for the film nonlinearity and the polychromy of the X-ray beam, and its effect on the wedge of Urografin 76%. The *ordinate* is the measured thickness in arbitrary units

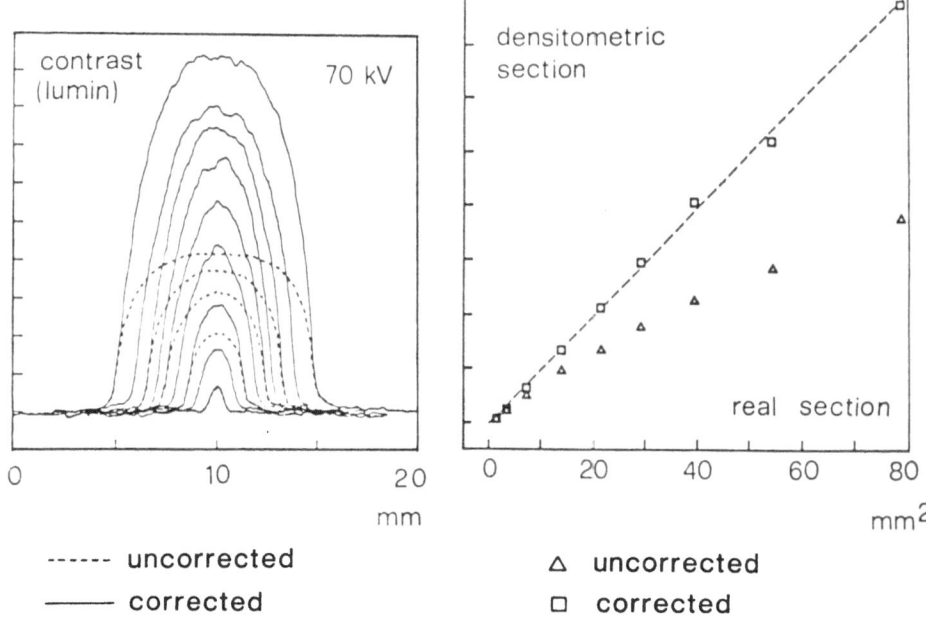

uncorrected (dashed)
corrected (solid)

△ **uncorrected**
□ **corrected**

Fig. 5. *Left panel,* scans across nine cylindrical holes filled with Urografin 76% after correction of the film nonlinearity *(dashed lines)* and after correction of the polychromy effect *(solid lines)*. The compression appears clearly already at 2-mm diameter. (True diameters in mm: 1, 2, 3, 4.15, 5.15, 5.95, 7, 8.25, 10.05). *Right panel,* densitometric cross sections obtained by integration of the areas under the scans

This nonlinearity was obviously negligible below 4 mm Urografin thickness, which means that the corresponding local exposures were confined to the rectilinear part of the characteristic curve of the film. Second, the nonlinearity resulting from polychromy is corrected using Eq. 8.

The correction has also been tested on images of cylindrical holes with diameters ranging from 1 to 10 mm drilled in a Plexiglas plate. Figure 5, left panel, shows in dashed lines the scans obtained across the holes before correction of the polychromy effect. Integration of the area under the curves yields the noncorrected densitometric cross sections of the holes, shown for comparison vs the true cross sections in the right panel. Application of the correction compensates the progressive compression of the scans with increasing diameter (solid lines) by the correct amount, as can be verified from the alignment of the corrected cross sections on the identity line in the right panel.

Conclusion

The designed correction procedure can be easily implemented in computer programs for video or cine densitometric applications. It improves the accuracy of flow and stenosis measurements by correcting the effect of beam polychromy, suppresses the need of copper filtration, and so permits analysis of well-contrasted images with preserved signal-to-noise ratio.

References

1. Rutishauser W (1969) Kreislaufanalyse mittels Röntgendensitometrie. Huber, Bern, pp 35 f.
2. Bürsch J, Johs R, Heintzen P (1971) Validity of Lambert-Beer's law in roentgen densitometry of contrast material (Urografin) using continuous radiation. In: Heintzen P (ed) Roentgen-, cine- and videodensitometry. Thieme, Stuttgart, pp 81–84
3. Pochon Y, Doriot PA, Rasoamanambelo L (1986) Roentgen densitometry by polychromatic X-ray beams (to be published)

Newer Developments in Photographic Materials and Processing

T. VON VOLKMANN

Kodak AG, Hedelfingerstrasse, D-7000 Stuttgart 60, FRG

First, I would like to make a few remarks about film and its characteristics as they relate to recording images. The second part of my paper deals with processing control and other factors necessary to produce images of consistently high quality. In the last part I will discuss a new film designed especially for use in cinefluorography, Kodak CFE film.

Film Properties

A film, any film that is, can be described by a variety of photographic and image structure characteristics. Three most important characteristics of a film for cinefluorographic use are: speed, contrast, and graininess. The reasons for this are obvious. Speed is needed because rapid movement is recorded using high camera speed, and also because it is always desirable to reduce patient radiation dosage as much as possible. Contrast is needed to distinguish between two structures of almost equal X-ray absorption. Lastly, fine grain is needed because graininess affects image visibility, especially of low contrast structures. It is interesting to note that film graininess is insignificant in general radiography under normal viewing conditions. In cinefluorography, however, it becomes visible because the film is viewed with magnification in a projector.

The relationships among these three factors are such that tradeoffs, based on the needs and preferences of the diagnostician, must be made when selecting a film for cinefluorographic studies.

I would like to illustrate this with an example. High speed films often have high graininess. Moreover, increased film speed reduces the number of X-ray quanta needed to produce an image of a given density, thereby leading to increased quantum mottle. Thus high speed, which has the desirable effects of

a) shortening exposure and thereby reducing image blurring resulting from motion and

b) decreasing radiation dose to the patient, also produces the undesirable effect of increased radiographic mottle from more graininess and quantum mottle.

Before proceeding further, let me say a few words about radiographic mottle or "noise." Radiographic mottle is the variation in optical density across a radiographic image made with a transducer which has been given a "uniform" X-ray exposure; i.e., an exposure made with an X-ray beam which does not contain an object to be radiographed. By transducer we mean a device such as an image intensifier or a fluorescent intensifying screen that converts X-ray energy to light. In the following discussion we will consider radiographic mottle to consist of two elements:

a) quantum mottle, and
b) film graininess. We well disregard density variations in the image which can arise from nonuniformity in structure of the transducer and from artifacts which can arise from improper film handling, processing, and/or house-keeping.

Quantum mottle is defined as the variation in density of a uniformly exposed radiographic image that results from the random spatial distribution of the X-ray quanta absorbed in the transducer. It is dependent on three factors in the following ways:

1. It is inversely related to the number of X-ray quanta absorbed in the trans-ducer to produce an image of a given density. Factors that decrease the number of quanta needed to form the image (e.g., an increase in film speed) tend to increase quantum mottle, and vice versa.
2. It is directly related to film contrast. Factors that increase film contrast tend to increase quantum mottle, whereas decreasing contrast tends to reduce quantum mottle.
3. It is inversely related to the blurring associated with light diffusion in the imaging system. Factors that increase light diffusion tend to decrease quan-tum mottle, and vice versa.

Film graininess is the visual impression of the density variation in a film uniformly exposed to light alone (not light from a transducer, because exposure by this kind of energy converter produces quantum mottle which usually over-whelms film graininess). Film graininess is due to the random distribution of the deposits of developed silver in the emulsion layer. The appearance depends on the type of film and how it is processed.

High contrast means that a film has a high sensitivity to every slight variation in brightness, including those caused by the random variation in the number of X-ray quanta absorbed by the input phosphor.

Every type of photographic film, and there are hundreds, represents an individual compromise depending on which of these three properties – speed, contrast, or graininess – is given the emphasis. The important fact is that some compromise must be made.

Let us go back to the quantum mottle. The severity of the quantum mottle observed in the image depends on the number of X-ray quanta required to produce a satisfactory image. The more X-ray quanta used, the less prominent will be the mottle caused by quantum fluctuation in the final image. Therefore, quantum mottle can be reduced by increasing the number of X-ray quanta used per frame. This can best be achieved by increasing the mAs which will reduce the density variations in the image. However, because of the higher mAs product, the overall density of the film will be increased and have to be brought back to the required level.

This is of course equivalent to making the whole system less sensitive, and obviously it is not acceptable in all cases. In cases where a higher dosage is accepted for the sake of improving the image quality the following courses are open:

1. The obvious solution is to use a slower film. If contrast is the same, the slower of the two films will produce less quantum mottle.
2. Another possibility is using a smaller diaphragm with the same film.
3. A neutral density filter can be placed in front of the camera lens to reduce the amount of light reaching the film.

Processing the Film

Speed, contrast, and graininess are determined by the type of film and they can, within limits, also be varied or manipulated by the processing conditions. Unlike in general radiography, it is common practice in cinefluorography to vary the contrast of the film according to the individual requirements of the diagnostician.

Before continuing, it should be noted that despite its apparent simplicity, photographic processing is a complex procedure. For satisfactory results, careful attention must be paid to many factors, including selection, preparation, and replenishment of solutions to achieve proper activity, control of temperature, agitation, and times of immersion in the various solutions and cleanliness to avoid solution contamination and processing artifacts. All of the five basic processing steps – development, stopping of development, fixation, washing, and drying – are important in producing the final image. Each of these steps can affect the speed, contrast, and graininess of the image. In the discussion which follows, we will assume that the last four steps have been appropriately standardized and will concentrate on development, which is the variable most commonly adjusted to change film speed and contrast.

Development depends essentially on three factors: time of development, temperature of the developer, and activity of the developer.

Within limits, as development is increased either by increasing the time or the temperature or by using a more active developer, film speed, contrast, and graininess increase – and vice versa. Therefore, because of their effect on film properties, some compromise must be made among these processing parameters that is suitable to the problem at hand.

Figure 1 shows the characteristic curves of a film developed for a series of times at constant temperature. It can be seen that, as development time increases, the characteristic curve moves progressively to the left (the speed increases). Also, as development time increases in the example shown, the slope of the characteristic curve grows progressively steeper (contrast increases) up to about 3-min development, after which increasing fog growth tends to reduce contrast. From this example we can see that when choosing processing conditions, consideration must be given to the speed, contrast, and fog levels which result, and the recommended conditions will necessarily entail compromises among these characteristics.

Figure 2 is an alternative way of showing the relationships among contrast, speed, and fog as derived from the characteristic curves in Fig. 1. The vertical dotted line indicates the recommended development time arising from that family of characteristic curves.

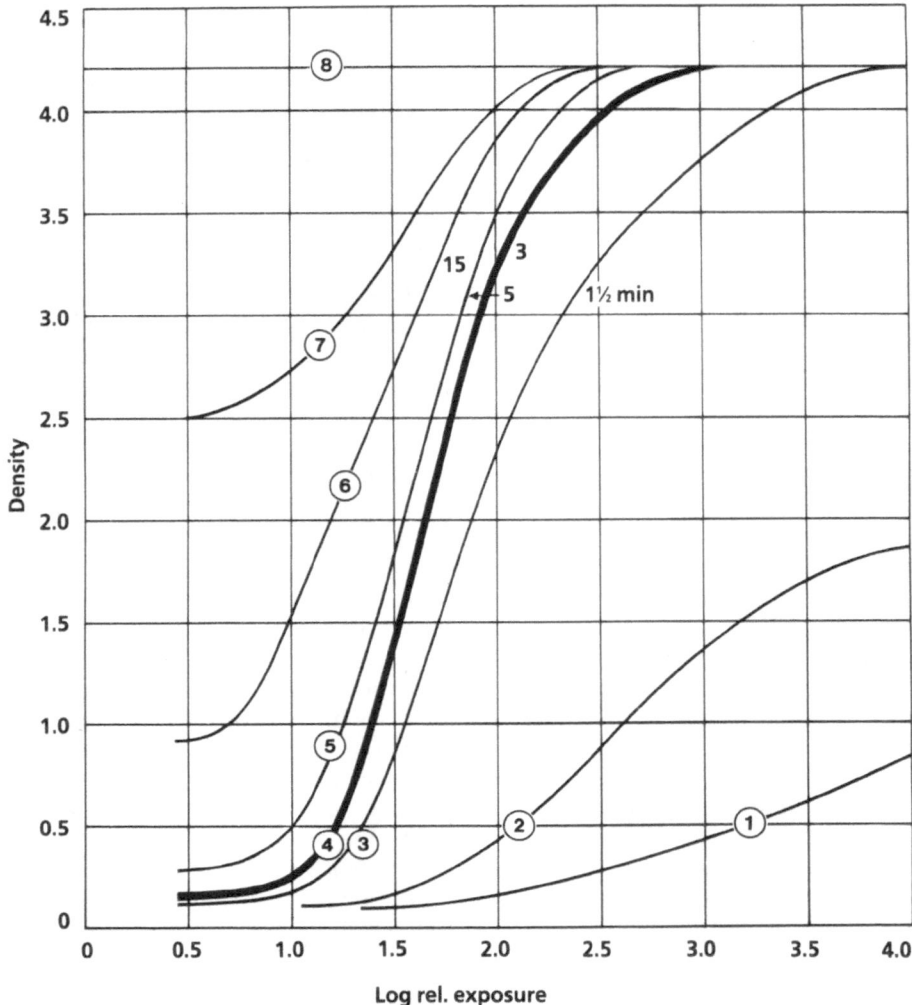

Fig. 1. Characteristic curves of a photographic film developed for a series of increasing times (*1–8*) at constant temperature

The Characteristic Curve

In the preceding discussion of film properties and development, the terms film contrast and film speed were used in a general qualitative sense. Although most people will agree on the meanings of phrases like "high contrast" or "low speed," it might be profitable to discuss in a more precise and quantitative way what is meant by "film contrast" and "film speed."

The response of a photographic film to exposure is usually represented by the characteristic curve, sometimes referred to as a sensitometric curve or an H and

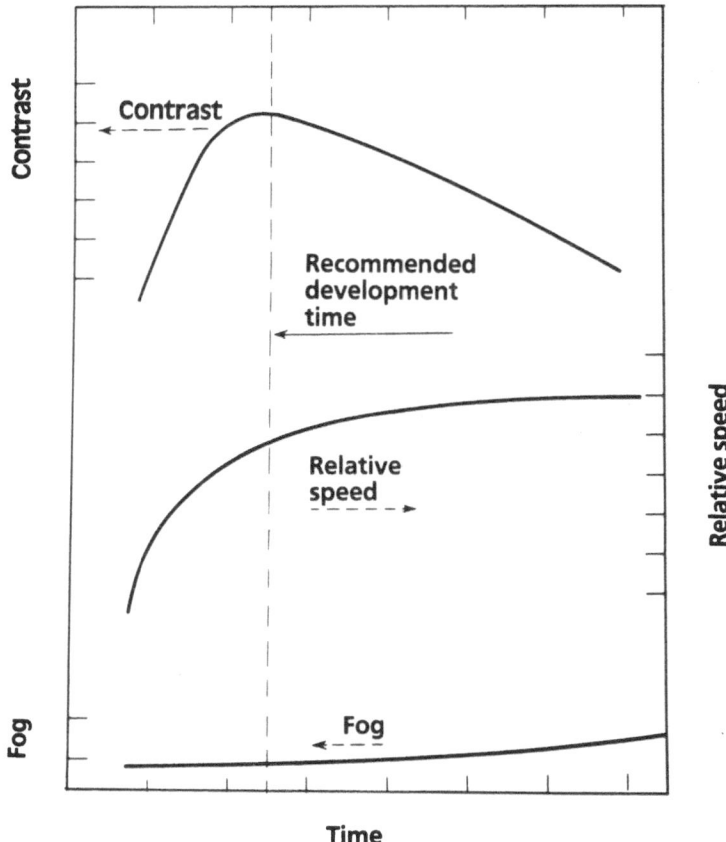

Fig. 2. Time-speed, time-contrast, and time-fog curves derived from the characteristic curves of Fig. 1. *Vertical dotted line,* recommended development time

D curve, named after Hurter and Driffield, who first used it. The characteristic curve expresses the relationship between the logarithm of the exposure applied to photographic material and the resulting optical density (Fig. 3).

Such curves are obtained by giving the film a series of known exposures, usually in a sensitometer, processing the film, measuring the resulting densities, and then plotting these densities against exposure, on a relative log scale.

The contrast of the film is related to the slope or steepness of the characteristic curve. The steeper the slope, the higher the contrast. Film contrast depends on the type of film, processing conditions, optical density, and fog. It should be emphasized that the shape of the characteristic curve does *not* depend on, for example, kV, mAs, or focus-to-film distance.

At this point it might be well to briefly enumerate some of the factors that affect radiographic contrast. By radiographic contrast we mean the density difference between two areas in the radiographic image. Radiographic contrast

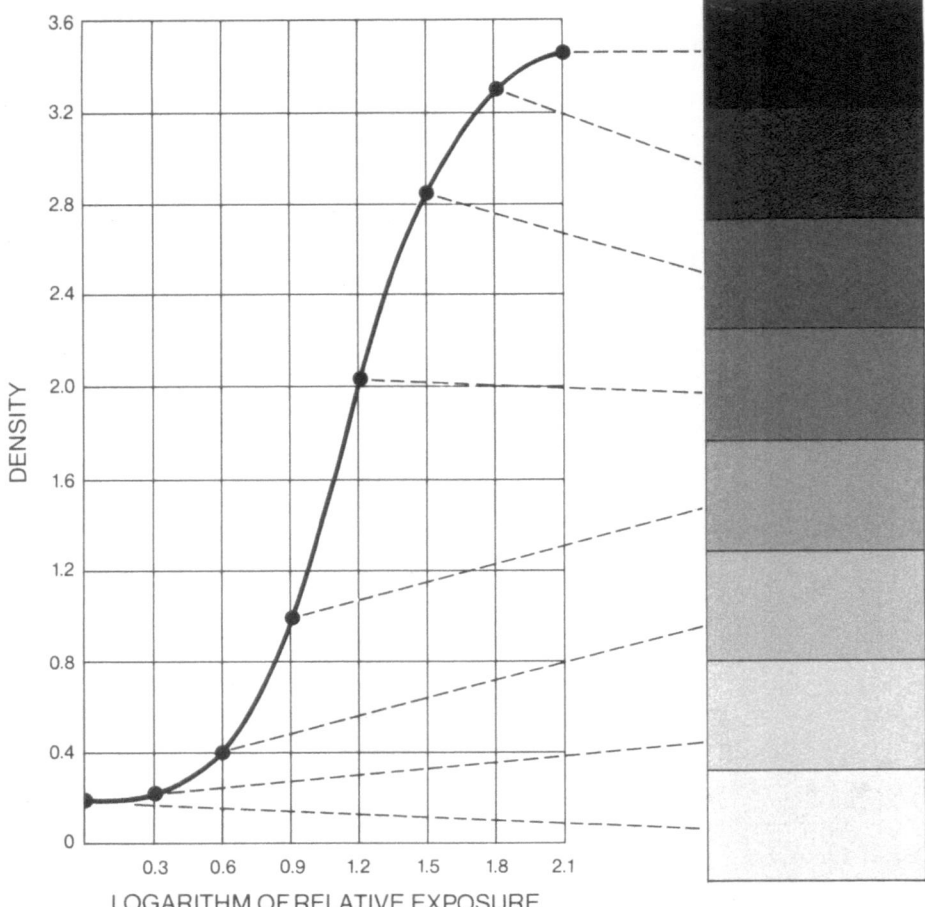

Fig. 3. Characteristic curve and sensitometric strip from which it was derived

is composed of subject contrast, the optical characteristics of the imaging system, and film contrast.

Subject contrast refers to the ratio of X-ray intensities emerging from two regions of the subject. It depends on absorption defferences in the subject, radiation quality, and scattered radiation. In addition to the effect of this distribution of X-ray intensities arriving at the input phosphor of the image intensifier, the contrast ratio of the image intensifier and the flare light associated with its optical system also influence radiographic contrast.

The contrast of the image is, as already noted, influenced by film contrast, too. However, it is important to remember that film contrast is a separate entity, distinct from and independent of subject contrast and image-intensifier contrast ratio, even though all of these factors contribute individually to radiographic contrast. In the following discussion we will restrict our attention to film con-

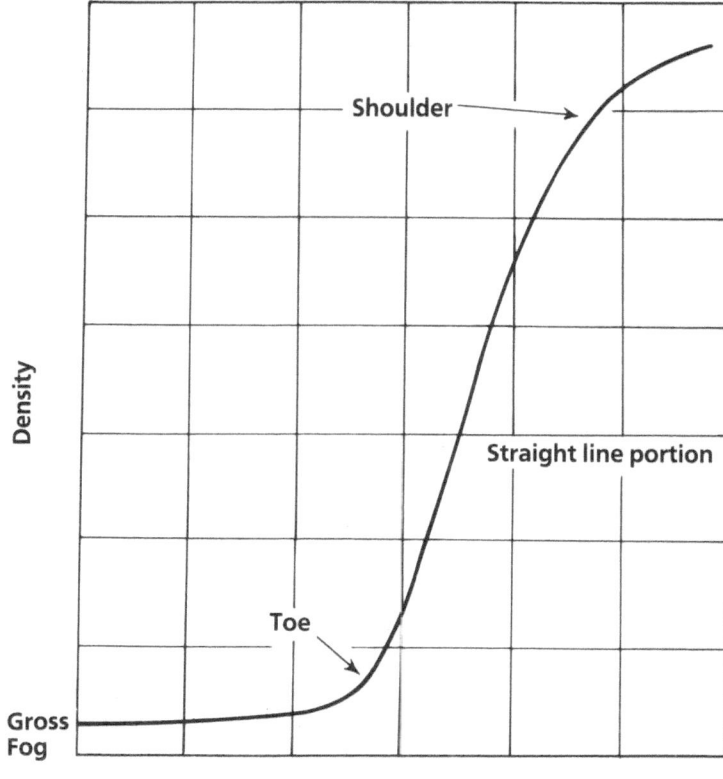

Fig. 4. Characteristic curve of a photographic film

trast and leave commentary on the other components of radiographic contrast for another occasion. As can be seen in Fig. 4, the contrast, that is, the slope of the characteristic curve, changes with increasing density: at first, in the toe region, the contrast is low; in the middle or straight line portion, it is high; and, in the shoulder, it is low again.

These changes in slope have a definite effect on the visibility of details in the cinefluorographic image. For example, two slightly different thicknesses in the subject radiographed will transmit slightly different exposures to the film. These exposures will have a certain small difference in log relative exposure between them. The difference in the densities corresponding to these two exposures will depend on just where on the characteristic curve they fall. The steeper the slope of the curve, the greater will be the density difference.

For example, let us assume that the two structures of interest differ in their X-ray transmission by an amount that will cause their brightness on the output phosphor to differ by 60% (Fig. 5).

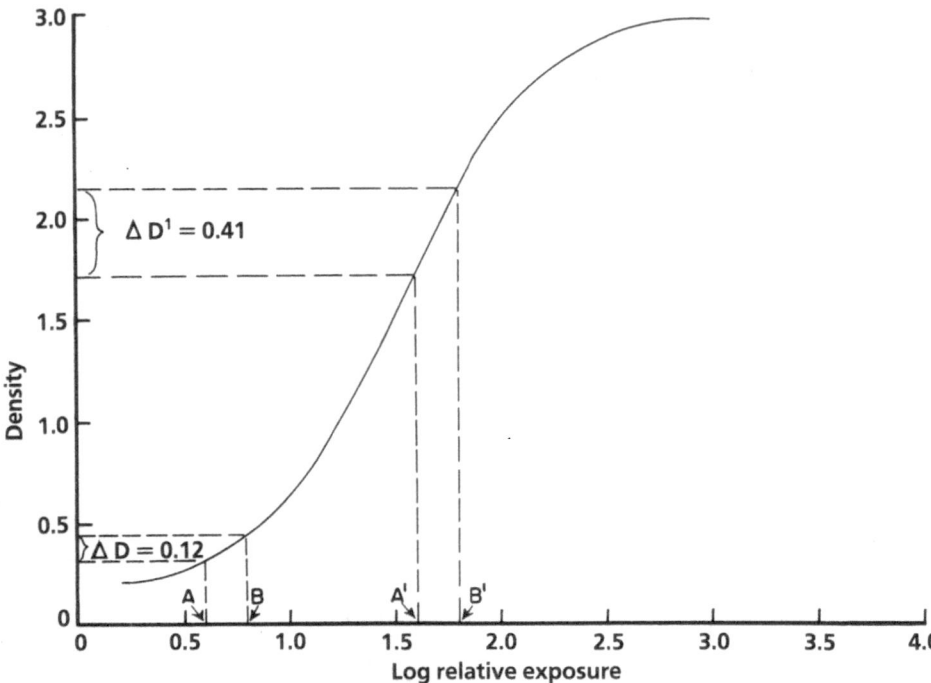

Fig. 5. Typical characteristic curve of a cinefluorographic film. The density difference to a given difference in logarithm of relative exposure depends upon the slope of the characteristic curve

If the subject is radiographed with an exposure that puts the densities on the toe of the characteristic curve (A to B in Fig. 5) the difference in density ΔD produced will be 0.12. If the exposure time or the milliamperage is now increased so that the exposures fall on the steeper part of the curve (A' to B'), ΔD will be greater, namely 0.41, and the two structures will be much more clearly distinguished in the image. Thus, the intensity ratio or subject contrast of the radiation emerging from the object are exaggerated in the cinefluorographic reproduction; and the steeper the slope of the characteristic curve, the greater the degree of exaggeration. In this sense the film acts as a "contrast amplifier." The ability of the film to exaggerate the subject contrast is of the utmost practical importance. Otherwise many small differences in the subject could not be made visible.

We should, however, be well aware that on every radiograph or cinefluorographic image we always have structures in the toe region with its lower contrast and in the straight line portion where the contrast and, thus, the visibility is much higher.

It is often useful to have a single number to indicate the contrast of a film. The terms commonly used are "average gradient" and "gamma." The average gradient is defined as the slope of a straight line joining two points of specified

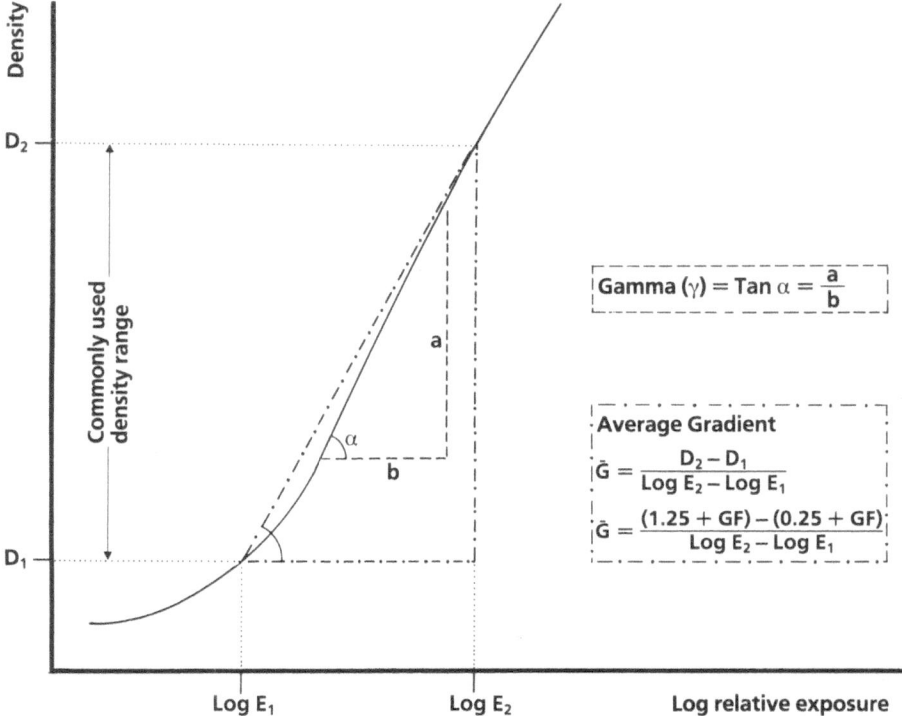

Fig. 6. Definition of average gradient and gamma

densities on the characteristic curve. These densities are usually the maximum and minimum useful densities under conditions of practical use. The average gradient, then, will indicate the average contrast properties of the film over the useful range. In cinefluorography these points have been assigned density values of 0.25 above gross fog and 1.25 above gross fog as illustrated in Fig. 6.

Gamma is defined as the slope of the straight line portion of the characteristic curve.

The other significant value, besides contrast, which can be obtained from the characteristic curve is the relative speed, which is indicated by the location of the curve along the exposure axis in relation to the curves of other films. The further to the left along the exposure axis the characteristic curve is located, the higher is the speed. Speed is inversely proportional to the exposure required to reach a certain density. The density value used for determining speed depends on the application of the film. In medical radiography, including cinefluorography, this is a density of 1.0 above gross fog.

Figure 7 shows the characteristic curves of two films. Film A has high contrast, film B has low contrast. Film A will differentiate more strikingly between structures of slightly differing X-ray transmission than will film B. Film B, however, will cover a much wider range of X-ray intensities within the useful

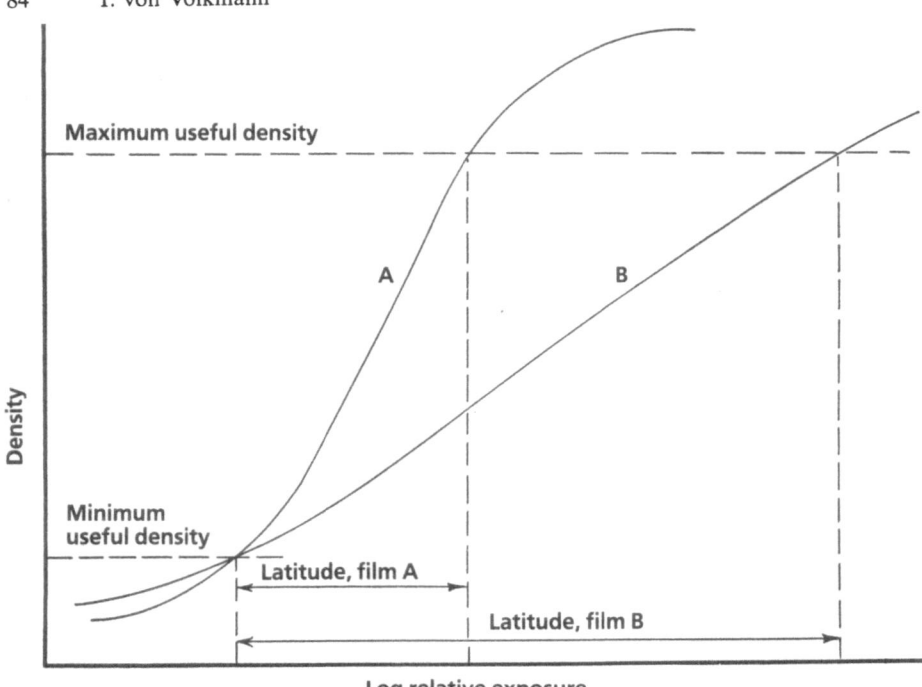

Fig. 7. Typical characteristic curves of a high-contrast film (*A*) and a low-contrast film (*B*). The range of exposures that can be covered within the useful range of density (i.e., latitude of the film) depends upon the average gradient

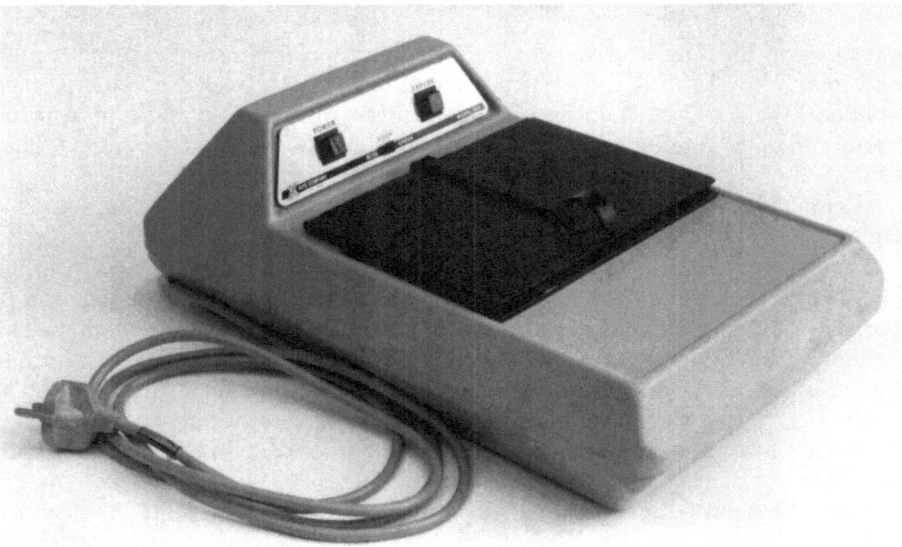

Fig. 8. Sensitometer for exposure to visible light

density range than will film A. Therefore, film B has the greater latitude. This illustrates still another photographic compromise that must be made. One can have either high contrast or wide latitude, and the choice depends on the specific problem at hand. The latitude which a film has to have depends, of course, on the range of intensities that must be recorded.

Processing Control

As mentioned previously, processing exercises a very important influence on the speed and contrast of the film. Consistent film processing is therefore one of the

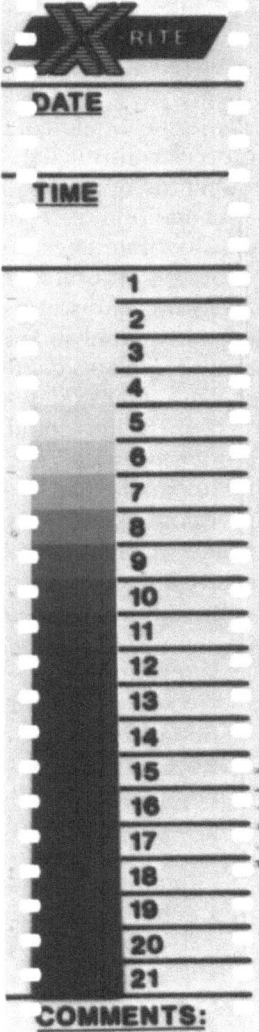

Fig. 9. Sensitometric strip

main requirements for maintaining the high quality standard required for cine-fluorographic images.

This uniformity in processing can be achieved through a program in which certain parameters are monitored at regular intervals. In cinefilm processing this program involves exposing film strips in a sensitometer (Fig. 8), then processing and evaluating these sensitometric strips (Fig. 9).

This evaluation could be done by plotting the whole curve and determining the values of speed and contrast as described above. However, that is usually too time consuming for everyday practice. Instead, the density values of two selected steps on the sensitometric strips can be used to monitor speed and contrast.

1. Speed index: a step with a density of about 0.85 above gross fog
2. Contrast index: the density difference between (a) a step which received four times the exposure of the speed step (0.6 logE above speed step) and (b) the speed step

These speed and contrast indices are given only for the purpose of simplifying process control; they should not be mixed up with the above-mentioned sensitometric definitions.

In addition, in a good control program, the gross fog is measured, that is, the density of an unexposed area on the film.

Because processing is a temperature- and time-dependent chemical reaction, these two parameters should also be monitored. The activity of the solutions depend not only on proper mixing of chemicals but also to a large extent on their proper replenishment to restore activity as they are used. The established replenishment rates should therefore be regularly monitored.

These values should be determined on a daily or weekly basis and are best plotted on a chart for ready reference to observe changes and trends among these parameters. A typical chart is shown in Fig. 10. The great advantage of a processing control as described here is that it can show when adjustment is needed so that corrective action can be taken before image quality is significantly affected.

In addition to processing control, regular attention should be given to other factors which can affect the quality of the cinefluorographic image, such as:

1. Safelighting
2. Good housekeeping and cleanliness to avoid artifacts on the film, contamination of solutions, and dirty optics in the image intensifier chain
3. Checking of exposing equipment for accuracy of kV, mAs, timer- and beam-limiting device settings, grid alignment and centering, optical systems focus, and automatic brightness control.

The monitoring of these parameters, along with those discussed above, adds up to a quality assurance program capable of producing consistently satisfactory images.

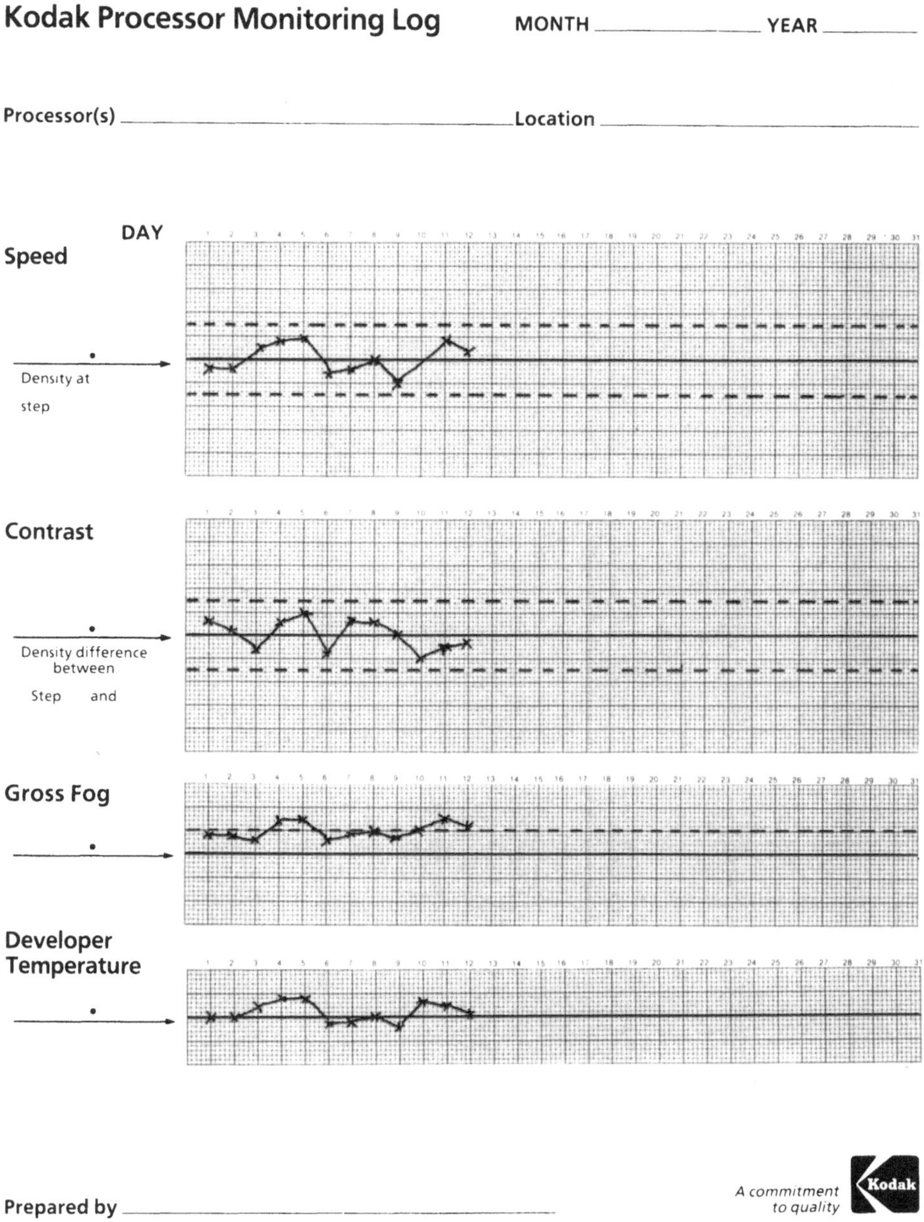
Kodak Processor Monitoring Log
MONTH
YEAR
Processor(s)
Location
DAY
Speed
Density at
step
Contrast
Density difference
between
Step
and
Gross Fog
Developer
Temperature
Prepared by
A commitment
to quality
Kodak

Fig. 10. Process control chart showing a daily control strip plot

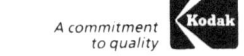

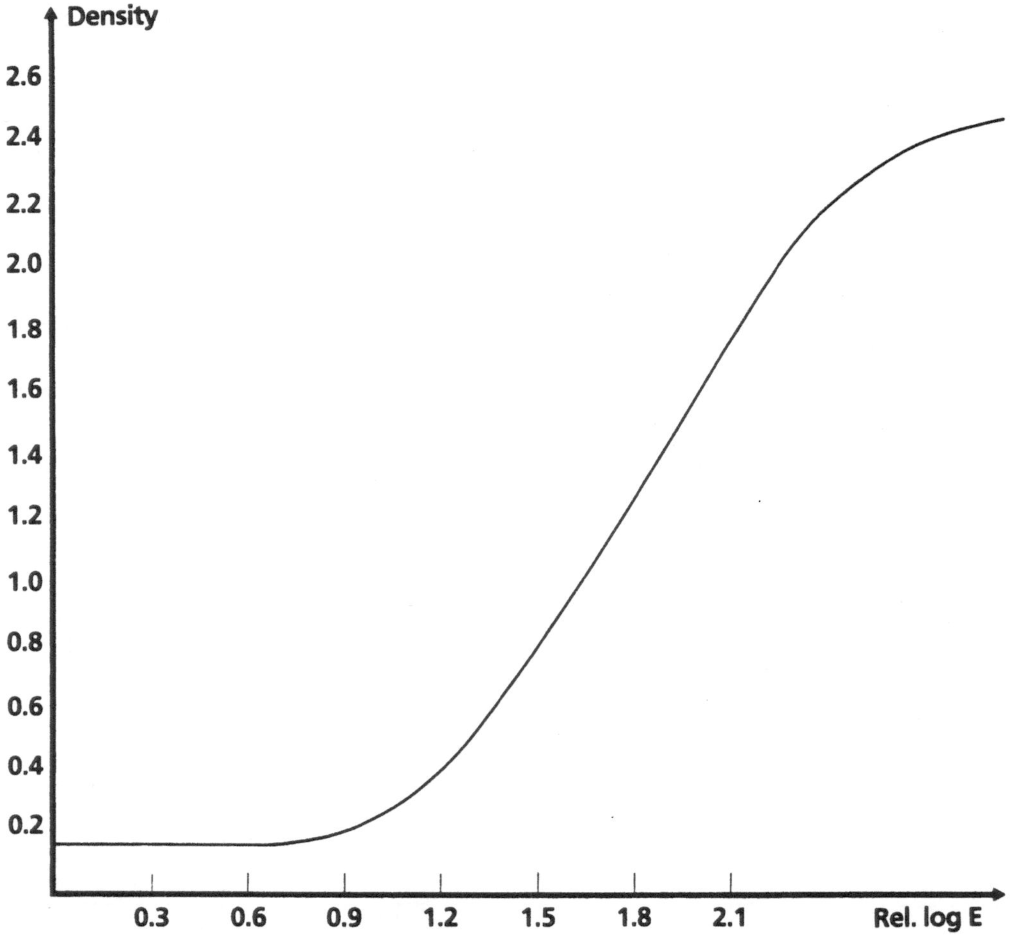

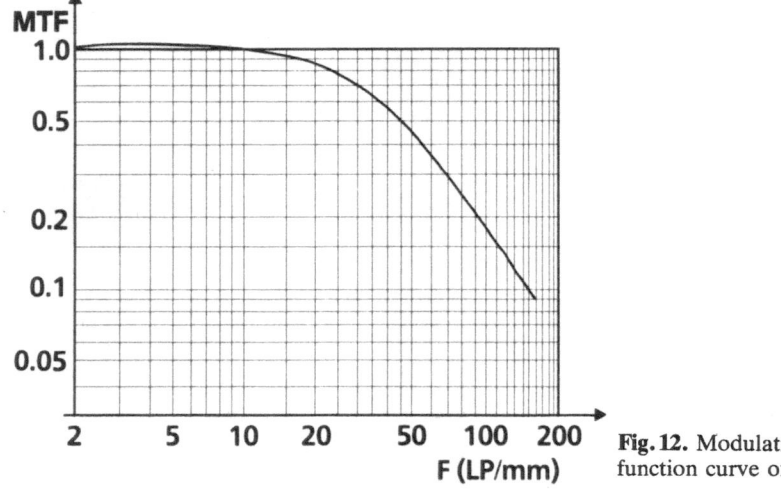

Fig. 11. Characteristic curve of Kodak CFE Film. Exposure: simulated P-20 phosphor; developer: Kodak X-Omat MX 496

Fig. 12. Modulation transfer function curve of Kodak CFE film

Kodak CFE Film

We at Kodak have been intensely involved in the development of a new film for cinefluorography taking into consideration the relationship between speed, contrast, and graininess, and the state of the art in film manufacturing. We have had numerous discussions with cardiologists, radiologists, and other specialists in the field. Judging by the needs these users expressed, we feel that the CFE film satisfies the special requirements of a film for angiocardiography.

Film	Rel. Speed	Gamma	RMS Granularity	Gross Fog
2496	80	1.9	16	0.10
CFA	180	1.9	23	0.16
CFE	100	1.8	14	0.14

Fig. 13. Comparison of Kodak CFE film with two other Kodak films used in cinefluorography (RAR 2496 and CFA)

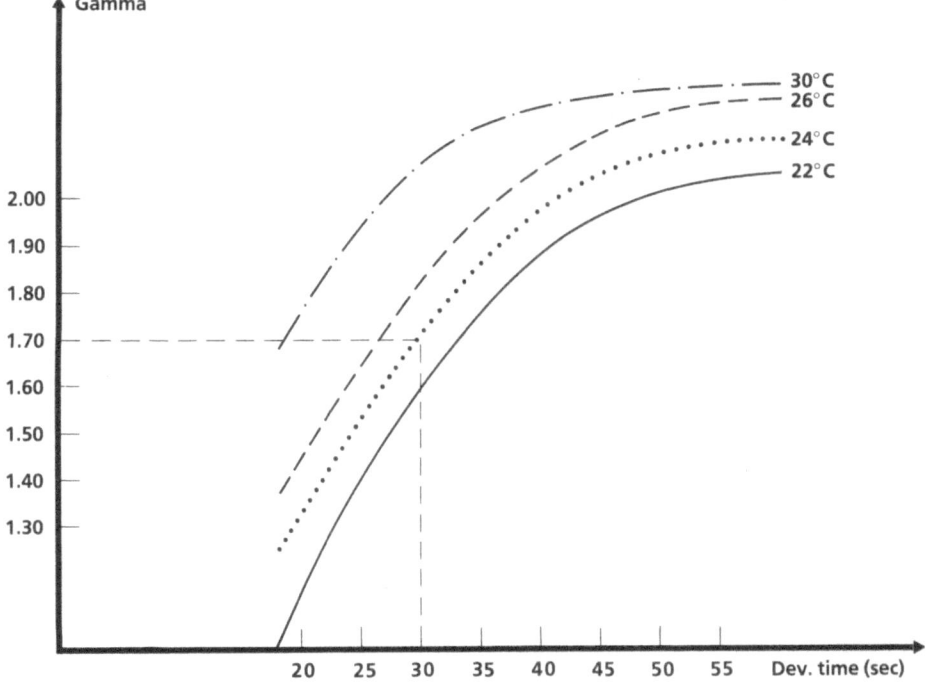

Fig. 14. Time-gamma curves of Kodak CFE film

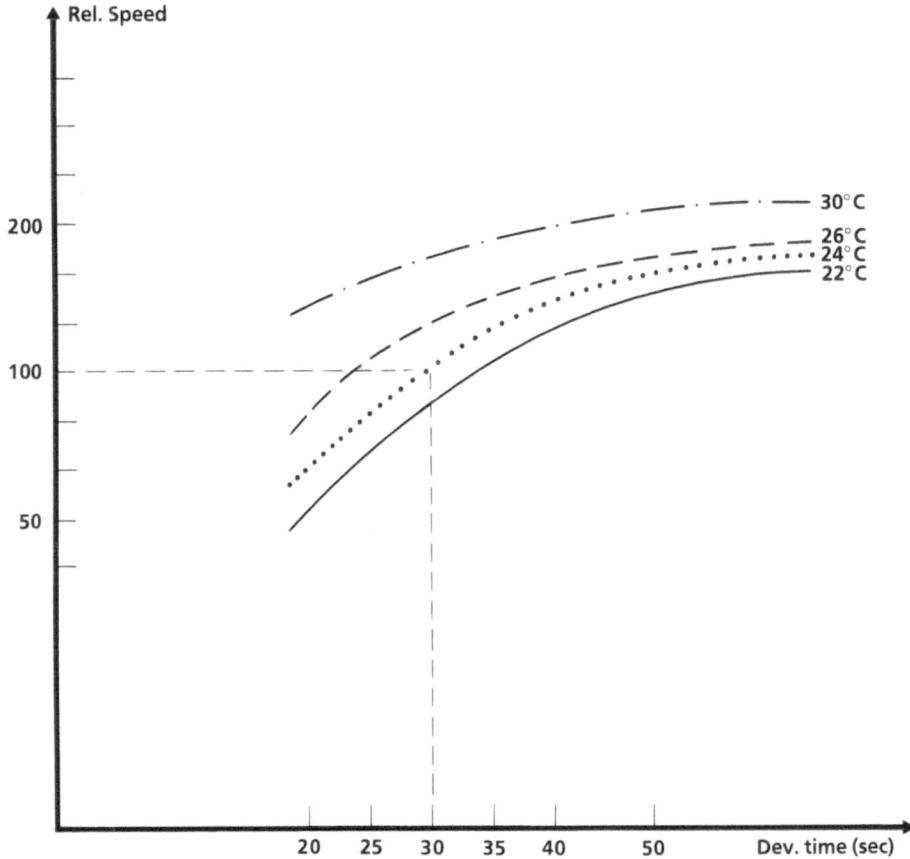

Fig. 15. Time-relative speed curves of Kodak CFE film

The Kodak CFE film has a medium speed. The gamma can be varied from 1.3 to 2.0 by changing the processing conditions. It has low granularity and a low gross fog (0.14). The emulsion is orthochromatic, matching the green output phosphor of the image intensifier, but it can also be handled under a red safelight in the darkroom. The emulsion is coated on a blue polyester base. The film has an antistatic backing (Figs. 11 and 12). The film can of course be processed in the rapid processors used in cinefluorography. The recommended processing conditions for a gamma of 1.7 are 24°C, 30 s in Kodak X-Omat developer MX 496.

Figure 13 compares Kodak CFE film to two other Kodak films used in cinefluorography with respect to various parameters (RAR film 2496 and CFA film). Figures 14 to 16 show the flexibility of the film with changing processing conditions.

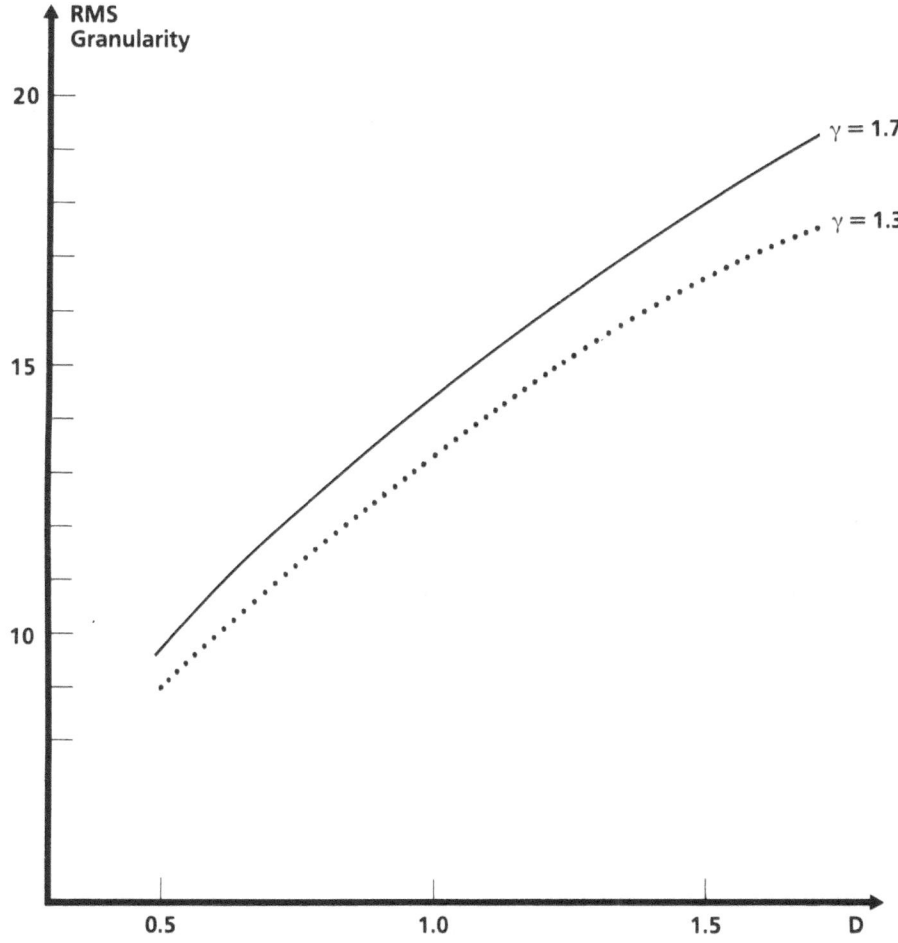

Fig. 16. Density-RMS granularity curves of Kodak CFE film

References

1. Eastman Kodak Company, Sensitometric properties of X-ray films
2. Lawrence DJ (1973) A simple method of processor control. Med Radiogr Photogr 49 (1):2–6

Recent Developments in Contrast Media*

G. HELLIGE

Abteilung für Experimentelle Kardiologie, Zentrum Physiologie und Pathophysiologie der Universität Göttingen, Humboldtallee 7, D-3400 Göttingen

The aim of research activities in angiocardiography is to improve diagnostic value while reducing the side effects and risk for the patient. This book focuses on the important developments in the field of engineering. The resulting advances in imaging and quantitation of function parameters will lead to better diagnoses and reduce side effects by reducing the required amounts of contrast material. There are also activities in the field of pharmacology seeking to develop new contrast media molecules. Reduction of toxicity will lead to reduction of side effects, and allow application of high amounts, which theoretically should improve the diagnostic value of angiocardiography. Characteristic of these parallel activities is the increasing number of symposia on contrast media – reflecting the intensity of research in this field.

More than 10 years ago in angiocardiography, particularly in coronary angiography, acute cardiovascular reactions (such as ventricular fibrillation) dominated over other side effects. Balancing the sodium content of the ionic contrast materials helped to reduce severe incidents to a tolerably low level. However, the limitations with regard to high risk cardiac patients and the general toxicity remained. The development of new materials enabling further reduction of side effects is based on research into the underlying pathophysiologic mechanisms.

The acute cardiac phenomena caused by common ionic contrast media are well known. Coronary angiography is accompanied by typical hemodynamic reactions: cardiodepression visible by increase of left ventricular diastolic pressure, decrease of peak pressure, and dP/dt followed by a delayed positive inotropic effect and a long-lasting increase of coronary blood flow caused by decrease of vascular resistance. Typical electrocardiographic effects are hypervoltage combined with a shift of the electrical axis of the heart, disturbance of electrical activation and repolarization waves, sinus slowing, and incidental initiation of fibrillation.

These reactions are mainly caused by the physicochemical properties of the common ionic contrast materials, which differ from blood by an extreme hyperosmolality of more than 2000 mosmol per kg water, an unphysiologic ion composition, hyperviscosity, and induction of a marked acidosis when mixed with blood. Subsequently, the mixture of blood and common ionic contrast

* Supported by the Deutsche Forschungsgemeinschaft, SFB 89

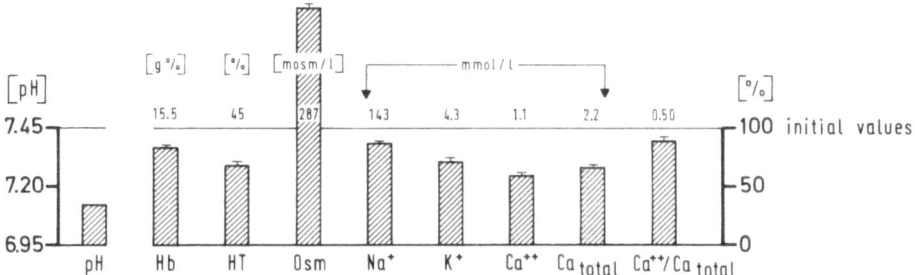

Fig. 1. Shifts of physicochemical parameters in blood caused by addition of 1 part diatrizoate to 5 parts blood (from Wolpers et al. 1981)

material is characterized, besides the pH shift already mentioned, by a disturbance of the main physicochemical parameters: decrease of hemoglobin content and disproportionate decrease of hematocrit, marked increase of osmolality, and decrease of sodium, potassium, and calcium, with disproportionate reduction of ionized calcium (Fig. 1). The electrolyte shifts results from dilution by the contrast medium itself, the water shifts from osmotic dehydration of blood cells and calcium binding properties. Corresponding changes are demonstrable following coronary angiography in the venous blood of the heart, with shifts of the sodium level dependent on the sodium composition of the contrast material, decrease of potassium, marked decrease of calcium, and increase of osmolality.

We have been able to demonstrate the effect of these alterations in the coronary blood on myocardial cells by use of intracellular microelectrodes in the beating, blood-perfused dog heart in situ. Under coronary angiography, we recorded a marked hyperpolarization of the cardiac cell membrane potential combined with prolongation of the action potential (Fig. 2), corresponding to the decrease of calcium and potassium levels in blood and interstitial fluid. In this case ventricular tachycardia is induced by a premature beat occurring in the vulnerable period of the prolonged action potential. The disturbances of electrophysiology on the cellular level by electrolyte shifts are responsible for the known ECG changes. The concomitant negative inotropic effect may also be explained by electrolyte shifts.

The disproportionate decrease of ionized calcium caused by its binding to the common ionic contrast media leads to an increase of the extracellular sodium to calcium ratio calculated from electrolyte levels in coronary venous blood. This ratio determines the amount of calcium entering the cell and taking part in the excitation-contraction coupling. High ratios, as produced by high sodium contrast media or strong calcium binding, cause marked cardiodepression. Addition of calcium to common contrast materials keeps the ratio balanced and reduces cardiodepression significantly.

Based on this knowledge about mechanisms of acute cardiac side effects of common ionic contrast media, the advantages of the newly developed so-called low osmolality contrast media are easily demonstrable.

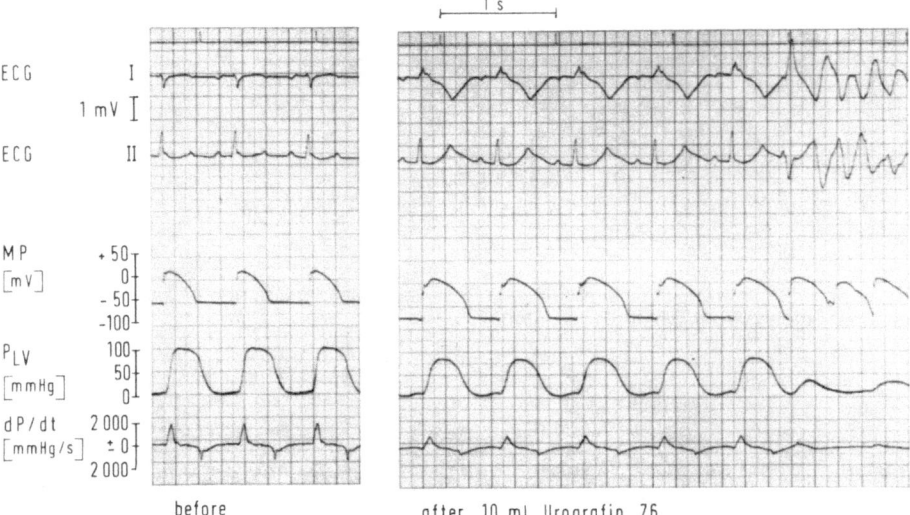

Fig. 2. Effects of coronary angiography on ECG, cellular membrane potential, ventricular pressure, and d*P*/d*t* in the blood-perfused dog heart in situ. Note the significant hyperpolarization and prolongation of action potential preceding initiation of ventricular tachycardia (from Wolpers et al. 1986)

The high osmotic pressures of common ionic molecules result from their chemical state. The generally used diatrizoates or metrizoates are salts of triodated aromatic acids consisting of two osmotically active compounds, the acid and a sodium or meglumine cation. Reduction of osmolality by half was aspired to by the construction of dimeric monoacid salts such as ioxaglate or monomeric nonionic derivatives of the acids like the first low osmolality contrast material, metrizamide (Fig. 3). These two low osmolality materials, ioxaglate,

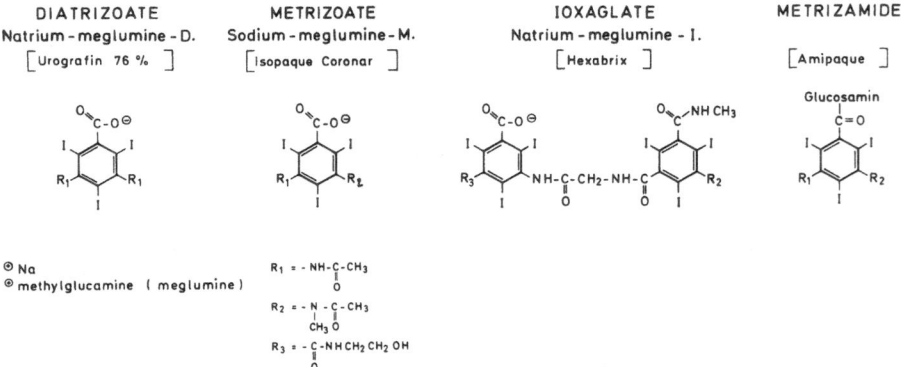

Fig. 3. Chemical structure of common ionic contrast materials diatrizoate and metrizoate and low osmolality materials ioxaglate and metrizamide

which is still ionic and very viscous at high concentrations, and metrizamide, which is unstable in solution and extremely expensive, have been supplemented by the first nonionic material to be stable in solution, iopamidol, and the two recently developed agents, iohexol and iopromide (Table 1).

Compared with commonly used materials, all of these preparations have a significantly reduced osmolality as well as a reduction or absence of calcium

Table 1. "Low osmolality" contrast media

INN and trade name	Type	Iodine content [mgI/ml]	Osmotic activity[a]
Ioxaglate Hexabrix	Ionic dimer	320	600 mosm/kg H_2O
metrizamide Amipaque	Nonionic unstable solution	e.g. 350	550 mosm/kg H_2O
Iopamidol Solutrast	Nonionic	370	799 mosm/kg H_2O
Iohexol	Nonionic	e.g. 370	980 mosm/kg H_2O
Iopromide	Nonionic	e.g. 370	790 mosm/kg H_2O

[a] Manufacturers' data

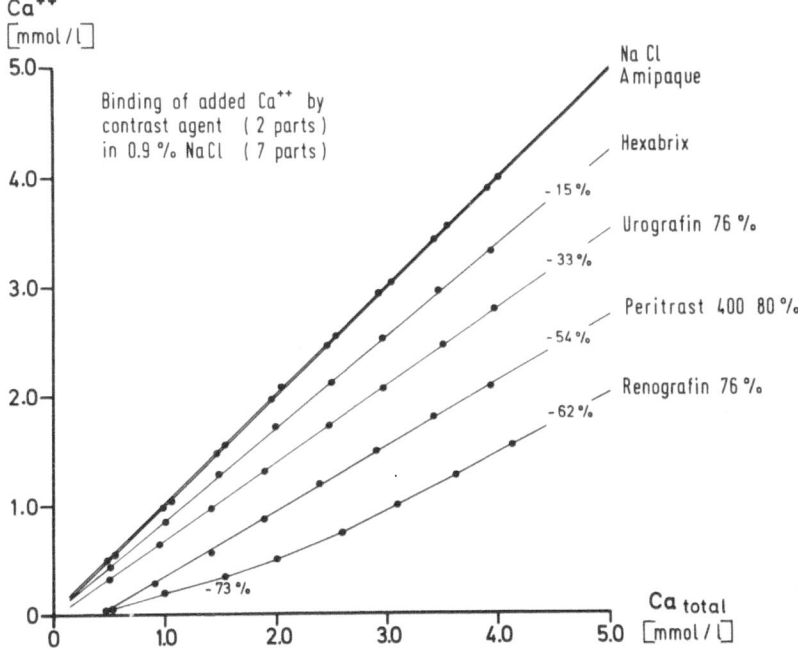

Fig. 4. Binding of ionized calcium by contrast media demonstrated by measurements of total and ionized calcium in the presence of contrast material (from Wolpers et al. 1981)

binding, which is demonstrable by titration experiments with parallel measurement of total calcium and ionized calcium level (Fig. 4). Whereas Renografin binds about 60% of the added ionized calcium, binding by ioxaglate is only about 15% and absent in the case of nonionic materials such as metrizamide. The same graduation is demonstrable in blood during angiography and correlates closely with the degree of the negative inotropic effects of the contrast media.

Nonionic materials even cause a positive inotropic effect, which is to be explained by the increase of intracellular calcium due to osmotic dehydration of muscle cells. This effect is also present in the case of common ionic contrast media, but is masked by the negative inotropic mechanisms.

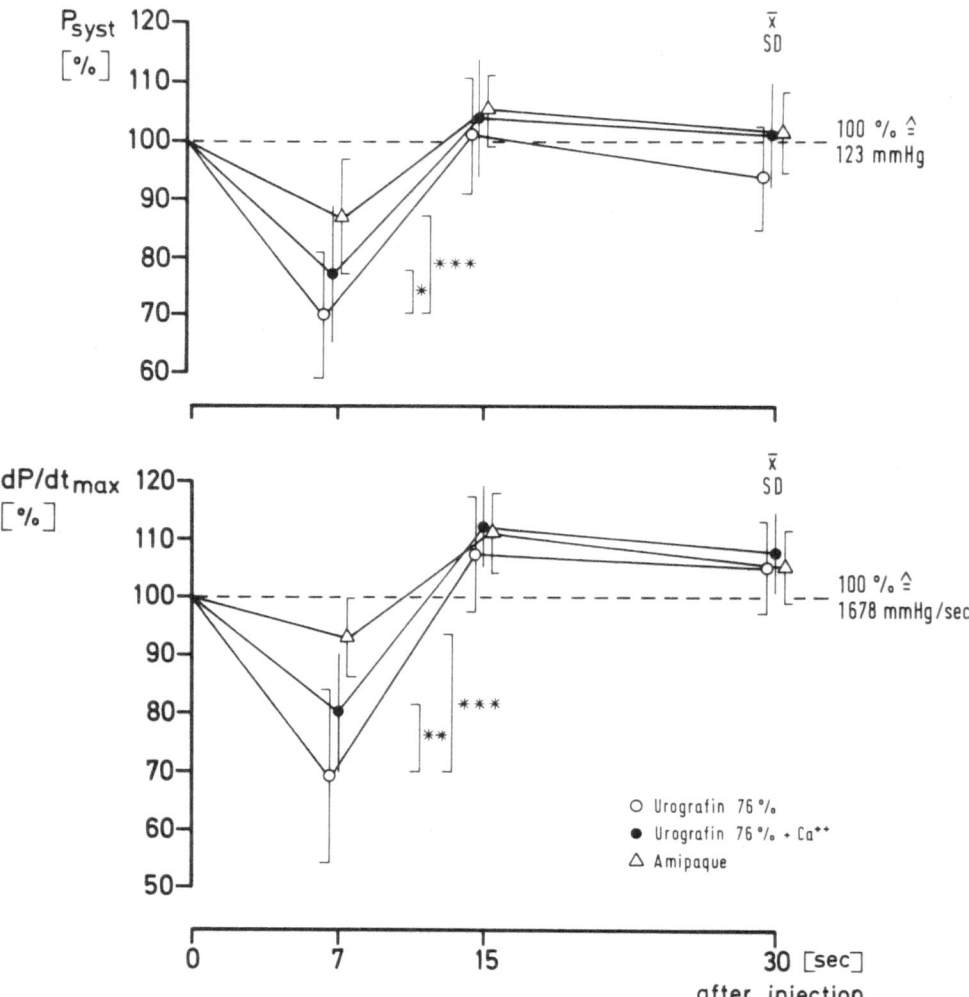

Fig. 5. Reduction of cardiodepressive effects of coronary angiography in patients by addition of calcium to diatrizoate and use of metrizamide (from Zipfel et al. 1980)

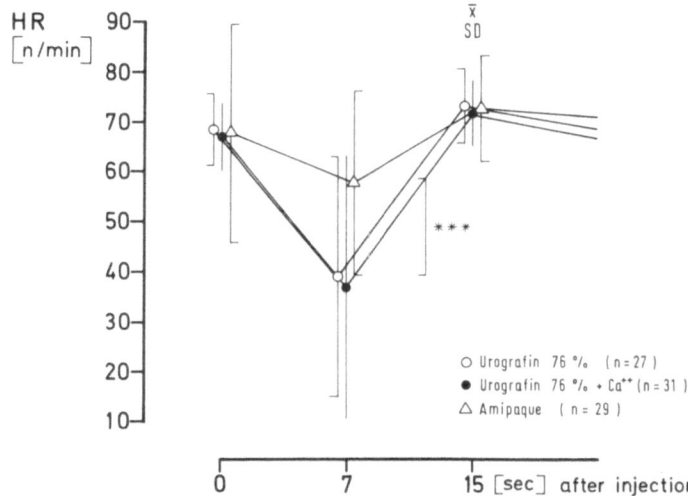

Fig. 6. Effects of diatrizoate, addition of calcium, and metrizamide on heart rate corresponding to Fig. 5 (from Zipfel et al. 1980)

Due to the reduced osmolality and the water and electrolyte shifts, the subsequent disturbances of the electrical activity of cells are reduced. Compared with the common ionic materials, changes in resting and action potential are diminished; excitation generation, conduction, and ECG parameters are less affected.

Clinical experience confirms the experimental findings. In two experiments we compared the side effects of coronary angiography using common diatrizoate, diatrizoate plus calcium, and metrizamide in patients with coronary heart disease and diatrizoate and ioxaglate in patients with chronic coronary heart disease or acute myocardial infarction. The results confirm the advantages of the low osmolality materials (Fig. 5). Cardiodepression, demonstrable by a drop of peak pressure and dP/dt, is significantly reduced by addition of calcium, but less completely than by the nonionic metrizamide. The superiority of the low osmotic metrizamide is demonstrated by a striking reduction of bradycardia, whereas the addition of calcium has no effect on sinus slowing (Fig. 6).

Similar results were obtained in comparing diatrizoate with ioxaglate. In both groups (patients with either chronic or acute coronary heart disease), pressure drop and bradycardia were significantly reduced.

Hemodynamic side effects under ventriculography are also diminished. Use of low osmolality contrast media leads to a significant reduction of arterial hypotension due to less peripheral resistance.

In summary, the *acute* cardiac side effects seem to be reduced to a nearly negligible level; *subacute* cardiovascular side effects seen also to be reduced. Low osmolality contrast media are reported to cause significantly less augmentation of the circulatory volume by water shift into the vascular system. Subsequent volume loading of the heart and risk of cardiac pump failure should thus be reduced.

The advantages of reduction of osmolality are also demonstrable with regard to extracardiovascular side effects. Hyperosmolality is said to be the main reason for release of histamine and other kinins which may be responsible for systemic reactions such as activation of the complement system, increase of capillary permeability, and subsequent generalized disturbance of organ function. The nonionic contrast media show significantly reduced protein binding, another major cause of toxicity in contrast material. The favorable influence on different factors is reflected by an overall reduction of toxicity, as is proved by a significant increase of the lethal dose being used in animal experiments. The final evaluation of general toxicity of the different low osmolality contrast media will need further animal experiments and, in particular, clinical experience.

To return to our introductory comments, we can confirm that the new generation of contrast media may help to reduce the side effects of cardiovascular angiography and permit examinations to be extended both to high risk patients and methods requiring high amounts of contrast media. The impressive progress made in the field of signal processing, through use of computers with improved imaging and quantitation of angiocardiographic parameters, should therefore be reinforced by these developments, the aim of which is improvement of diagnosis and reduction of side effects.

References

Wolpers HG, Baller D, Ensink FBM, Schröter W, Zipfel J, Hellige G (1981) Influence of arteriographic contrast media on the Na^+/Ca^{++}- ratio in blood. Cardiovasc Intervent Radiol 4:8–13

Wolpers HG, Baller D, Ensink FBM, Hoeft A, Korb H, Hellige G (1986) Einfluß von Röntgenkontrastmittel auf das Membranpotential am schlagenden Herzen. Z Kardiol (to be published)

Zipfel J, Baller D, Blanke H, Karsch KR, Rentrop P, Wiegand VW, Wolpers HG, Hellige G (1980) Reduktion kardialer Nebenwirkungen von Röntgenkontrastmitteln in der Angiokardiographie durch Zusatz von Kalzium und Verwendung eines nichtionischen Kontrastmittels. Klin Wochenschr 58:1339–1346

Estimation of Ventricular Volume, Fractional Ejected Volumes, Stroke Volume, and Quantitation of Regurgitant Flow

H. T. Dodge, F. H. Sheehan and D. K. Stewart

Division of Cardiology RG-20, University of Washington School of Medicine, Seattle, WA 98195, USA

Imaging of the left ventricle by angiography has made it possible to develop methods for determining dimensions, volume, stroke volume, and wall thickness of the left ventricular (LV) chamber. The first measurements of LV chamber volumes in man were reported over 25 years ago [1] and this was followed by a number of studies in both experimental animals and man to further develop and validate methods [2–7], to establish normal values for LV volume [8, 9], and to determine volume changes that occur with various types of heart diseases [1, 7, 10–20]. The demonstration that the change of computed chamber volume from end-diastole to end-systole agreed closely with stroke volume in subjects without arrhythmias, shunts, or valvular regurgitation [21] provided the basis for a method to quantify mitral and/or aortic valvular regurgitant flow [22]. The various methods for determining volume have been tested and adapted to improved high speed filming techniques using cine angiography in differing projections [23–26].

This paper will be a review of methods for determining LV chamber volumes, stroke volume, and ejection fraction from LV ventriculograms, with an assessment of the accuracy of the methods. The review will include the application of these methods to quantify regurgitant flow resulting from valvular insufficiency of left heart valves.

To determine LV chamber volumes from contrast ventriculograms there are three major problems which must be overcome:

a) image distortion from nonparallel X-ray beams, from pin-cushion distortion in image intensifier systems, and image distortion in cine projection;
b) varying LV image projections on the X-ray films resulting from the LV spatial position and projections used for filming, and
c) selection of a suitable reference figure for purposes of volume calculation.

In the early studies which we conducted to develop and evaluate methods for computing LV chamber volumes, the left ventricles of human hearts were distended with known volumes of barium sulfate paste and at increasing known increments of volume with biplane orthogonal filming at the known volumes in differing projections [3]. The images were corrected for X-ray distortion and the dimensions and projected areas were determined [3]. Volumes were calculated by a number of methods and compared with the known volumes. These studies demonstrated that chamber volumes computed from the projected area of the

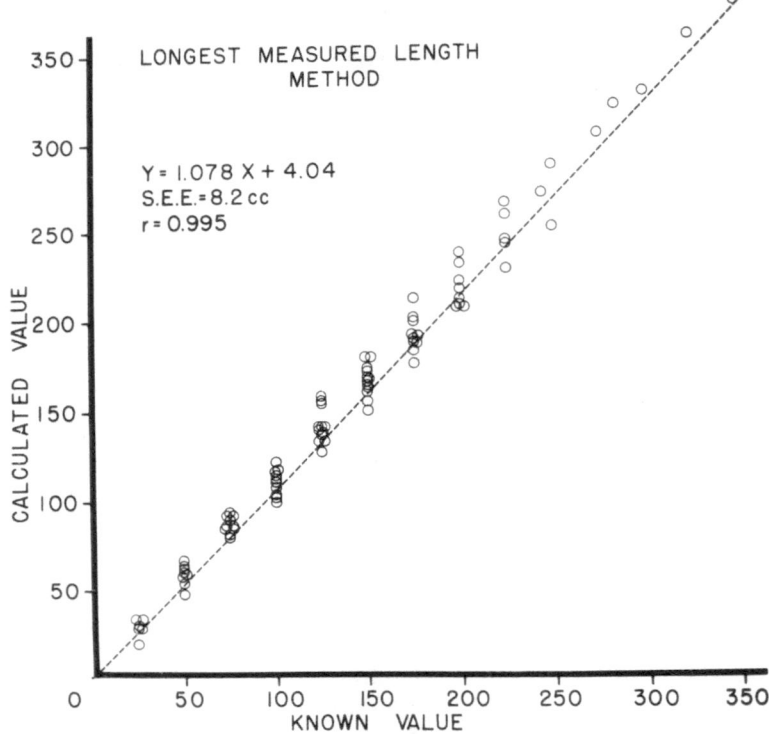

Fig. 1. Relationship between known LV chamber volumes and volumes calculated from the projected areas and lenghts on biplane films

chamber and the longest projected length (so-called area-length method), and by assuming an ellipsoid reference figure, were closely correlated with known volumes ($r = 0.995$) and had a standard error of estimate of $\pm$ 8.2 cc [3], as is shown in Fig. 1.

With this method volumes (V) were computed as:

$$V = \tfrac{\pi}{6} L \cdot Da \cdot Db,$$

where L is the longest measured chamber length on either of the biplane films. Da and Db equal the transverse diameters in the orthogonal projections computed from the respective projected chamber areas (A) and semilengths by assuming an ellipse reference figure such that $D = \tfrac{4A}{\pi L}$. This is illustrated in Fig. 2.

Comparisons of known chamber volumes with volumes with volumes computed using the calculated spatial length of the chamber and also by Simpson's rule were not significantly different from those calculated by the area-length method and required more complex calculations [3]. A method in which the chamber axes were measured directly showed a larger overestimation of volume and a larger standard error of estimate than was observed for the other methods

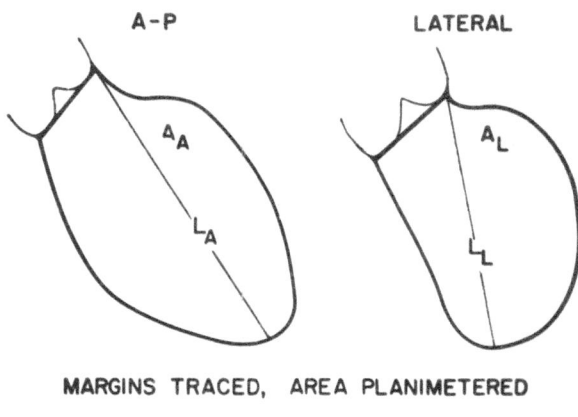

Fig. 2. Volume computed using the area-length method

A-P   LATERAL

MARGINS TRACED, AREA PLANIMETERED

$$D_A = \frac{4A_A}{\pi L_A} \; ; \; D_L = \frac{4A_L}{\pi L_L}$$

$$L_M = L_A \text{ OR } L_L \text{ WHICHEVER LARGEST}$$

$$V = \frac{\pi}{6} (D_A \cdot D_L \cdot L_M)$$

[3]. However, for all of the methods there was a systematic overestimation of volume, probably due to chordae tendinae and papillary muscles occupying a portion of the chamber and because of the assumption of an ellipsoid reference figure which is only an approximation for the shape of the LV chamber.

Studies by other investigators who have calculated LV chamber volumes from films of radiopaque casts of the left ventricle have also shown a close correlation between calculated and known volumes and standard errors of estimates similar to those described above [2, 5–7, 25, 26]. More recently, volumes have been computed of casts filmed in simulated right and left anterior oblique (RAO, LAO) projections, with calculated and known volumes having a close relationship similar to those described in the earlier studies [25, 26]. Rogers and coworkers have shown a close agreement of volumes computed from films taken in the anteroposterior (AP), lateral, and RAO-LAO projections [26].

The early studies for determining LV chamber volume in man were done with biplane filming in the AP and lateral projections. From an analysis of biplane ventriculograms of 55 subjects with heart disease of various etiologies, it was shown that the minor diameters of the LV chamber in the two projections were similar [23]. The mean direction of the long axis of the left ventricle was directed anterior 20.3° and leftward 39.8°, and usually changed only a few degrees in direction during systole, with a mean of 3.8° ± 1.6° in the AP and 6.2° ± 2.5° in the lateral direction [23]. Therefore, the projection of the LV long axis is relatively constant during systole and diastole. The spatial length of the left ventricle (calculated as midaortic valve-to-apex distance) agreed closely with the maximum projected length of the chamber and was usually represented in the

AP projection. It was then demonstrated that chamber volumes could be calculated from films taken in a single AP projection as follows:

$$V = \frac{\pi}{6} L \cdot D^2,$$

where L is the maximum chamber length in the AP projection, and D is the diameter of the LV in the AP film.

There was a close correlation between volumes and stroke volumes calculated from AP films and from AP and lateral biplane films, but with a slight overestimation of volume computed from the AP films because the minor diameter in the AP projection was usually slightly larger than in the lateral projection [23].

The direction of the long axes of the left ventricle indicated that a more consistent representation of this length might be obtained from films taken in the right anterior oblique (RAO) projection. The study by Kennedy and coworkers demonstrated that LV chamber volumes computed from films taken in the single RAO as well as the single AP projection were closely correlated with volumes computed from biplane films, but with a systematic overestimation of volume [24].

Because of the known systematic overestimation of volume using these methods, the computed volumes (V) in our laboratory are adjusted (V') by the following regression equations, which have been determined in these earlier studies [27]:

$$V'(\text{ml}) = 0.928 \, V(\text{ml}) - 3.8 \tag{1}$$
$$V'(\text{ml}) = 0.951 \, V(\text{ml}) - 3.0 \tag{2}$$
$$V'(\text{ml}) = 0.81 \ \ V(\text{ml}) + 1.9 \tag{3}$$

Equation 1 is used for volumes computed by the area-length method from biplane films taken in the AP and lateral projections. Both Wynne and coworkers and Rogers and coworkers have demonstrated that Eq. 1 can also be applied to adjust volumes computed from biplane films taken in the RAO and LAO projections [24, 25]. Equation 2 is used to adjust volumes computed from films taken in the single AP projection and Eq. 3 for volumes computed from the single RAO projection.

Normal values for LV chamber volume as determined by these methods have been established [8, 9]. The figures for normal values used in our laboratory are as follows: end-diastolic volume 70 ± 20 (one standard deviation) ml/m^2 and end-systolic volume 24 ± 10 ml/m^2. The ejection fraction, or portion of the end-diastolic volume ejected and computed as SV/EDV, is 0.67 ± 0.08. These values for normal are similar to those found by other investigators [17, 25, 28]. Normal values are summarized in Table 1. This table also includes normal values for children under the age of 2 years, for whom smaller values relative to body surface are obtained [9]. This is presumably because of a higher heart rate in infants and young children. Normal adults with slow heart rates tend to have larger volumes relative to body size [8].

Studies have been reported of interobserver and intraobserver variability in determining volumes and ejection fractions when manual analysis of films is done [26]. Rogers and coworkers have reported an interobserver mean variability for two trained observers of 10 ± 2 ml (5.3%) for end-diastolic volume,

Table 1. Normal volume values for adults and children

	End diastolic volume (ml/m^2)	End systolic volume (ml/m^2)	Ejection fraction
Adults	70 ± 20	24 ± 10	0.67 ± 0.08
Children and infants < 2 years ($n = 8$)	42 ± 10	13.4	0.68 ± 0.05
Children > 2 years ($n = 8$)	73 ± 11	27 ± 7	0.63 ± 0.05

8 ± 1 ml (8.2%) for end-systolic volume, and 0.05 ± 0.01 (10%) for ejection fraction [26]. In our laboratory we have evaluated the intraobserver variability for two separate analyses of the same films by the same technician and interobserver variability of two separate analyses of the same films by two different technicians who have had special training for this work. The intraobserver and interobserver variability for end-diastolic and end-systolic volume are shown in Fig. 3 and 4, respectively. The findings for both intra- and interobserver variability are also given for stroke volumes and ejection fractions in Table 2. These results are similar to those reported by Rogers and coworkers [26] and show good agreement on repeated analysis by the same or different trained observers.

The difference between the end-diastolic volume and end-systolic volume provides a measure of LV stroke volume. This can be estimated from computations of volume of single end-diastolic and end-systolic films, but probably more accurately from an average of volumes computed from several films taken at end-diastole and end-systole or from volume curves when rapid cine filming rates are used. Several studies have shown that stroke volumes computed from the ventriculograms agree closely with stroke volumes computed by the independent Fick or indicator-dilution methods [4, 5, 18, 21, 28–30]. There has been concern that the volume of contrast medium injected for the angiography

Table 2. Inter- and intraobserver variability

Variable	Intraobserver variability ($n = 26$)		Interobserver variability ($n = 28$)	
	r	SEE	r	SEE
EDV	0.99	4.47 ml	0.99	8.3 ml
ESV	0.97	4.16 ml	0.99	7.3 ml
LV vol	0.99	4.32 ml	0.99	8.0 ml
EF	0.89	0.03	0.93	0.04
SV	0.95	6.97 ml	0.97	7.15 ml

r, correlation coefficient; SEE, standard error of estimate; EDV, end-diastole volume; ESV, end-systole volume; EF, ejection fraction; SV, stroke volume

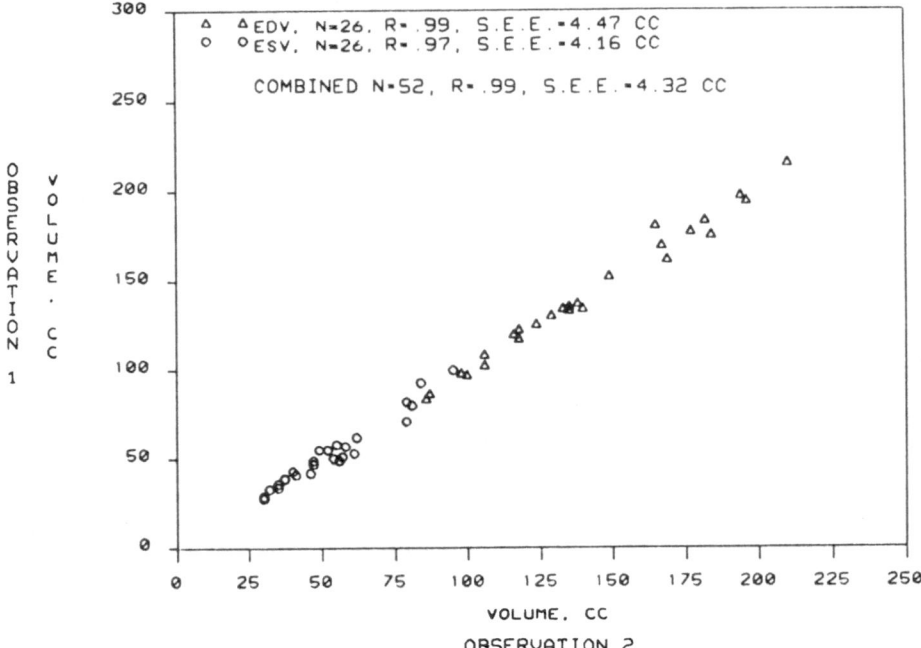

Fig. 3. Intraobserver variability for computing LV chamber volumes with the first determination on the vertical axis and second on the horizontal axis. *EDV,* end-diastolic volume; *ESV,* end-systolic volume; *SEE,* standard error of estimate

artificially elevates LV chamber volume and stroke volume. However, stroke volumes determined by angiography in man have been only slightly larger than stroke volumes determined by indicator-dilution and/or Fick methods [21, 30]. Furthermore, a study in which cardiac dimensions in man were followed by measurements from epicardial radiopaque markers prior to, during, and after injection of angiographic contrast medium failed to demonstrate a systematic change of end-diastolic volume or stroke volume until at least the seventh beat following injection [31].

The above studies have demonstrated that by applying quantitative angiographic methods, the volume of blood displaced from the left ventricle from end-diastole to end-systole, or LV stroke volume, can be determined directly. Accordingly, this has provided a method for determining the LV stroke volume (LVSV) in patients with aortic and/or mitral valve insufficiency [22]. Furthermore, measurement of the difference between the LVSV and the effective stroke volume, or forward stroke volume, as determined by the Fick and/or indicator-dilution methods, has provided a method for quantifying mitral and/or aortic valve regurgitant flow as follows [22, 27]:

LVSV = LVEDV − LVESV
Regurgitant flow/beat = LVSV − effective SV
Regurgitant flow cc/min = regurgitant flow cc/beat × heart rate

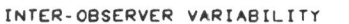

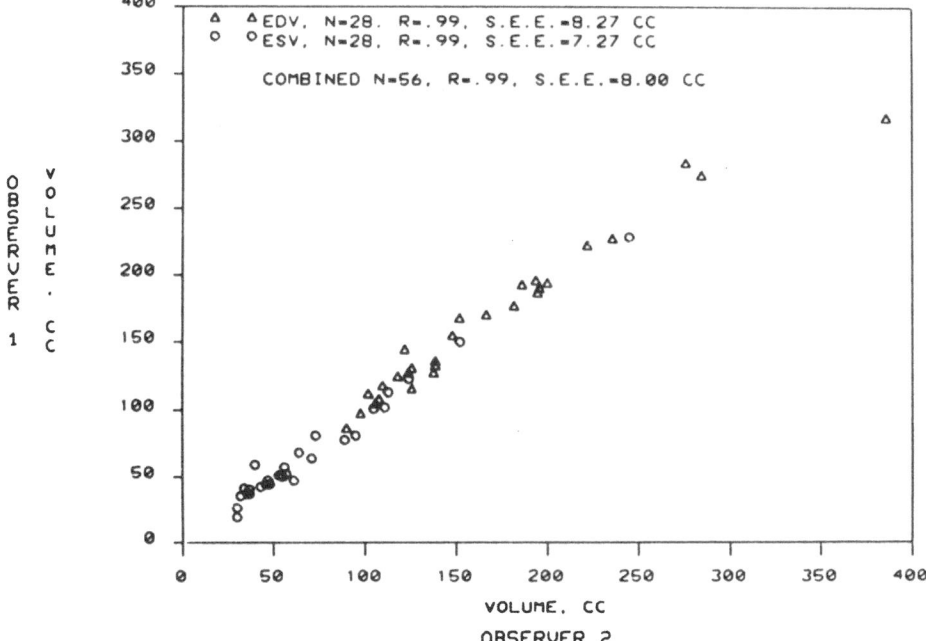

Fig. 4. Interobserver variability with observer 1 on the vertical axis and observer 2 on the horizontal axis. *EDV,* end-diastolic volume; *ESV,* end-systolic volume; *SEE,* standard error of estimate

The results of such an analysis in a group of patients with mitral valve disease are shown in Fig. 5. These techniques then provide a method for quantifying the volume load placed on the left ventricle by left heart valvular regurgitant lesions.

The relationship between the LV stroke volume and the end-diastolic volume ($\frac{SV}{EDV}$) has been termed the LV ejection fraction. As previously described, the normal left ventricle ejects approximately two-thirds of the end-diastolic volume with systole. With depressed LV myocardial function the stroke volume becomes inappropriately small relative to the end-diastolic volume, the left ventricle usually dilates and the ejection fraction is reduced [13, 19, 20]. Ejection fractions below 0.5 are usually considered abnormal. With severe cardiomyopathy or myocardial damage from ischemic heart disease, the end-diastolic volume may enlarge to 400–500 ml and the ejection fraction may be depressed to below 0.1. It has been found that even in the presence of valvular heart disease, when there is ventricular compensation through dilation and hypertrophy in response to pressure and volume overloads, and when myocardial performance is not depressed, values for ejection fraction are similar to those found in normal hearts [27]. This is illustrated in Fig. 6, which shows the

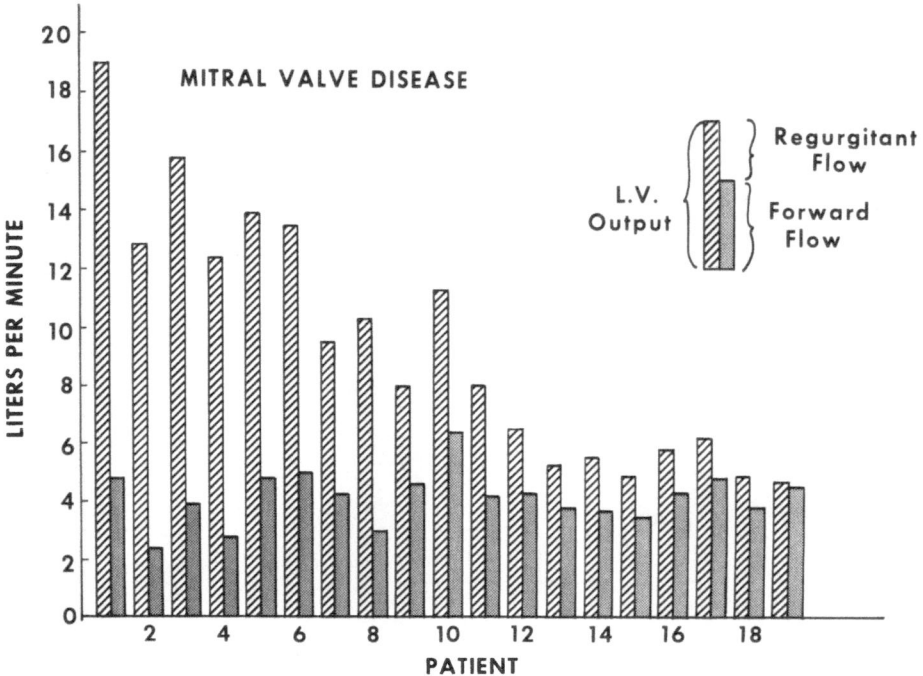

Fig. 5. Quantified LV/min output and regurgitant flow in patients with mitral valve disease

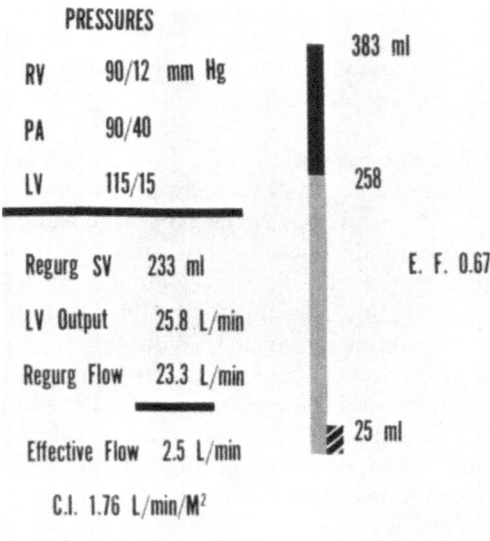

Fig. 6. Hemodynamic findings from a patient with severe mitral valve insufficiency. Volumetric data were derived from a cine ventriculogram and the effective flow and cardiac index using the Fick method

hemodynamic findings from a patient with severe mitral valve insufficiency. The left ventricle is greatly dilated, the end-diastolic pressure elevated, and the cardiac index very reduced. There is a large LV stroke volume and normal ejection fraction, consistent with relatively normal LV myocardial function. However, the ejection fraction is influenced by changes of preload and afterload [32–34]. Accordingly, in patients with aortic valve stenosis and a systolic pressure overload, a low ejection fraction may mislead to an overestimation of the extent of LV myocardial depression. In patients with mitral valve insufficiency and consequently a low LV afterload, an ejection fraction which is only slightly depressed may mislead to an underestimation of the extent of LV myocardial depression. Because of these problems, the LV end-systolic volume and pressure relationships have been suggested and used to evaluate the status of myocardial performance [34]. However, the ejection fraction is relatively simple to measure, can now be measured relatively noninvasively by several techniques, and has proved to provide a useful index of myocardial performance in patients with LV myocardial disease, such as cardiomyopathy or damage from ischemia or infarction, as well as in patients who have mechanical defects, such as valvular heart disease.

With the further development and application of digital angiography methods, we can anticipate further automation of quantitative volumetric methods and development of new techniques for quantifying measurement of ventricular volumes and wall motion of angiographic images [35, 36].

References

1. Dodge HT, Tanabaum HL (1956) Left ventricular volume in normal man and alterations with disease. Circulation 14:927
2. Chapman CB, Baker O, Reynolds J, Bonte FJ (1958) Use of biplane cinefluorography for measurement of ventricular volume. Circulation 18:1005
3. Dodge HT, Sandler H, Ballew DH, Lord JD (1960) The use of biplane angiocardiography for the measurement of left ventricular volume in man. Am Heart J 60:776
4. Gribbe P (1961) Comparison of the angiocardiographic and direct Fick methods in determining cardiac output. Cardiologia 36:20
5. Arvidsson H (1961) Angiographic determination of left ventricular volume. Acta Radiol 56:321
6. Davila JC, Sanmarco ME (1966) An analysis of the fit of mathematical models applicable to the measurement of left ventricular volume. Am J Cardiol 18:31
7. Goerke RJ, Carlsson E (1967) Calculation of right and left ventricular volumes. Method using standard computer equipment and biplane angiograms. Invest Radiol 2:360
8. Kennedy JW, Basley WA, Figley MM, Dodge HT, Blackmon JR (1966) Quantitative angiocardiography. 1. The normal left ventricle in man. Circulation 34:272
9. Graham TP Jr, Jarmakani JM, Canent RV Jr, Morrow MN (1971) Left heart volume estimations in infancy and childhood: reevaluation of methodology and normal values. Circulation 43:895
10. Arvidsson H (1958) Angiocardiographic observations in mitral valve disease, with special reference to the volume variations in the left atrium. Acta Radiol (Suppl):158
11. Bunnell IL, Ikkos D, Rudhe JG, Swan HJC (1961) Left heart volumes in coarctation of the aorta. Am Heart J 61:165
12. Dodge HT, Hay RE, Sandler H (1962) Pressure-volume characteristics of the diastolic left ventricle of man with heart disease. Am Heart J 64:503

13. Bartle SH, Sanmarco ME, Dammann JF Jr (1965) Ejected fraction: an index of myocardial function. Am J Cardiol 15:125
14. Bunnell IL, Grant C, Greene DG (1965) Left ventricular function derived from the pressure-volume diagram. Am J Med 39:881
15. Jones JW, Rackley CE, Bruce RA, Dodge HT, Cobb LA, Sandler H (1964) Left ventricular volumes in valvular heart disease. Circulation 29:887
16. Miller GAH, Brown R, Swan HJC (1964) Isolated congenital mitral insufficiency with particular reference to left heart volumes. Circulation 29:356
17. Miller GAH, Swan HJC (1964) Effect of chronic pressure and volume overload on left heart volumes in subjects with congenital heart disease. Circulation 30:205
18. Miller GAH, Kirklin JW, Rahimtoola SH, Swan HJC (1965) Volume of the left ventricle in tetralogy of Fallot. Am J Cardiol 16:488
19. Miller GAH, Rahimtoola SH, Ongley PA, Swan HJC (1965) Left ventricular volume change in endocardial fibroelastosis. Am J Cardiol 15:631
20. Dodge HT, Sandler H, Baxley WA, Hawley RR (1966) Usefulness and limitations of radiographic methods for determining left ventricular volumes. Am J Cardiol 18:10
21. Dodge HT, Ray RE, Sandler H (1962) An angiocardiographic method for determining left ventricular stroke volume in man. Circ Res 11:739
22. Sandler H, Dodge HT, Hay RE, Rackley CE (1963) Quantitation of valvular insufficiency in man by angiocardiography. Am Heart J 65:501
23. Sandler H, Dodge HT (1968) The use of single plane angiocardiograms for the calculation of left ventricular volume in man. Am Heart J 75:325
24. Kennedy JW, Trenholme SE, Kasser IS (1970) Left ventricular volume and mass from single-plane cineangiocardiograms: a comparison of anteroposterior and right anterior oblique methods. Am Heart J 80:343
25. Wynne J, Green LH, Mann T, Levin D, Grossman W (1978) Estimation of left ventricular volumes in man from biplane cineangiograms filmed in oblique projections. Am J Cardiol 41:726
26. Rogers WJ, Smith LR, Hood WP Jr, Mantle JA, Rackley CE, Russell RO Jr (1979) Effect of filming projection and interobserver variability on angiographic biplane left ventricular volume determination. Circulation 59:96
27. Dodge HT, Kennedy JW, Petersen JL (1973) Quantitative angiocardiographic methods in the evaluation of valvular heart disease. Prog Cardiovasc Dis 16:1
28. Bartle SH, Sanmarco ME (1966) Comparison of angiographic and thermal washout techniques for left ventricular volume measurement. Am J Cardiol 18:235
29. Hugenholtz PG, Wagner HR, Sandler H (1968) In vivo determination of left ventricular volume: comparison of the fiber-optic-indicator dilution and angiocardiographic methods. Circulation 37:489
30. Hunt D, Baxley WA, Kennedy JW, Judge TP, Williams JE, Dodge HT (1973) Quantitative evaluation of cineaortography in the assessment of aortic regurgitation. Am J Cardiol 31:696
31. Vine DL, Hegg TD, Dodge HT, Stewart DK, Frimer M (1977) Immediate effect of contrast medium injection on left ventricular volumes and ejection fraction: a study using metallic epicardial markers. Circulation 56:379
32. Wikken DEL, Chalier AA, Hoffman JEI et al. (1964) Effects of alterations in aortic impedence on the performance of the left ventricle. Circ Res 14:283
33. Weber KT, Janicki JS, Reeves RC, Hefner LL (1976) Factors influencing left ventricular shortening in isolated canine heart. Am J Physiol 230:419
34. Grossman W, Braunwald E, Mann T, McLaurin LP, Green LH (1977) Contractile state of the left ventricle in man as evaluated from end-systolic pressure-volume relations. Circulation 56:845
35. Ritman EL, Sturm RE, Wood EH (1973) Biplane roentgen videometric system for dynamic (601 sec) studies of the shape and size of circulatory structures, particularly the left ventricle. Am J Cardiol 32:180
36. Heintzen PH, Malerszyk V, Pilarczyk J, Scheel KW (1971) On-line processing of the video image for left ventricular volume determination. Comput Biomed Res 4:474

Estimation of Left Ventricular Muscle Mass

H. JUST

Cardiology Department, Medizinische Universitätsklinik, Freiburg im Breisgau, FRG

Angiographic estimation of ventricular mass has been applied to the left ventricle. The right ventricular myocardium has not been subject to such studies due to the complex structure of the right ventricle and its relatively thin, coarsely trabeculated wall. Estimation of volume of the right ventricle has indeed been attempted, but no meaningful estimates of right ventricular muscle mass obtained through angiocardiography have been published. The following considerations, therefore, are concerned with means of improvement of angiocardiographic determination of left ventricular muscle mass.

The usefulness of estimation of left ventricular myocardial mass (2,3) is seen in the recognition and quantitation of left ventricular hypertrophy, as well as in establishing the "adequacy" of left ventricular hypertrophy (mass-to-volume ratio). Furthermore, ventricular function analysis (8) requires calculation of left ventricular wall stress and tension, requiring measurement of wall thickness.

At present wall thickness is measured in the right anterior oblique (RAO) projection in the central third of the anterior wall contour. Calculation of total left ventricular mass then utilizes the volume method, assuming that the left ventricle is an ellipsoid of rotation of symmetrical configuration [1, 4, 9]. Volume measurement of an ellipsoid of rotation with the axis A, B, and C is done according to the following formula:

$$V = \frac{\pi}{6} \cdot A \cdot B \cdot C$$

where A indicates the long axis and B and C the transverse axes, which in the case of an ellipsoid of symmetrical configuration are equal. If the long axis is called L and the short axis D, then

$$V = \frac{\pi}{6} \cdot L \cdot D^2$$

The area-length method utilizes the calculation of the volume of an ellipsoid of rotation as well. The long axis in the RAO projection is rather easily measured. Short axis measurement, however, frequently meets with difficulties, mainly in situations where an asymmetrical shape of the left ventricle is encountered. By measuring the area through planimetry, the short axis can be calculated and inaccuracies due to irregular shape of the ventricle thereby reduced. In this case, where the long axis and the cross-sectional area of the ventricular cavity are being measured, the formula for calculation of the short axis is as follows:

$$D = \frac{4}{\pi} \cdot \frac{F}{L}$$

Here D indicates the short axis, F the left ventricular cross-sectional area, and L the long axis.

For calculation of the volume of the ellipsoid of rotation, then, the following formula applies:

$$V = \frac{8}{3 \cdot \pi} \cdot \frac{F^2}{L}$$

If the area of the left ventricle and the short axis is measured, then the formula is written:

$$V = \frac{2}{3} \cdot F \cdot D$$

For determination of left ventricular myocardial mass by application of the area-length method, the long axis is increased by addition of the wall thickness. The area is determined by measuring the complete outer contour, including wall thickness, at a representative point. Alternatively, in the more commonly applied version, the short axis is augmented by addition of one wall thickness to the radius. Calculation of volume of an inner ellipsoid of rotation is then performed, utilizing area and long axis of the opacified left ventricular chamber, and

$$V_M = (V_{\text{tot}} - V) \cdot 1.05$$

V_M is the left ventricular myocardial mass, V_{tot} the volume of the ellipsoid of rotation utilizing the outer contour, and V_I the "inner" volume of the left ventricle in end-diastole; 1.05 is the specific gravity of myocardial tissue. Measurements of left ventricular mass are usually performed in end-diastole. Here the endocardial contour is more easily defined due to flattening of the trabecular structure. The complete formula for calculation of left ventricle mass is given in Fig. 1.

$$LVM = (V_{c+w} - V_c) \times 1.050$$

$$V_{c(ED)} = 4/3\pi \times d_1/2 \times d_2/2 \times L/2$$

$$V_{c+w} = 4/3\pi \times (d_1/2 + w) \times (d_2/2 + w) \times (L/2 + w)$$

(adapted from Rackley et al. 1964)

Fig. 1. Modified formula for the calculation of myocardial mass from semi-angiocardiograms. *LVM*, left ventricular mass; Vc, Vc *(ED)*, left ventricular cavity volume at end-diastole; Vc + w, volume of the left ventricle including the wall (outer contour); 1.050, specific gravity of myocardial tissue; d_1 and d_2, short axis of the ellipsoid of rotation; L, long axis of the left ventricle; w, wall thickness. The formula is applicable to both RAO and LAO projections, provided the long axis is optimally defined and the outer contour clearly delineated (for sites of measurement, see text)

The area-length method as described above, although widely employed, is open to several sources of error, which attain particular significance if the left ventricular contour is irregular. In these cases the application of Simpson's rule to the estimation of left ventricular mass would appear to be more suitable. Here volume is calculated as the integral of all cylindrical slices that can be placed through the left ventricle along its long axis. This method lends itself to application with television systems. It shows definite advantages over the area-length method, especially in irregular ventricular contours. It does, however, require computer assistance. This method again utilizes the difference between the outer and the inner volume of the left ventricle, thereby requiring measurement of wall thickness.

Both the area-length method and Simpson's rule can be applied to the biplane technique. Both rely on accurate measurement of wall thickness if left ventricular myocardial mass is to be determined. Accuracy is thereby significantly improved. Table 1 gives an evaluation of the faithfulness of different oblique and angulated views in representing long axis, short axis, myocardial wall thickness, and left ventricular end-diastolic volume in different biplane, bihemiaxial projections. As can be seen, angulated views prolong long axis representation and reduce left ventricular end-diastolic volume. Myocardial wall thickness measurement, however, does not seem to be significantly influenced by angulation of view.

The measurements as obtained from full size cut film images, from projected cine-angiocardiograms, or from the television system require correction through an calibration factor, compensating for magnification due to the divergent X-ray beam, emanating from an X-ray source within finite distance. Only recently have we developed an integrated mathematical model and angiographic system which can be applied to biplane, bihemiaxial views, obviating the need for calibration (10).

Sources of Error

There are three major sources of error:
1. It is well known that application of the area-length method, and also of Simpson's rule with currently employed calibration techniques in RAO single plane, anteroposterior and lateral biplane techniques, overestimates the natural volume (6, 7). Therefore a correction factor needs to be introduced.
2. Failure to obtain the true long axis, especially in systems without angulation, i.e., hemiaxial views, introduces significant error.
3. Measurement of wall thickness is difficult, and from routine films it is often impossible. The reason for this is inadequate delineation of the outer myocardial contour due to exaggerated contrast (lung vs myocardium) (Fig. 2). Furthermore, the anterior midwall position for measurement of a "representative" myocardial wall thickness, as usually accepted, cannot necessarily be considered truly representative (see below).

Means of Improvement

There are five means of improving estimation of left ventricular muscle mass:
1. Angiographic delineation of ventricular contours for estimation of muscle mass should routinely be done in biplane fashion. With optimal image quality both the area-length method and Simpson's rule can be applied.
2. The projections chosen for biplane filming should be selected in such a way as to represent the longest axis in both RAO and in LAO projection, and to furnish sufficient points for measurement of left ventricular myocardial wall thickness.
3. Calibration techniques should be improved as potential sources of error.
4. Great care has to be taken with the improvement of quality of image as regards delineation of the inner and the outer myocardial contours through contour shading and film processing to a low gamma (approximately 1.4).
5. In ventricles of irregular shape, multiple measurements of wall thickness should be taken and/or Simpson's rule should be applied from the beginning.

Suggestions for Improvement of Techniques of Estimation of Myocardial Mass

The formula for calculation of ventricular mass based on the volume model is given in Fig. 1. The following are four suggestions for improvement of techniques of estimation of myocardial mass:
1. For optimal delineation of endocardial and epicardial ventricular contours and faithful reconstruction of the three-dimensional configuration of the left ventricle, biplane, bihemiaxial projections are to be recommended. Optimal angles for filming of the left ventricle as normally situated are 30° RAO plus 10° caudal angulation, and 60° LAO with 20°–30° cranial angulation. These angulated views provide enhancement of accuracy of volume estimation by 10%–20% (Table 1).

Table 1. Estimation of left ventricular mass: Comparison of conventional and bihemiaxial biplane technique ($n = 31$)

Parameter	Comparison	Mean 1	Mean 2	Difference	P Value	$S_{\bar{x}}1$	$S_{\bar{x}}2$
Long axis	RAO/LAO$_C$	10.1	7.7	−23.2%	0.0001	1.2	0.8
Long axis	LAO$_C$/LAO$_a$	7.7	8.3	+ 9.3%	0.0001	0.8	0.9
Long axis	RAO$_C$/RAO$_a$	10.1	10.0	− 0.4%	0.5737	1.2	1.2
Long axis	RAO$_a$/LAO$_a$	10.0	8.3	−16.0%	0.0001	1.2	0.9
Short axis	RAO/LAO$_C$	6.5	6.27	− 2.8%	0.0534	0.9	0.7
Short axis	RAO$_a$/LAO$_a$	6.56	6.0	− 7.6%	0.0025	0.9	0.9
Myoc. wall	RAO$_C$/RAO$_a$	0.9	0.9	0	0.3304	0.2	0.2
Myoc. wall	M$_C$/M$_a$	0.9	0.9	0	0.1109	0.1	0.2
LVEDV	Conv./ang.	219.0	211.0	− 2.9%	0.0284	77.0	71.0
LVM	Conv./ang.	211.0	220.0	+ 4.9%	0.2154	60.0	69.0

C, conventional; a, angulated views

2. Delineation of the outer contour of the left ventricle can be improved through use contour-adapted diaphragms, which can be rotated within the X-ray image so as to attenuate the contrast between myocardial and pulmonary tissue density (Fig. 2). At the same time, angiocardiographic films should be processed to a low gamma of around 1.42, for better description of the outer contour, even though the inner, trabeculated ventricular contour will lose in accuracy of contour definition.

3. Error introduced through calibration can be avoided by using computer-based, calibration-free systems, as developed by Wollschläger et al. (1984) (10). These procedures are ideally suited for application with biplane systems. They do utilize three-fold rectangular configuration for optimal structural quantitation. Here, both tube-image intensifier systems are oriented at approximately 90° towards the long axis of the ventricle *and* maintain a spatial angle of 90° between themselves.

4. Measurement of wall thickness must be taken with great care. The measurement should be taken vertically to the tangent applied to the outer contour of the ventricle at the point of measurement (Fig. 2). Selection of the point of measurement is difficult and has not been validated so far.

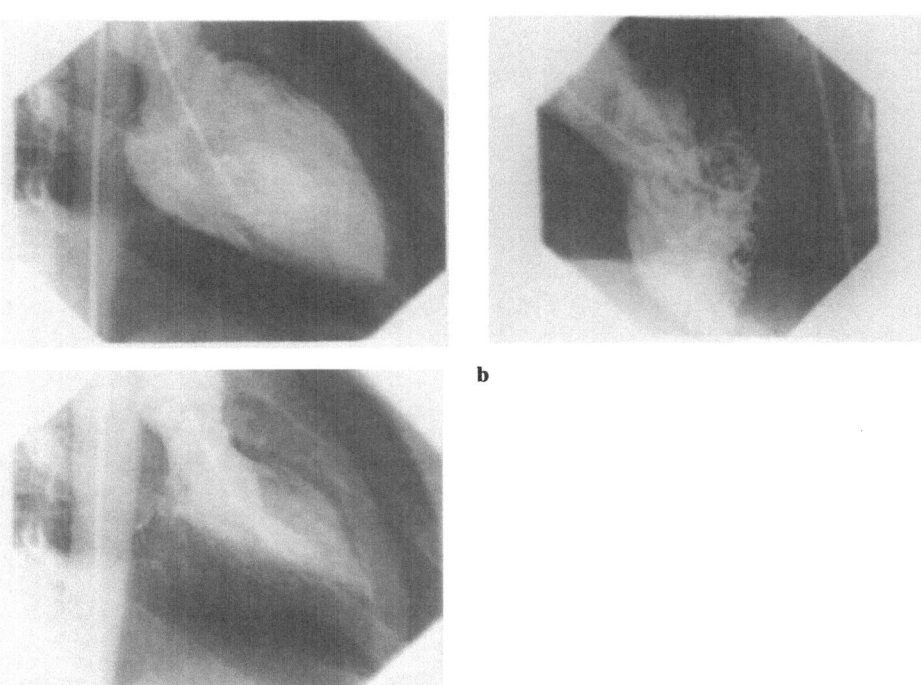

b

a

Fig. 2a, b. Cine – roentgenogram of the left ventricle at **a** 30° RAO projection with 10° caudal angulation, and **b** 60° LAO with 20° cranial angulation. The contour diaphragm, improving recognition of the outer ventricular wall, is easily visible in both projections

Evaluation of Site of Measurement for Left Ventricular Wall Thickness

In order to improve the accuracy of wall thickness measurement and thus of determination of left ventricular myocardial muscle mass, we evaluated nine different points of measurement of the left ventricular wall in the study of biplane, bihemiaxial ventriculograms.

The angiographic system used was a Siemens Elema Angioscop C with two identical systems positioned in triple orthogonal view, with the RAO projection at 30° with 10° caudal angulation, and the LAO system at 55° plus 20°–28° cranial angulation. Thirty-four patients with widely varying ventricular size and muscle mass were studied. Patients with irregular myocardial contour and regional myocardial disease (coronary artery disease) were excluded.

Films were taken in end-diastole during relaxed respiratory arrest with injection of 15–25 ml contrast fluid (Solutrast) at an injection rate of 8–12 ml/s. Filming was done with 50 frames/s. The 35-mm films were processed to a gamma of 1.42. Contour diaphragms were routinely used in both projections (Fig. 2).

The points of measurement of wall thickness were selected as shown in Fig. 3. At each point of measurement the tangent was placed on the outer contour of the ventricle and wall thickness measured vertical to this tangent (Fig. 4).

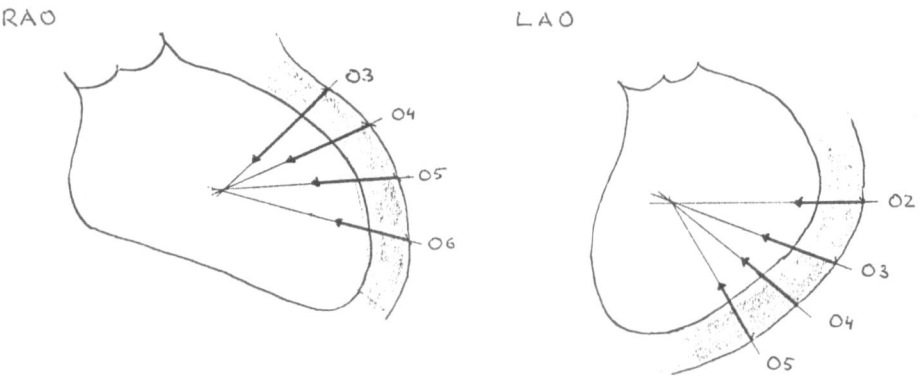

Fig. 3. Sites of measurement utilized for determination of ventricular wall thickness in RAO (*above*) and LAO projection (*below*). For values for oblique and angulated views, see text

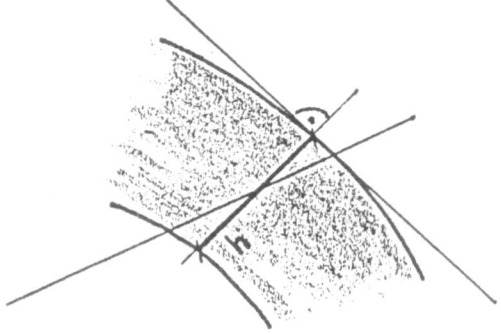

Fig. 4. Method of measurement of wall thickness as used in this study. At the point of exit of the radius from the myocardial shell at the epicardium a tangent is applied. A vertical line arising from this tangent running through the myocardial wall meets the radius in the midwall area; *h* is the measured value of wall thickness

The measurements were taken by two independent observers. Each obtained three measurements and gave the mean value for further calculations. The sum of the mean values at each site of measurement (five in RAO and four in LAO) were used to calculate a mean or 100% value. The measurements at each individual site were then related to this 100% value. The resulting figures 5 and 6 are derived from the numerical values given in Table 2 (RAO projection) and Table 3 (LAO projection). With these calculations deviations from the mean

Table 2. Left ventricular end-diastolic wall thickness (RAO), in 5 different points of measurement in mm

Patient	Sites				
	02	03	04	05	06
1	115.0	105.0	92.0	95.0	92.0
2	115.0	118.0	118.0	97.0	50.0
3	106.0	97.0	89.0	92.0	115.0
4	91.0	78.0	91.0	115.0	124.0
5	104.0	87.0	94.0	106.0	108.0
6	113.0	109.0	113.0	95.0	69.0
7	142.0	103.0	82.0	77.0	95.0
8	122.0	92.0	99.0	94.0	92.0
9	104.0	96.0	93.0	102.0	104.0
10	131.0	113.0	100.0	83.0	72.0
11	100.0	94.0	107.0		
12	149.0	74.0	87.0	89.0	
13		130.0	107.0	87.0	75.0
14	144.0	107.0	92.0	78.0	78.0
15	125.0	100.0	91.0	88.0	95.0
16	133.0	103.0	88.0	88.0	88.0
17	155.0	88.0	79.0	86.0	91.0
18					
19	118.0	97.0	92.0	92.0	
20	111.0	104.0	93.0	87.0	104.0
21	110.0	99.0	96.0	99.0	94.0
22	128.0	104.0	83.0	85.0	
23	116.0	102.0	96.0	90.0	96.0
24	95.0	88.0	97.0	108.0	112.0
25	132.0	106.0	88.0	80.0	94.0
26	89.0	102.0	109.0		
27	102.0	96.0	93.0	102.0	105.0
28		104.0	104.0	96.0	96.0
29	103.0	96.0	101.0		
30	107.0	95.0	95.0	114.0	88.0
31	129.0	93.0	83.0	93.0	
32	95.0	89.0	86.0	114.0	114.0
33	121.0	106.0	98.0	78.0	96.0
34	125.0	96.0	96.0	91.0	91.0
Mean	117.1	99.1	94.9	93.4	93.8
SD	17.1	10.7	8.9	10.5	15.9
n	31.0	33.0	33.0	30.0	26.0
Median	115.0	99.0	93.0	92.0	94.5

value can be taken as an indicator of the accuracy or inaccuracy of measurement at a given site.

Table 2 gives the measurements of wall thickness deviation from the mean (mean of all sites of measurement in the RAO projection) in 34 patients with different kinds of heart disease (cardiomyopathy, valvular heart disease, normals) with a wide range of wall thicknesses. Patients with regional myocardial disease (asymmetrical hypertrophy, coronary disease) were excluded. In several instances meaningful measurements were not possible. In Table 3, end-diastolic

Table 3. Left ventricular end-diastolic wall thickness (LAO), in 4 different points of measurement in mm

Patient	Sites			
	02	03	04	05
1	99.0	92.0	102.0	107.0
2	100.0	100.0	97.0	102.0
3	117.0	103.0	85.0	94.0
4	101.0	105.0	107.0	87.0
5	126.0	96.0	92.0	85.0
6	118.0	98.0	91.0	93.0
7				
8				
9	93.0	98.0	103.0	106.0
10	107.0	94.0	100.0	100.0
11		101.0	101.0	98.0
12	89.0	118.0	108.0	86.0
13	107.0	104.0	96.0	93.0
14	122.0	94.0	85.0	
15	102.0	107.0	102.0	90.0
16				
17		104.0	102.0	93.0
18				
19				
20	110.0	102.0	97.0	91.0
21	117.0	98.0	88.0	98.0
22	105.0	99.0	101.0	95.0
23				
24				
25				
26	80.0	107.0	101.0	113.0
27	98.0	118.0	100.0	84.0
28	154.0	106.0	63.0	77.0
29				
30	105.0	97.0	97.0	100.0
31	89.0	106.0	100.0	106.0
32				
33				
34				
Mean	106.9	102.1	96.3	95.1
SD	16.2	6.8	9.7	8.9
n	20.0	22.0	22.0	21.0
Median	105.0	101.5	100.0	94.0

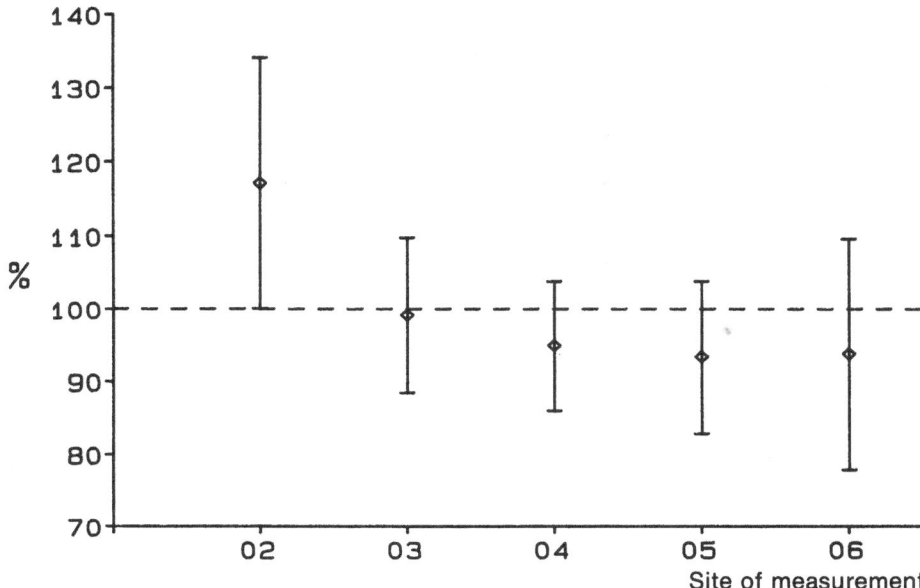

Fig. 5. Wall thickness measurement at five different sites in RAO projection (Fig. 3) together with standard deviations. On the *abscissa* the wall thickness measurement is given in percentage of the mean value of all measurements. On the *ordinate* the site of measurement is indicated. The *dashed line* shows the 100% value. As can be seen, positions 03, 04, and possibly 05 are well suited for wall thickness measurement, although 03 has to be preferred. Positions 02 and 06 (apical area) can not be considered valid

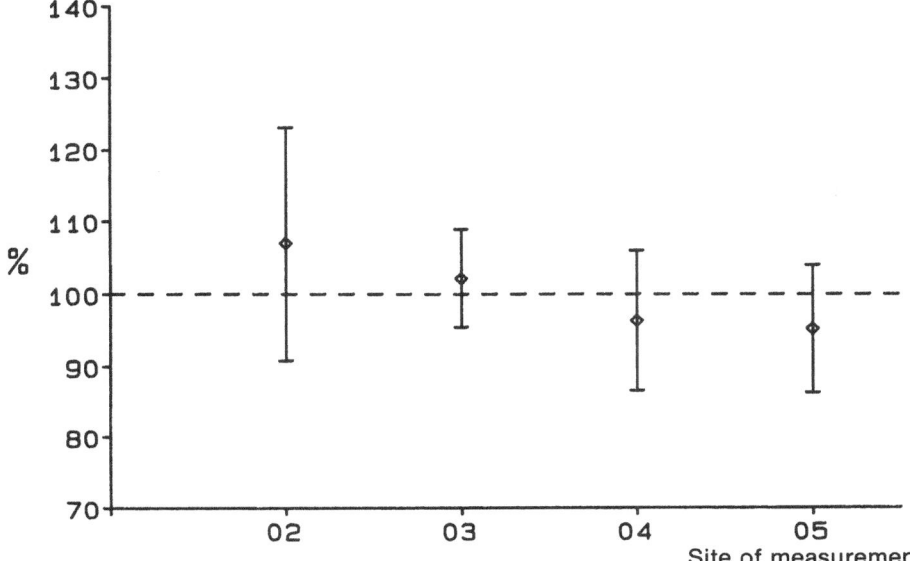

Fig. 6. Graphic representation of wall thickness measurement in LAO projection at four different sites. The *dashed line* represents the 100% value, that is, the mean of all measurements taken in this projection. The *abscissa* gives the percentage values, the *ordinate* the four sites of measurement. As can be seen, position 03 is the best for wall thickness measurement in LAO projection. Position 02 is probably altered through epicardial fat, positions 04 and 05 through the difficulty of excluding posterior papillary muscle tissue

wall thickness in LAO projection is given as a percentage of the mean value (sum of all wall thickness measurements in LAO projection), in the four different sites measured; the representation is the same as in Table 2. Note the higher incidence of inability to measure wall thickness.

As can be seen from the Tables 2 and 3 and Fig. 5 and 6, the least deviation from the mean, together with the smallest standard deviation, is obtained at measurement sites 03 and 04 – possibly also in 05 in RAO, and in 03 and maybe 04 in the LAO projection. 02 in RAO deviates, probably due to inclusion of epicardial fat of unpredictable size, which also may be the reason for the large standard deviation in the more apically oriented 06 position in the RAO and the 02 site in the LAO projection.

The tables also show that meaningful measurements were not always possible. Especially in the LAO projection, contour definition maybe hampered by overprojection of spine or liver, especially in the more strongly angulated views.

It can be said, however, that the entire midwall of the left ventricle in RAO projection in positions 03 to 05, as well as position 03 and maybe 04 in the LAO projection may be considered accurate and reliable.

If the above-mentioned suggestions are observed, then biplane, bihemiaxial quantitative angiocardiography will remain the "gold standard" for estimation of left ventricular volume and mass, providing optimal conditions for calculation of wall stress parameters.

For the future, it can be predicted that biplane angiocardiographic systems will become predominant. They will use semi- or fully automatic positioning into optimal oblique and/or angulated views for delineation of the inner and the outer shell of the left ventricle. In this situation, even intravenous contrast application or the use of other imaging procedures, such as computer tomography or magnetic resonance imaging, will be applicable to the aforementioned modalities of calculation of left ventricular mass.

With the development of automated contour detection facilities, even the determination of left ventricular muscle mass may become a figure available for everyday analysis of left ventricular function in the diagnosis and treatment of heart disease.

References

Dodge HT, Sandler H, Ballew DW, Lord JD Jr (1960) The use of biplane angiocardiography for the measurement of left ventricular volume in mass. Am Heart J 60:762

Dodge HT, Baxley WA (1963) Left ventricular volume and mass and their significance in heart disease. Am Heart J 23:528

Efer LM, Greenberg HM, Cooke JJ, Galin R (1969) Dynamic changes in left ventricular free wall thickness in the human heart. Circulation 39:455

Greene D, Carlisle R, Grant C, Bunnell L (1967) Estimation of left ventricular volume by one-plane cineangiocardiography Circulation 34:61

Kennedy JW, Baxley WA, Figley MM, Dodge HT, Blackmon JR (1966) Quantitative angiocardiography. I. The normal left ventricle in man Circulation 34:272

Kennedy JW, Reichenbach DD, Baxley WA, Dodge HT (1967) Left ventricular mass. A comparison of angiocardiographic measurements with autopsy weights. Am J Cardiol 19:221

Kennedy JW, Trenkline SE, Kasser IS (1970) Left ventricular volume and mass from single-plane cineangiocardiogram. A comparison of anteroposterior and right anterior oblique methods. Am Heart J 80:343

Kennedy JW, Twiss RD, Blackmon JR, Dodge HT (1968) Quantitative angiocardiography. III. Relationships of left ventricular pressure, volume and mass in aortic valve disease. Circulation 38:838

Rackley CE, Dodge HT, Coble YD, Hay RE (1964) A method for determining left ventricular mass in man. Circulation 24:666

Wollschläger H, Lee P, Bonzel T, Zeiher A, Just H (1984) Quantitative Koronarangiographie: Neue Vermessungsmethode durch Bestimmung des Vergrößerungsfaktors bei Anwendung der Geometrie biplaner isozentrischer Röntgensysteme. Biomed Tech 29 [Suppl 53]: pp 53–54

Roentgen-Anatomic Assessment of Left and Right Ventricular Spatial Orientation in Congenital Heart Disease*

P. E. Lange, D. G. W. Onnasch, G. H. Schaupp, C. Zill, and P. H. Heintzen

Department of Pediatric Cardiology and Bioengineering, Schwanenweg 20, D-2300 Kiel, FRG

Introduction

With increasing use of axial angiocardiography [1, 2], especially in patients with congenital heart disease, knowledge of left and right ventricular spatial orientation is of practical value. However, no systematic study exists of ventricular position during normal growth and in patients with typical congenital heart diseases. We therefore developed a computerized method to assess three-dimensional ventricular orientation on the basis of anatomical landmarks, which can be defined reproducibly on biplane projections. This report presents the results of subjects with normal ventricles and those of patients with congenital heart disease.

Methods

The patients were studied in a fasting state in supine position. Infants up to 12 months of age received Luminal (phenobarbital) (10 mg/kg body wt.), and older children Dolantin (pethidine) (1–1.5 mg/kg body wt.), Luminal (10 mg/kg body wt., maximum 200 mg), and Atropin (0.01–0.015 mg/kg body wt.) premedication, given 1 h before the diagnostic cardiac catheterization.

Before the first angiocardiogram was taken, shunts were quantified by oxymetry. Left and right ventricular pressures were recorded using a side hole catheter (NIH no. 5F–7F), connected to a Statham P23db transducer (Statham Instruments, Oxnard, California, USA). Zero pressures were referenced to the level of the venae cavae in the lateral projection. The basis for the determination of volume data and ventricular spatial orientation were biplane videoangiographic projections of the ventricles (posterior-anterior and lateral), displayed on a TV monitor side by side and recorded with 50 frames after selective injection of 76% Urografin (Schering AG, Berlin) into the left ventricle (1 ml/kg body wt.) or right ventricle (1.5 ml/kg body wt.). For calibration purposes a steel sphere of 60 or 30 mm (zoom) diameter was filmed at the location the

* Supported by the Deutsche Forschungsgemeinschaft and the Bundesministerium für Forschung und Technologie

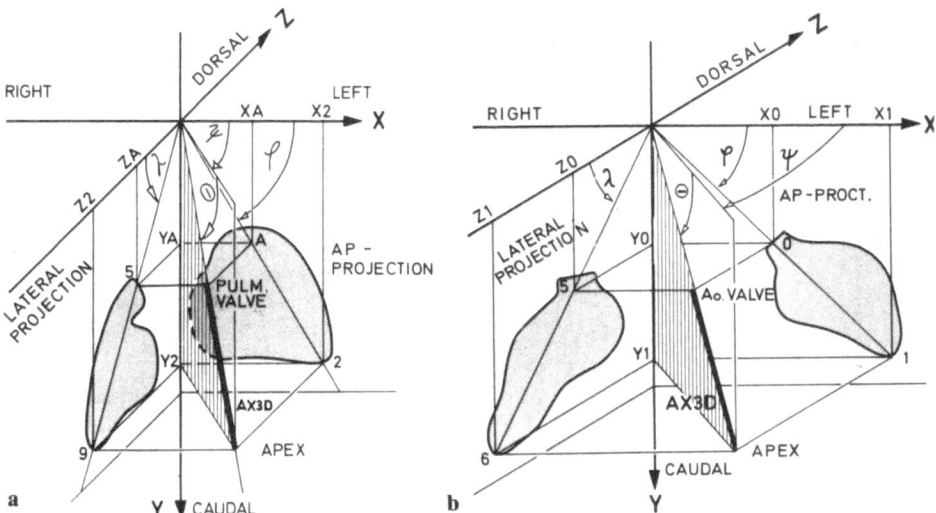

Fig. 1a,b. Definition *a* of the right and *b* of the left ventricular axis (*AX3D*). It was determined on the basis of the anatomical landmarks apex (*1* and *6* for the left, *2* and *9* for the right ventricle) and semilunar valve (*0* and *5* for the aortic, *5* and *A* for the pulmonic valve). The axis is characterized by the angles φ and λ in the anteroposterior and the lateral projection, and by the spatial angles θ (latitude) and ψ (longitude)

respective ventricle occupied. The borders of the biplane projections (steel sphere and ventricles in sinus beats) were traced manually using a resistance foil and stored in a digital computer [3]. The largest ventricular projection was assumed to represent end-diastole and the smallest end-systole. Since the vertical extent of both projections should be the same, the input program controlled it and permitted an interactive adjustment of the height on the basis of the computer-stored outlines of the calibration sphere. In addition to biplane outlines, up to ten anatomically defined landmarks were marked, whereby the ventricular spatial axes between the center of the semilunar valve ring and apex (Fig. 1) as well as the thickness of the left ventricular wall were determined [4].

Ventricular volumes at end-diastole and end-systole were calculated with the multiple slices method for the right ventricle and the area-length method for the left ventricle. The volumes were corrected with factors appropriate for position and cardiac phase [5, 6].

The spatial ventricular axis between the aortic or pulmonary valve ring, respectively, and the apex was defined and related to the body axes of the patient in supine position within the coordinate system of the Frank ECG. Its orientation was described by the angles φ and λ in the anterior-posterior and lateral projection, respectively, as well as by the angles θ (latitude) and ψ (longitude) (Fig. 1).

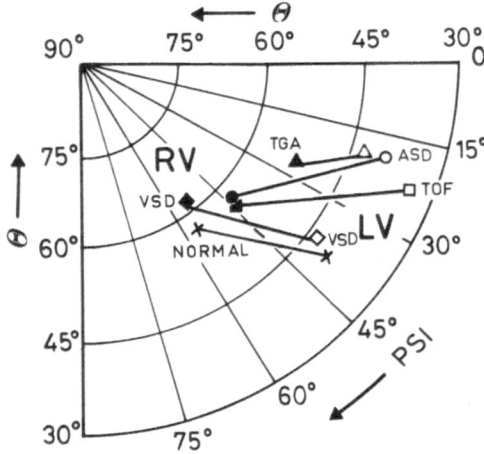

Fig. 2. Spatial orientation of right (*RV, closed symbols*) and left (*LV, open symbols*) ventricular axis defined by the spatial angles θ (latitude) and ψ (longitude) (see also Fig. 1). Mean values for normal, ventricular septal defect (*VSD*), tetralogy of Fallot (*TOF*), atrial septal defect (*ASD*), and transposition of the great arteries with intact septum (*TGA*)

Results

Mean values and standard deviations of projection (φ and λ) and spatial angles (θ and ψ) are summerized in Fig. 2 and Tables 1 and 2.

There was a growth related change of direction of the long axis of normal ventricles, which was most distinct for the angle θ (Fig. 3). For the left ventricle it changed from 30° in infants to 50° in adolescents. For the right ventricle the increase of this angle was similar during growth. There was no systematic growth-dependent change of the angle ψ being 39.2° ± 9.8° for the left ventricle and 56.2° ± 9.5° for the right ventricle in a normal heart.

However, the angle ψ of a normal left ventricle may be altered by a volume-overloaded right ventricle, as in atrial septal defect. For an average shunt of 86% ± 33% of systemic flow, the posterior shift was 20° (Fig. 4, Table 2). There

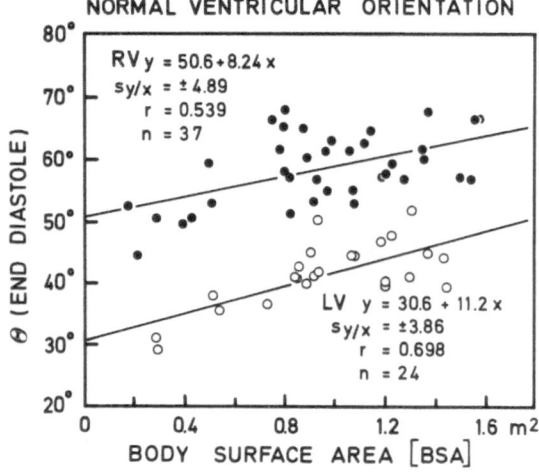

Fig. 3. Relationship between the end-diastolic spatial angle θ of normal right (*RV, closed circles*) and left (*LV, open circles*) ventricles and the body surface area. There is a significant increase of θ, indicating a decrease of the ventricular apices in relation to the pulmonic and aortic valves respectively

Table 1. Right ventricular spatial orientation

		φ	λ	ψ	θ	α
Normal (*n* = 37)						
ED	Mean	71.1	63.3	56.2	58.4	16.7
	SD	6.3	5.3	9.5	5.7	5.5
ED–ES	Mean	−2.4	−2.9	−0.1	−3.2	−1.8
	SD	3.4	2.3	4.9	2.8	4.1
Pulmonary stenosis (*n* = 19)						
ED	Mean	72.1	66.0	53.3	60.5	16.6
	SD	4.8	6.4	12.3	4.9	6.0
	Sign.	NS	NS	NS	NS	NS
ED–ES	Mean	−2.1	−2.1	−0.3	−2.4	−1.1
	SD	4.2	2.7	9.6	2.3	3.9
	Sign.	NS	NS	NS	NS	NS
Atrial septal defect (*n* = 19)						
ED	Mean	65.8	67.2	43.8	57.7	12.8
	SD	6.3	5.1	12.3	4.1	4.3
	Sign.	<0.01	<0.05	<0.01	NS	<0.01
ED–ES	Mean	−0.1	−2.6	3.8	−1.5	1.6
	SD	3.9	4.1	5.0	4.4	3.8
	Sign.	<0.05	NS	NS	NS	<0.01
Ventricular septal defect (*n* = 15)						
ED	Mean	75.2	67.6	56.8	63.5	15.7
	SD	4.1	5.6	12.0	4.4	4.4
	Sign.	<0.01	<0.05	NS	<0.01	NS
ED–ES	Mean	−1.6	−3.2	1.4	−2.9	−2.7
	SD	3.3	2.2	8.2	2.0	3.3
	Sign.	NS	NS	NS	NS	NS
Tetralogy of Fallot (*n* = 19)						
ED	Mean	65.5	64.9	45.0	56.5	8.1
	SD	7.2	8.8	11.8	8.0	5.5
	Sign.	<0.01	NS	<0.01	NS	<0.01
ED–ES	Mean	2.2	−2.8	6.5	0.1	0.0
	SD	7.4	7.3	12.0	7.2	4.8
	Sign.	<0.05	NS	<0.01	NS	NS
Transposition of the great arteries (*n* = 41)						
ED	Mean	58.6	69.6	30.8	53.8	9.8
	SD	8.1	10.4	13.8	8.5	7.6
	Sign.	<0.01	<0.01	<0.01	<0.01	<0.01
ED–ES	Mean	1.3	−5.6	8.0	−0.3	0.1
	SD	5.4	4.0	7.6	5.1	4.1
	Sign.	<0.01	<0.01	<0.01	<0.01	NS

SD, standard deviation; sign., statistically significant at given *P* level compared with normal; NS, not significant; ED, end-diastolic spatial orientation; ED–ES, end-diastolic–end-systolic change of spatial orientation; for definition of projection angles φ, λ, and α, and spatial angles ψ and θ see Fig. 1

Table 2. Left ventricular spatial orientation

		φ	λ	ψ	θ
Normal (n = 37)					
ED	Mean	49.2	55.1	39.2	41.5
	SD	7.0	7.3	9.8	5.3
ED–ES	Mean	3.7	2.4	1.2	3.1
	SD	3.7	3.3	4.3	3.0
Aortic stenosis (n = 16)					
ED	Mean	46.8	50.1	41.7	38.3
	SD	9.1	5.6	7.2	6.6
	Sign.	NS	<0.05	NS	NS
ED–ES	Mean	5.5	1.8	3.9	3.7
	SD	4.4	5.1	5.2	3.1
	Sign.	NS	NS	NS	NS

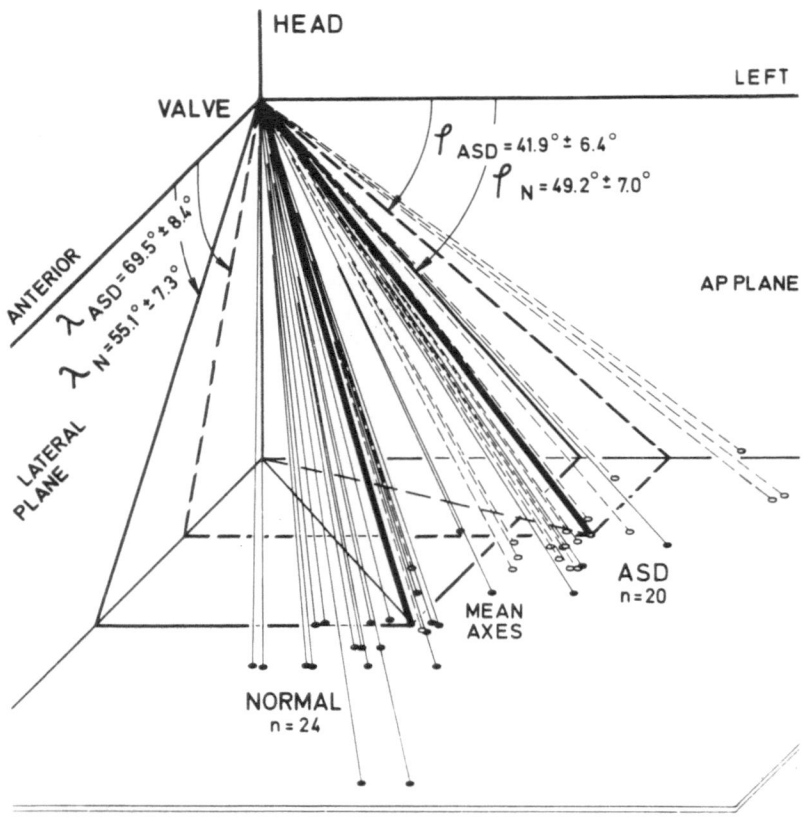

Fig. 4. Spatial orientation of the left ventricular axis (mean and individual values) in normal hearts and in patients with atrial septal defects (*ASD*). The apex of the functional normal left ventricle is significantly (*P*<0.01) shifted posteriorly by 20° in comparison to normals

Table 2. (continued)

		θ	Λ	γ	φ
Atrial septal defect ($n = 20$)					
ED	Mean	41.9	69.5	19.2	39.9
	SD	6.4	8.4	9.4	5.4
	Sign.	<0.01	<0.01	<0.01	NS
ED–ES	Mean	1.9	−0.8	1.4	1.7
	SD	2.4	7.5	5.4	2.6
	Sign.	NS	NS	NS	NS
Ventricular septal defect ($n = 8$)					
ED	Mean	50.6	56.7	38.8	43.3
	SD	5.3	6.2	7.8	4.3
	Sign.	NS	NS	NS	NS
ED–ES	Mean	5.3	−0.5	5.7	3.1
	SD	4.5	3.4	3.1	3.7
	Sign.	NS	<0.05	<0.05	NS
Hypertrophic cardiomyopathy ($n = 7$)					
ED	Mean	40.8	63.6	26.1	36.5
	SD	9.3	17.2	17.0	7.0
	Sign.	<0.05	NS	NS	NS
ED–ES	Mean	4.5	−0.1	4.0	3.3
	SD	3.7	7.6	6.8	3.5
	Sign.	NS	NS	NS	NS
Congestive cardiomyopathy ($n = 14$)					
ED	Mean	37.3	65.0	20.2	34.6
	SD	6.8	16.3	14.8	5.4
	Sign.	<0.01	<0.05	<0.01	<0.01
ED–ES	Mean	1.0	−3.3	3.2	0.4
	SD	3.8	4.8	3.4	3.3
	Sign.	<0.05	<0.01	NS	<0.05
Tetralogy of Fallot ($n = 11$)					
ED	Mean	37.0	62.8	22.5	34.0
	SD	8.9	10.6	13.1	6.5
	Sign.	<0.01	<0.05	<0.01	<0.01
ED–ES	Mean	7.1	2.2	3.5	5.9
	SD	5.0	7.4	6.6	4.9
	Sign.	<0.05	NS	NS	NS
Transposition of the great arteries ($n = 15$)					
ED	Mean	44.1	60.9	29.9	38.6
	SD	10.0	12.8	16.8	6.9
	Sign.	NS	<0.01	<0.05	NS
ED–ES	Mean	4.3	−3.2	−1.5	4.7
	SD	5.7	6.5	6.1	5.0
	Sign.	NS	NS	NS	NS

For abbreviations, see Table 1.

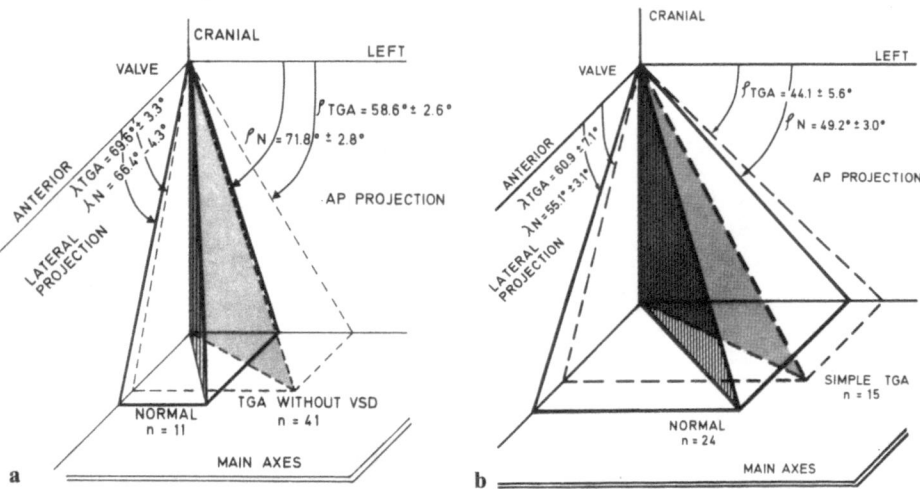

Fig. 5 a, b. Spatial orientation *a* of the right and *b* of the left ventricular axis in normal hearts and in patients with transposition of the great arteries (*TGA*) with intact interventricular septum

was no significant correlation between any angle of the left or right ventricular long axis and the shunt size.

During contraction, the apex rose (decrease of θ) by $3.1° \pm 2.9°$ for the left ventricle and by $3.2° \pm 2.8°$ for the right ventricle, but did not move significantly posteriorly or anteriorly to the aortic and pulmonary valve ring, respectively.

In pulmonic and aortic stenosis and hypertrophic cardiomyopathy, the spatial orientation of the long axis of the ventricle affected was not significantly different from normal (Tables 1 and 2). In ventricular septal defect, right ventricular θ was significantly ($P < 0.01$) increased (63.5 ± 4.4) compared with normal (Table 2), while in congestive cardiomyopathy both θ (34.6 ± 5.4) and ψ (20.2 ± 14.8) of the left ventricle were significantly ($P < 0.01$) decreased. In tetralogy of Fallot, and especially in transposition of the great arteries with intact septum, both θ and ψ were significantly ($P < 0.01$) reduced for the left and right ventricular long axes (Tables 1 and 2; Fig. 5).

Discussion

During the period of growth the apices of normal left and right ventricles decrease significantly with respect to their semilunar valve planes (Fig. 3). This may be related to the changing body proportions during growth. No significant rotation around the head-to-foot axis or posterior shift of the apices was observed. During contraction, the apices of both ventricles shift slightly but significantly ($P < 0.01$) superior with respect to the semilunar valve planes (Tables 1 and 2). A shift of similar extent has been observed in adults [7–10]. However, its spatial direction could not be determined since those measurements were based on monoplane projections. A similar movement in children and adults, however, appears likely.

The spatial orientation of a normal ventricle may also be influenced by an abnormal opposite ventricle. The apex of the functionally normal left ventricle in patients with atrial septal defect, for example, is shifted posteriorly (Fig. 4). Because of large scatter of data, there was poor correlation between any angle and the degree of left-to-right shunting. Nevertheless, the enlarged right ventricle appears to be the cause for this shift, pushing the left ventricle posteriorly. Mild to moderate increase of myocardial muscle mass without concomitant increase of chamber size, e.g., in the patients with aortic and pulmonic stenosis, does not seem to alter the spatial orientation of the affected ventricle (Tables 1 and 2). With marked hypertrophy of the left ventricular myocardium, as in hypertrophic myocardiopathy, the mean values for the angles ψ and θ are below normal (Table 2). This alteration, however, is not statistically significant because of the small number and large scatter.

If, however, an increased muscle mass is accompanied by enlarged end-diastolic and end-systolic ventricular size, as in atrial septal defect [11, 12], the apex of the right ventricle is significantly ($P<0.01$) shifted to the left with respect to the pulmonary valve plane (Table 1, Fig. 4). In addition, the inclination of the right ventricular diaphragmatic plane (Fig. 1) is significantly less than normal (Table 2). The most marked and highly significant posterior and superior shift of the left ventricular apex was noted in congestive cardiomyopathy (Table 2). These enlarged ventricles were the most spherical, probably accounting for alteration of left ventricular spatial orientation. If a severely hypertrophied right ventricle is associated with a relatively small left ventricle, as in tetralogy of Fallot [12–14] characteristically a marked shift of both ventricular apices to the left is observed. The angle ψ is significantly ($P<0.01$) smaller than normal. In transposition of the great arteries this effect is even more pronounced. Muscle volume of the left ventricle seems to be diminished with respect to its end-diastolic volume [15], while the end-diastolic size may be reduced, normal, or enlarged, depending on the pulmonary flow [12]. By contrast, the right ventricle is enlarged and hypertrophied [12, 16, 17].

Whether the malalignment of the great arteries in tetralogy of Fallot and transposition of the great arteries contribute to the observed alterations of ventricular spatial orientation remains to be determined.

Alterations of ventricular spatial orientation result mainly in a posterior and, rarely, in an inferior shift of the apices. The general trend appears to be related to the limitations of space in the thorax.

Conclusions

1. The method described allows the characterization of left and right ventricular spatial orientation.
2. The spatial orientation of the normal left and right ventricles changes significantly during growth.

3. The spatial orientation of a functional normal ventricle can be significantly varied by a diseased opposite ventricle.
4. In many congenital heart diseases the spatial orientation of the left and right ventricle is typically altered.
5. Alterations of ventricular spatial orientation seem to be limited to posterior and, rarely, inferior shifts of the affected and the opposite ventricle.

References

1. Bargeron LM Jr, Elliot LP, Soto B, Bream PR, Curry GC (1977) Axial angiography in congenital heart disease. I. Concept, technical and anatomical considerations. Circulation 56:1075–1083
2. Ceballos R, Soto B, Bargeron LM Jr (1981) Angiographic anatomy of the normal heart through axial angiography. Circulation 64:351–359
3. Onnasch DGW (1985) Computerized geometric evaluation of angio- and echocardiographic images. Herz 10:228–237
4. Onnasch DGW, Lange PE, Heintzen PH (1984) Left ventricular muscle volume in children and young adults. Ped Cardiol 5:101–106
5. Lange PE, Onnasch D, Farr F, Heintzen PH (1978) Angiocardiographic left ventricular volume determination. Accuracy, as determined from human casts, and clinical application. Eur J Cardiol 8:449–476
6. Lange PE, Onnasch D, Farr F, Heintzen PH (1978) Angiocardiographic right ventricular volume determination. Accuracy, as determined from human casts, and clinical application. Eur J Cardiol 8:477–501
7. Sniderman AD, Marpole D, Fallen EL (1973) Regional contraction patterns in the normal and ischemic left ventricle in man. Am J Cardiol 31:484–489
8. Brower RW, Meester GT (1976) Computer based methods for quantifying regional left ventricular wall motion from cine ventriculograms. Proc Computers in Cardiology, IEEE Computer Society, Long Beach, pp 55–62
9. Rickards A, Seabra-Gomes R, Thurston P (1977) The assessment of regional abnormalities of the left ventricle by angiography. Eur J Cardiol 5:167–182
10. Ingels NB, Daughters GT, Stinson EB, Alderman EL (1979) Dynamic geometry of the left ventricle in intact unanesthetized man: motion of specific midwall sites in the 30° right anterior oblique projection. Proc Computers in Cardiology, IEEE Computer Society, Long Beach, pp 153–156
11. Nakazawa M, Jarmakani JM, Gyepes MT, Prochazka JV, Yabek SM, Marks RA (1977) Pre- and postoperative ventricular function in infants and children with right ventricular volume overload. Circulation 55:479–484
12. Lange PE (1983) Quantitative Dextro-Video-Angiokardiographie. Methodik und klinische Anwendung. Habilitationsschrift. University of Kiel
13. Jarmakani JM, Graham TP, Canent RV, Jewett PH (1972) Left heart function in children with tetralogy of Fallot before and after palliative or corrective surgery. Circulation 46:478–490
14. Jarmakani JM, Nakazawa K, Isabell-Jones J, Marks RA (1976) Right ventricular function in children with tetralogy of Fallot before and after aortic-to-pulmonary shunt. Circulation 53:555–561
15. Lange PE, Onnasch, DGW, Stephan E, Wessel A, Radley-Smith R, Yacoub M, Regensburger D, Bernhard A, Heintzen PH (1981) Two-stage anatomic correction of complete transposition of the great arteries: ventricular volumes and muscle mass. Herz 6:336–343
16. Jarmakani JM, Canent RV (1974) Pre- and postoperative right ventricular function in children with transposition of the great vessels. Circulation 49/50 II:39–45
17. Graham TP, Atwood GF, Boucek RJ Jr, Boerth RC, Nelson JH (1975) Right heart volume characteristics in transposition of the great arteries. Circulation 51:881–889

Systems for Quantitative Analysis of Left Ventricular Wall Motion*

W. J. ROGERS, L. R. SMITH, W. P. HOOD, J. A. MANTLE, S. E. PAPAPIETRO, R. O. RUSSELL, JR., and C. E. RACKLEY

Division of Cardiology, Department of Medicine, University of Alabama in Birmingham, Birmingham, Alabama 35294, USA

Introduction

Tennant and Wiggers [1] were perhaps the first to demonstrate the phenomenon of segmental left ventricular dysfunction when, in 1935, they ligated a coronary artery in a dog and at once observed paradoxic motion of the underlying myocardium. Subsequently, Harrison [2] recognized disordered patterns of contraction in the kinetocardiograms of patients with ischemic heart disease and applied the term "asynergy," and, later, "dyssynergy," [3] to this condition. More recently, Herman et al. [4], in an elegant quantitative ventriculographic study of patients with coronary artery disease, introduced the now familiar terms "hypokinesis," "akinesis," and "dyskinesis" for description of left ventricular contraction abnormalities.

Although an experienced cardiac radiologist can often recognize and quantify disordered left ventricular wall motion by simple visual inspection, several studies have shown that such visual subjective analysis may be prone to considerable interobserver variability [5, 6]. For example, Zir et al. [6] reported a study in which four experienced cardiac radiologists analyzed five discrete segments of 20 right anterior oblique (RAO) left ventriculograms and assigned to each segment one of six grading categories, ranging from "normal" to "dyskinesis." Surprisingly, disagreement by at least one grading category was found in 42% of the 100 segments analyzed, disagreement by two or more categories was found in 16%, and disagreement by three or more categories was found in 11% of the segments. "In some cases," Zir et al. stated, "one man's dyskinesis was another man's normal motion."

Clearly then, objective methods are needed to quantify left ventricular wall motion. Such objective methods would have the following theoretical advantages:
a) more precise quantitation of individual wall segments;
b) increased reproducibility;
c) decreased interobserver and intraobserver variability;
d) easier comparisons between patients; and

* This research was supported in part by the National Heart, Lung, and Blood Institutes (Specialized Center of Research for Ischemic Heart Disease, contract no. 5P50HL17667-08)

e) more accurate serial assessment of the same patient's ventricular function at
    different points in time.

Many such objective wall motion analysis techniques have evolved over the
past 15 years. Unfortunately, none has gained universal acceptance, and considerable controversy surrounds the methodology of these techniques. This paper
will briefly review the merits of the major analytical systems now in use and will
also describe the validation of a system currently in clinical use at the University
of Alabama in Birmingham.

Basic Requirements for Wall Motion Analysis

A ventriculogram on which wall motion analysis is to be performed should be of
superior radiographic quality, since no system of analysis, regardless of its
sophistication, can provide more information than that obtained in the ventriculogram itself. The cardiac cycle chosen for analysis should be one in which
there is adequate chamber opacification, but should not represent the cycle
containing a premature depolarization or the following cycle.

In patients with ischemic heart disease, either simultaneous or sequential
biplane ventriculography is desirable, since important wall motion abnormalities may be visible only in one plane and absent in the other. Even with
biplane ventriculography, visualization of wall motion may be supoptimal, since
some radiographic views [for example, the anteroposterior, lateral, and left
anterior oblique (LAO)] result in considerable left ventricular foreshortening.
In order to minimize left ventricular foreshortening, we now routinely use
special angled or "axial" biplane ventriculographic projections for all routine
clinical studies in our laboratories [7, 8].

These projections employ a 45° RAO view coupled with a 60° LAO 25°
cranial angulated view (Fig. 1). The 45° RAO projection provides a significantly
longer axial view of the left ventricle than does the traditional 30° RAO
projection, giving a true tangential view of the mitral valve as well as a large
"clear area" between the mitral valve and descending aorta, and thus improving
the ability to quantify mitral regurgitation. The 60° LAO 25° cranial view
projects the left ventricular apex inferiorly, projects the left ventricular outflow
tract superiorly, reduces left ventricular foreshortening, and "uncovers" the left
ventricular outflow tract. Segmental wall motion abnormalities of the ventricular septum, apex, and posterior wall were found to be significantly better
demonstrated by the cranial angulated 60° LAO view in patients who were
studied by both axial and nonaxial ventriculography [7] (Fig. 2).

Once obtained, optimal quality ventriculograms can be analyzed for wall
motion by systems which are either

a) manual,
b) semiautomated, or
c) fully automated.

The simplest but most time-consuming system is the manual system, in which a
trained individual, either physician or technician, traces the contour of the end-

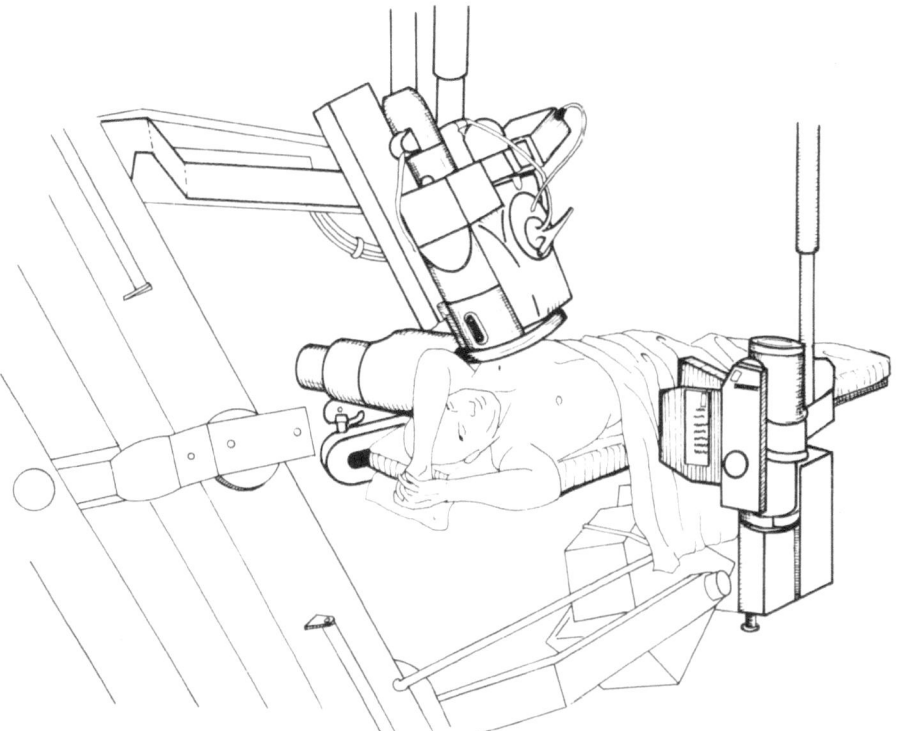

Fig. 1. Patient and equipment positioning for axial oblique left ventriculography. In order to obtain the axial 45° RAO, 60° LAO 25° cranial ventriculogram, we elevate the patient's left shoulder 45°, we angulate the vertical imaging system 25° cranially and 15° to the patient's left. The horizontal system is not rotated; it images a 45° RAO view (actually a 45° left posterior oblique view). (Reproduced with permission from [7])

diastolic and end-systolic ventriculographic silhouettes and then manually employs the analytic steps detailed below in the next section. With the semi-automated wall motion analysis systems, now common in many institutions [9], the operator traces the ventriculographic silhouettes utilizing a graphic X–Y digitizer pen interfaced to a computer, which in turn is programmed to automatically perform wall motion analysis and to generate a display of the results. Fully automated analytic systems are still in the developmental stage and employ computer techniques first to detect the angiographic chamber boundaries and then to perform wall motion analysis on these data [10].

Commonly Employed Systems for Wall Motion Analysis

Analysis of left ventricular wall motion is confounded by the potential for complex "background" motion, which may be either extracardiac or cardiac in etiology.

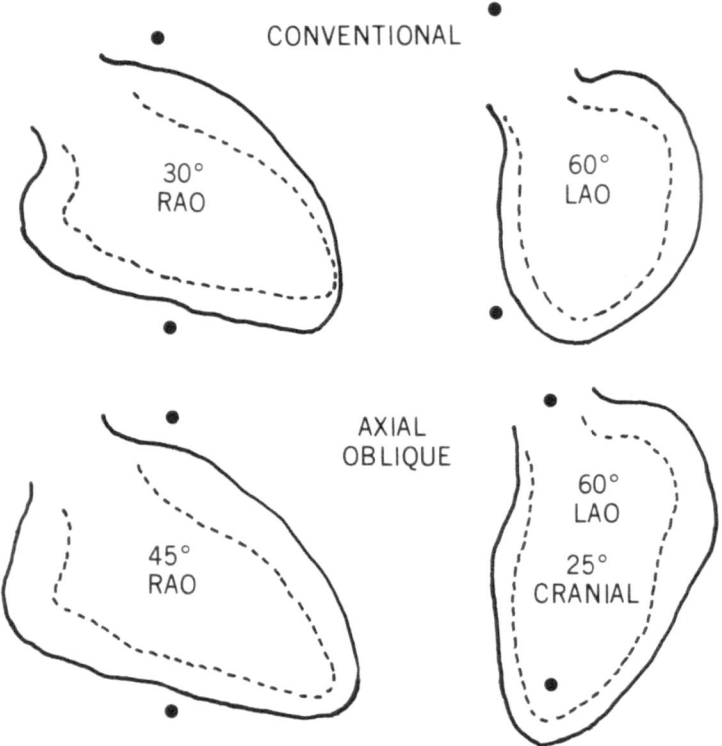

Fig. 2. Comparison of left ventricular silhouette pairs in the conventional (30° RAO/60° LAO) and axial (45° RAO/60° LAO 25° cranial) projections. Data shown are from a single representative patient with normal wall motion. Note the foreshortening evident in both "conventional" views in comparison to their "axial" counterparts. (Reproduced with permission from [7])

Extracardiac motion may consist of diaphragmatic (respiratory) or whole body motion, or motion of the radiographic imaging system (panning). The extracardiac variables can be essentially eliminated if the patient is motionless at end-inspiration during filming, and if the entire ventricle can be imaged without panning. The presence of diaphragmatic movement can be ascertained in individual cases by tracing the diaphragmatic position in relation to other fixed extracardiac structures (for example, the vertebrae) on end-diastolic and end-systolic frames [11].

"Background" cardiac motion, of course, cannot be eliminated and consists of a counterclockwise rotation of the left ventricular long axis of 3°–5° in the frontal plane as well as a counterclockwise 5°–10° rotation of the left ventricle around its long axis in the sagittal plane [12, 13]. Attempts to compensate for these complex movements account for many of the differences between current methods for wall motion analysis.

Although several dozen techniques for wall motion analysis are currently in use, most of them can be described in terms of thress basic variables:
a) the reference system,
b) the coordinate system, and
c) the measurement system employed.

Reference Systems

Most wall motion analysis systems consider only the end-diastolic and the end-systolic cineventriculographic frames, recognized by simple inspection and traced onto paper. A matter of great controversy and considerable importance is the method by which these silhouettes are then superimposed in order to "visualize" and quantify ventricular wall motion (Fig. 3). The relative merits of the most widely employed reference systems will be discussed below in terms of the RAO projection.

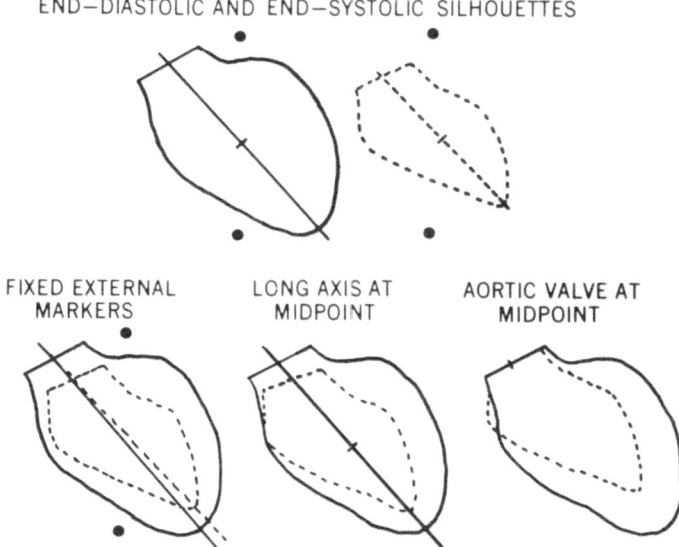

Fig. 3. Common reference systems for silhouette superimposition. End-diastolic (*solid lines*) and end-systolic (*dashed lines*) silhouettes for a normal patient are shown. The *large dots* above and below the silhouettes are markers produced on each cine frame by two lead markers attached to the input phosphor of the image intensifier in our laboratory. Also shown is the long axis, defined by the midpoint of the aortic valve and the ventricular apex, and the long-axis midpoint. When the fixed external marker system is employed (*lower left*) the end-systolic long axis is tilted upward several degrees from the end-diastolic long axis. Wall motion appears uniform. When the long axis and midpoint system is utilized for silhouette superimposition (*lower middle*), the display shows exaggerated anterolateral wall motion and reduced inferior wall motion. When the aortic valve and midpoint reference system is used (*lower right*), basal motion is reduced and apical motion is greatly exaggerated

Fixed External Markers

Fixed extracardiac structures (ribs, vertebrae, or radiographic markers) may be utilized for superimposition of the silhouettes [11, 14]. This technique is in current use at our institution and employs two small lead markers attached to the input phosphor of the image intensifier (Fig. 3). These markers are traced along with the end-diastolic and end-systolic silhouettes and then superimposed to make a composite tracing. The technique is simple, rapid, easily performed manually, and makes no assumptions about left ventricular geometry. A disadvantage of the method is its great sensitivity to both cardiac and extracardiac movement. In particular, the method does not account for the usual 3°–5° upward apical tilt of the left ventricular long axis with systole (Fig. 3). Some authorities maintain that this systolic apical rotation tends to artifactitiously enhance diaphragmatic wall motion at the expense of anterolateral wall motion [15] when the fixed external reference system is used. Others feel that the degree of apical rotation is almost always minimal, is easily measured, and that quantitation of anterior and inferior wall motion is not artifactitiously altered [11, 16].

Long Axis at Midpoint

In order to correct for the systolic apical tilt, many investigators superimpose the long axes of the end-systolic and end-diastolic left ventricular silhouettes [17–19]. The long axis may be defined in a variety of ways – for example, by the midpoint of the aortic valve and the apex [17], by the aortic-mitral valve intersection and the apex [12], or by the apex and some point in the aortic valve plane so that the long axis divides the LV silhouette into two halves of equal area [19].

The method of superimposing long axes may also differ. For example, the fixed external reference system may be first utilized, the long axes drawn, and then the end-systolic silhouette rotated about the point of intersection of the long axes until the long axes are superimposed [19]. Alternatively, and more commonly, the long axes are simply superimposed at their midpoints.

Disadvantages of this method are the following:
a) it assumes that the ventricle contracts uniformly inward toward the long axis (and its midpoint), while
b) it is highly dependent on the method of definition of the long axis. Changes in the configuration of the apex in systole in patients with abnormal ventricles can dramatically shift the long axis, sometimes artifactitiously, so that
c) if long axis midpoint superimposition is used, apical wall motion abnormalities may be minimized or obliterated altogether.

Aortic Valve at Midpoint

Since the aortic valve contains no contractile tissue, some investigators have elected to utilize the aortic valve plane as a motionless reference point [4] (Fig. 3), superimposing the aortic valve plane of end-diastolic and end-systolic silhouettes along with another reference such as the aortic valve midpoint or the long axis. This method, now used infrequently, has many disadvantages:

a) it contradicts independent data that the aortic valve does actually move downward with systole [13];

b) it makes the assumption that the entire left ventricle is moving symmetrically toward the aortic valve;

c) it minimizes basal motion; and

d) it obliterates apical akinesis and dyskinesis [11, 12, 15].

Coordinate Systems

An early system for quantitation of wall motion abnormalities was introduced by Feild et al. [14] at our institution. This system employed silhouette pairs superimposed according to a fixed external reference system (Fig. 4). The portion of the end-diastolic perimeter which was akinetic or dyskinetic was measured manually by a map-measuring device and expressed as a percentage of the total end-diastolic circumference and averaged for the two biplane views. The major limitation of this technique was its inability to quantitate hypokinesis.

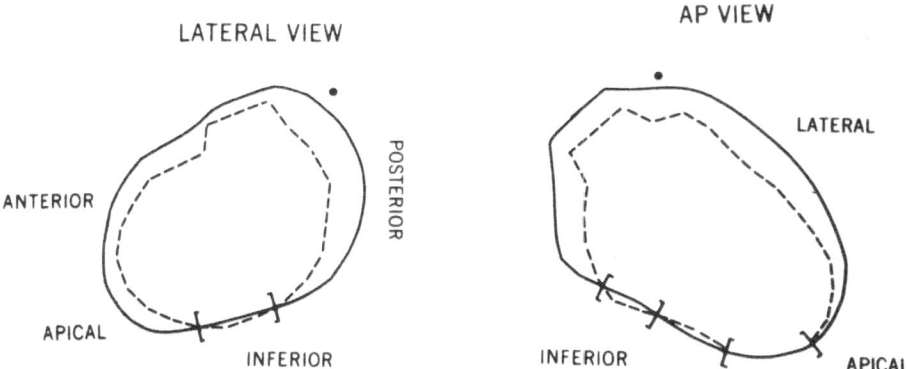

Fig. 4. Quantification of left ventricular asynergy. The end-systolic and end-diastolic silhouettes are superimposed using a fixed external reference system. The portion of the end-diastolic perimeter which is either dyskinetic or akinetic is measured and expressed as a percentage of the entire end-diastolic circumference [14]. This measurement, the percent abnormally contracting segment (% ACS), is averaged for the biplane views. It fails to assess hypokinesis. (Reproduced with permission from [14])

Hypokinesis as well as akinesis and dyskinesis may be quantified by constructing a grid over the superimposed silhouette pairs. The coordinate grid may be either a rectilinear or a polar system (Fig. 5) [20, 21].

RECTILINEAR   POLAR

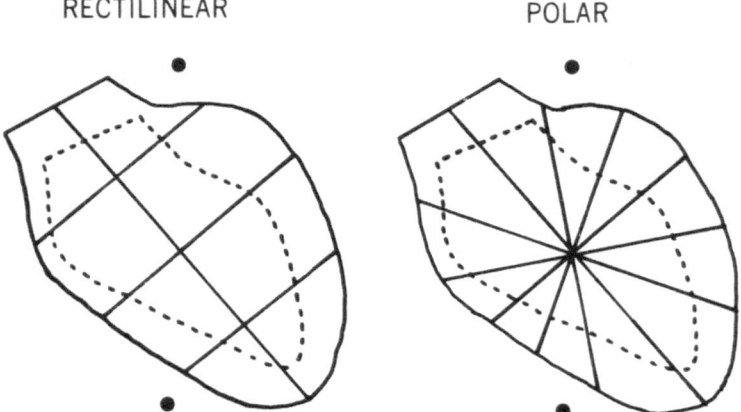

Fig. 5. Common coordinate systems. In this example, the fixed external reference system has been arbitrarily chosen. On the *left* is an example of a rectilinear coordinate system in which chords are erected perpendicular to the end-diastolic long axis dividing it into four equal segments. In the polar coordinator system shown on the *right*, the center of the end-diastolic long axis was arbitrarily chosen as the center point for construction of radii at 30° intervals, using the long-axis-aortic intersection as the zero point

Rectilinear Coordinate System

The rectilinear system employs a central long axis (variably defined as described above) with perpendicular chords extending from the long axis to the silhouette borders. The chords (or hemichords) may overlap for the silhouette pairs or may be defined independently at discrete intervals along each long axis and thus be nonoverlapping. The technique is simple and easily implemented manually. The problem is that all inward motion is expressed as perpendicular to the long axis – this may be true for the body of the left ventricle, but is certainly not true for the apex or base.

Polar Coordinate System

The polar coordinate system attempts to overcome the physiological shortcomings of the rectilinear system by expressing wall motion as inward motion from the periphery toward a central point within the ventricular chamber. This central point has been variably defined as the end-diastolic center of mass, the end-systolic center of mass [22], or as some point along the ventricular long axis, such as its midpoint [16, 18]. Radii from the midpoint to the periphery are constructed at discrete angular intervals, for example 30° intervals as shown in Fig. 5. Disadvantages of this system include its relative complexity in comparison to the rectilinear system and the currently unresolved controversy as to the choice of the central point.

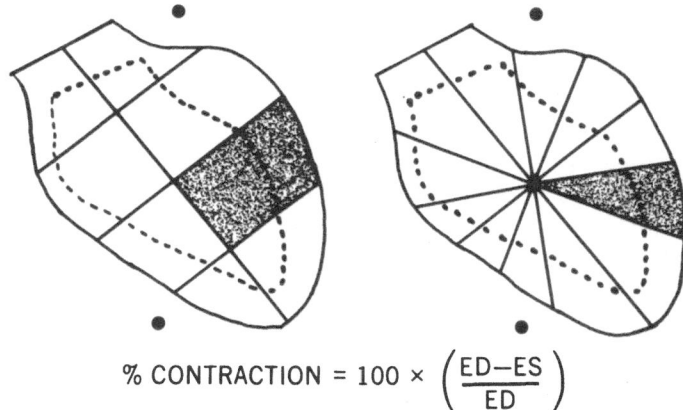

$$\% \text{ CONTRACTION} = 100 \times \left(\frac{\text{ED}-\text{ES}}{\text{ED}} \right)$$

Fig. 6. Linear vs area measurement. With linear measurement the length of end-diastolic and end-systolic hemichords or radii are assessed and the percentage contraction expressed as shown in the formula above. With area measurement, end-diastolic and end-systolic sectors (*shaded*) are planimeted and "area ejection fractions" are calculated

Measurement Systems

Either *linear* or *area* measurement techniques may be utilized [20] (Fig. 6). Both techniques assess regional contraction, usually as a percentage change from end-diastolic dimension. The simplest technique is linear measurement whereby the difference in hemichord or radius length between end-diastole and end-systole is expressed as a percentage of the end-diastolic dimension for each hemichord or radius.

Proponents of area measurement argue that it gives a more representative average assessment of ventricular motion than arbitrarily placed chords or radii. The area measurement is more tedious, requiring planimetry techniques, and is best performed with computer assistance.

Validation of Wall Motion Analysis Systems

Gold Standards

In order to ascertain which wall motion analysis technique is best, several investigators have performed "validation studies" in which several of the most commonly used analysis systems have been compared in selected patients. Several "gold standards" have been chosen for these studies.

First, the subjective impression of an experienced observer has been utilized as a gold standard [12]. If the experienced observer disagreed with analysis of wall motion using the objective technique, the objective technique was judged inadequate. Previously mentioned data [5, 6] on the wide variability in subjective interpretation of wall motion by experienced observers suggest that this method of validation may be subject to gross error.

Secondly, patients with normal coronary anatomy and no evidence of valvular disease or cardiomyopathy have been utilized as standards [23–25]. The reasoning has been that a technique properly analyzing such patients should display relatively uniform and normal inward wall motion. Likewise, postinfarction patients have been utilized as standards, particularly those having single vessel coronary artery disease with the stenosed vessel supplying the infarct zone. A valid wall motion analysis system should properly display disordered wall motion in the infarct zone in these patients.

Finally, radiopaque markers have been implanted in the ventricles of patients undergoing cardiac surgery and have been utilized to follow the actual motion of discrete points in the ventricular wall and to define more precisely the central point of ventricular contraction in these patients [16].

Validation Studies at the University of Alabama in Birmingham

In order to ascertain which of several wall motion analysis systems was most representative, we analyzed biplane left ventricular cineangiograms in 34 patients with normal coronary anatomy and no evidence of cardiac disease, and in 25 patients with prior documented myocardial infarction and single vessel coronary artery disease, with the diseased vessel supplying the infarct zone [23]. Three reference systems were examined:
a) fixed external radiographic markers;
b) long axis at midpoint; and
c) aortic valve at midpoint (see Fig. 3).

Five segmental wall motion areas were defined in each biplane silhouette pair by radial lines, and segmental area ejection fraction was determined for each of the 10 segments using a computerized system (Fig. 7). Three origins for the radial lines were considered:
a) the end-diastolic center of mass;
b) the end-systolic center of mass; and
c) the midpoint of the long axis. The long axis was defined by the midpoint of the aortic valve and the apex.

In the normal patients, segmental area ejection fractions were rather similar and uniform in magnitude when we used reference systems employing fixed external markers or the midpoint of the long axis. However, the aortic valve midpoint reference system yielded segmental area ejection fractions in normals that varied markedly in magnitude, even in adjacent segments (Figs. 8, 9).

In the subgroup of patients with prior isolated anterior or inferior infarction, all of the methods depicted significantly diminished segmental area ejection fractions in the infarct zones. However, the only system showing abnormalities exclusively in these zones was the system employing fixed external radiographic markers with radii emanating from the diastolic center of mass. We have therefore chosen to use this system routinely for wall motion analysis at our institution.

ORIGIN OF THE
RADIAL LINES   ANTEROPOSTERIOR   LATERAL

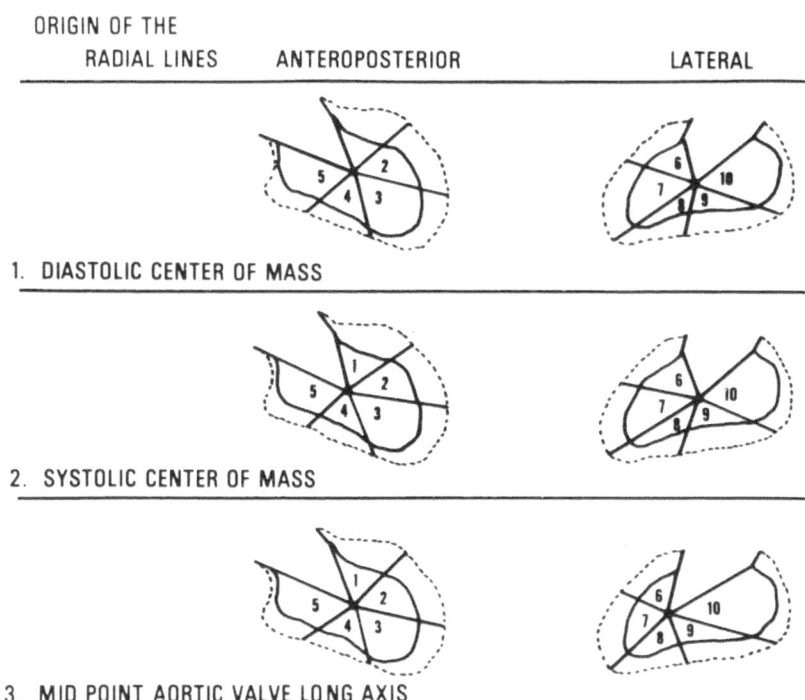

1. DIASTOLIC CENTER OF MASS

2. SYSTOLIC CENTER OF MASS

3. MID POINT AORTIC VALVE LONG AXIS

Fig. 7. Radial system employed at the University of Alabama in Birmingham. In the validation study, we tested the following origins for the radial lines: diastolic center of mass, systolic center of mass, and midpoint of the long axis. The ventricular apex is detected manually. For the anteroposterior or RAO projections we divide the angle between the left margin of the aortic valve and the apex into fifths – segments 1 and 2 represent two-fifths. Likewise the angle between the right margin of the aortic valve and apex is divided into fifths – segments 4 and 5 each represent two-fifths. The apex represents the remaining area. For the lateral or LAO projections we divide the angle between the anterior margin of the aortic root and apex into two parts and the angle between the posterior margin of the aortic root and apex into three parts, thus detecting five segments. (Reproduced with permission from [23])

The fixed external reference system, found to be most representative in our study, has also been recommended in similar studies by others [11, 12, 24]. However, as yet, the method is still not uniformly accepted by all investigators, and much controversy continues over the optimal technique for wall motion analysis.

Future Directions

The controversy over the best system for analyzing ventricular wall motion will probably never be resolved by isolated studies on small populations from single institutions and may ultimately require a multiinstitutional collaborative study,

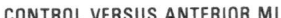

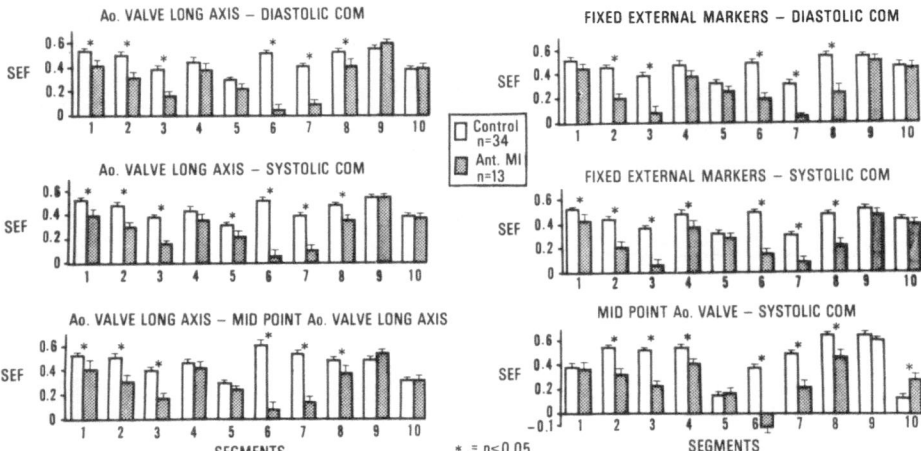

Fig. 8. Segmental ejection fractions (SEF) for normal patients (controls) and for patients with prior anterior infarcts for the six systems tested. We anticipated that the most representative system would display uniformly normal SEF in the normal controls and significantly reduced SEF exclusively in segments 2, 3, 6, and 7 in anterior infarcts. Only the system utilizing fixed external markers with diastolic center of mass (as the center for the radial lines) met both these requirements. (Reproduced with permission from [23])

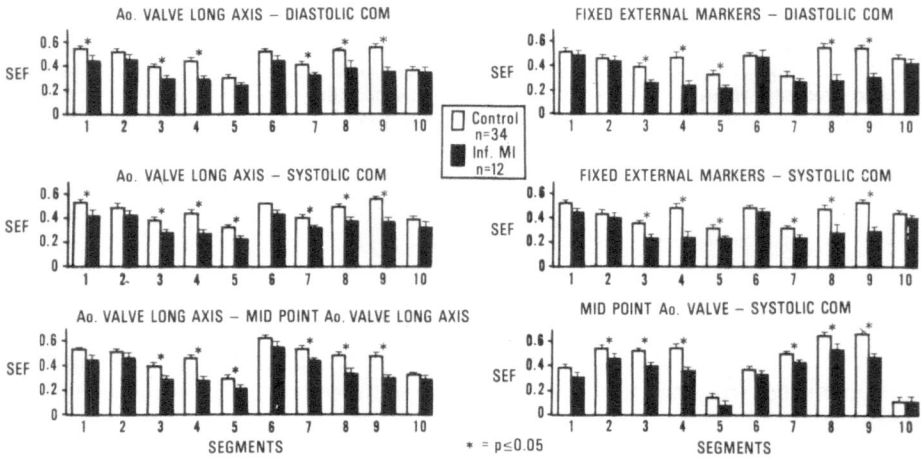

Fig. 9. Segmental ejection fractions (SEF) for normal patients (controls) and patients with prior inferior infarcts for the six systems tested. We anticipated that the most representative system would display uniformly normal SEF in normal controls and significantly diminished SEF in normal controls and significantly diminished SEF exclusively in segments 3, 4, 8, and 9 in the inferior infarct patients. Only the system utilizing fixed external markers with diastolic center of mass (as the center for the radial lines) met both of these requirements. (Reproduced with permission from [23])

employing a large population data base. The future will likely see increased implementation of angiographic systems utilizing computer digital enhancement techniques, automatic border recognition, and fully automated wall motion analysis [26].

Wall motion analysis systems have recently been implemented in radionuclide ventriculograms [27–29]. Although radionuclide ventriculograms do not as yet have the resolution and definition of contrast ventriculograms, they do have the distinct advantages of being essentially noninvasive and easily repeatable. The two-dimensional radionuclide ventriculographic silhouettes possess a third dimension, "count density," which is proportional to ventricular volume. Thus, radionuclide segmental ejection fractions assume the character of segmental *volumetric* ejection fractions, in comparison with the segmental *area* ejection fractions of contrast ventriculograms. Furthermore, radionuclide ventriculograms, being themselves the end-product of computer analysis, are easily subjected to further sophisticated computations. One such example is temporal Fourier phase analysis, a technique which promises to be an important tool in the detection and quantification of regional left ventricular asynergy [30].

Acknowledgements. The authors gratefully acknowledge the secretarial assistance of Mrs. Louise Patterson in the preparation of this manuscript.

References

1. Tennant R, Wiggers CJ (1935) Effect of coronary occlusion on myocardial contraction. Am J Physiol 112:351
2. Harrison TR (1955) Some unanswered questions concerning enlargement and failure of the heart. Am Heart J 69:100
3. Harrison TR, Reeves TJ (1968) Principles and problems of ischemic heart disease. Year Book Medical Publishers, Chicago, p 23
4. Herman MV, Heinle RA, Klein MD, Gorlin R (1967) Localized disorders in myocardial contraction. N Engl J Med 277:222
5. Chaitman BR, DeMots H, Bristow JD, Rosch J, Rahimtoola SH (1975) Objective and subjective analysis of left ventricular angiograms. Circulation 52:420
6. Zir LM, Miller SW, Dinsmore RE, Gilbert JP, Harthorne JW (1976) Interobserver variability in coronary angiography. Circulation 53:627
7. Rogers WJ, Smith LR, Bream PR, Elliott LP, Rackley CE, Russell RO Jr (1982) Quantitative axial oblique contrast left ventriculography: validation of the method by demonstrating improved visualization of regional wall motion and mitral valve function with accurate volume determinations. Am Heart J 103:185
8. Elliott LP, Green CE, Rogers WJ, Hood WP, Mantle JA, Papapietro SE (1982) The advantages of the caudo-cranial left anterior oblique left ventriculogram in adult heart disease. Am J Cardiol 49:369–380
9. Smith LR, Zisserman D, Cunningham W, Wixson SE, Bishop SP, Hood WP Jr, Mantle JA, Rogers WJ, Russell RO Jr, Logic JR, Rackley CE (1976) Measurement of cardiac parameters from cardiovascular images. Computers in Cardiology, IEEE Computer Society, Long Beach, pp 49–54
10. Smalling RW, Skolnik MH, Myers D (1976) Digital boundary detection, volumetric and wall motion analysis of left ventricular cine angiograms. Comput Biol Med 6:73–83
11. Chaitman BR, Bristow JD, Rahimtoola SH (1973) Left ventricular wall motion assessed by using fixed external reference systems. Circulation 48:1043

12. Probst P, Moore R, Kim SW, Zollikofer C, Amplatz K (1981) Comparison of various quantization methods of segmental ventricular wall motion in ischemic heart disease. Fortschr Rontgenstr 134:376
13. McDonald IG (1970) The shape and movements of the human left ventricle during systole. Am J Cardiol 26:221
14. Feild BJ, Russell RO Jr, Dowling JT, Rackley CE (1972) Regional left ventricular performance in the year following myocardial infarction. Circulation 46:679
15. Brower RW, Meester GT (1976) Computer based methods for quantifying regional left ventricular wall motion from cine ventriculograms. Computers in Cardiology, IEEE Computer Society, Long Beach, pp 55–62
16. Ingels NB, Daughters GT II, Stinson EB, Alderman EL (1980) Evaluation of methods for quantitating left ventricular segmental wall motion in men using myocardial markers as a standard. Circulation 61:966
17. Hamilton GW, Murray JA, Kennedy JW (1972) Quantitative angiocardiology in ischemic heart disease. Circulation 40:1065
18. Harris LD, Clayton PD, Marshall HW, Warner HR (1974) A technique for detection of asynergistic motion in the left ventricle. Comput Biomed Res 7:380
19. Leighton RF, Wilt SM, Lewis RP (1974) Detection of hypokinesis by a quantitative analysis of left ventricular cineangiograms. Circulation 50:121
20. Gelberg HJ, Brundage BH, Glantz S, Parmley WW (1979) Quantitative left ventricular wall motion analysis: a comparison of area, chord, and radial methods. Circulation 59:991
21. Daughters GT, Alderman EL, Stinson EB, Ingels NB (1979) Methods for ventricular wall motion assessment: towards a uniform terminology. Computers in Cardiology, IEEE Computer Society, Long Beach, pp 145–148
22. Rickards A, Seabra-Gomes R, Thurston P (1977) The assessment of regional abnormalities of the left ventricle by angiography. Eur J Cardiol 5:167
23. Papapietro SE, Smith LR, Hood WP Jr, Russell RO Jr, Rackley CE, Rogers WJ (1978) An optimal method for angiographic definition and quantification of regional left ventricular contraction. Computers in Cardiology, IEEE Computer Society, Long Beach, pp 293–296
24. Alderman EL, Schwarzkopf A, Ingels NB, Daughters GT, Stinson EB, Sanders WJ (1979) Application of an externally referenced, polar coordinate system for left ventricular wall motion analysis. Computers in Cardiology, IEEE Computer Society, Long Beach, pp 207–210
25. Karsch KR, Lamm U, Blanke H, Rentrop KP (1980) Comparison of nineteen quantitative models for assessment of localized left ventricular wall motion abnormalities. Clin Cardiol 3:123
26. Smalling R, Cole JS, Skolnick M (1979) Comparison of digital boundary detection and semi-automated analysis of left ventricular cine angiograms. Cathet Cardiovasc Diagn 5:331
27. Jengo JA, Mena I, Blaufuss A, Criley JM (1978) Evaluation of left ventricular function (ejection fraction and segmental wall motion) by single pass radioisotope angiography. Circulation 57:326
28. Okada RD, Pohost GM, Nichols AB, McKusick KA, Strauss HW, Boucher CA, Block PC, Rosenthal SV, Dinsmore RE (1980) Left ventricular regional wall motion assessment by multigated and end-diastolic, end-systolic gated radionuclide left ventriculography. Am J Cardiol 45:1211
29. Papapietro SE, Yester MV, Logic JR, Tauxe WN, Mantle JA, Rogers WJ, Russell RO Jr, Rackley CE (1981) Method for quantitative analysis of regional left ventricular function with first pass and gated blood pool scintigraphy. Am J Cardiol 47:618
30. Rogers WJ, Logic JR, Yester MV, Papapietro SE, Mantle JA, Smith LR, Rackley CE (1982) Temporal Fourier analysis of gated radionuclide ventriculograms – a tool for visualizing and quantifying left ventricular contraction abnormalities. Am J Cardiol [Abstract] 49:1045

Improved Detection of Wall Motion Abnormalities by Quantitative Spatial and Temporal Analysis: Application in Normal and Infarcted Ventricles*

Ch. Chen,[1] T. Bonzel,[1] H. Just,[1] G. Seiffert,[2] A. Zeiher,[1] W. Kasper,[1] and H. Wollschlaeger[1]

[1] Medical Clinic, Department of Cardiology, University of Freiburg,
 D-7800 Freiburg im Breisgau, FRG
[2] Institute for Medical Statistics, University of Freiburg, D-7800 Freiburg im Breisgau, FRG

Introduction

Regional wall motion abnormalities are a significant feature of coronary artery diesease [1, 2], so that the quantitative analysis of these abnormalities has become an important tool for the evaluation of ventricular function [3–42]. Until now attention has been focused primarily on hypokinesis, akinesis, and dyskinesis based on the superimposition of end-diastolic and end-systolic ventricular cavity outlines [3–13]. However, it is well known that the maximal systolic myocardial expansion in infarcted or ischemic myocardium occurs in the early rather than the late phase of systole. Therefore, essential characteristics of wall motion abnormalities will be missed if only analysis of end-diastolic and end-systolic ventricular contours is made [14–24]. In spite of these observations, the temporal properties of wall motion [2, 16] have received less attention. The most important reason has been the lack of sufficiently simple methods available for quantitative analysis of regional contraction throughout systole [15, 24–26]. The purpose of this study was to develop a relatively simple method applicable to cineventriculography for quantitation of temporal and spatial wall motion heterogeneity and to apply this method for the study of normal and infarcted ventricles.

Methods and Patients

Angiographic Data Acquisition

The ventriculograms of 15 normal subjects and 26 patients with coronary artery disease were analyzed. Cineventriculography was performed before coronary angiography using the Judkins technique. A biplane cinegraphic X-ray system with 27-cm image intensifiers (Bi-Angioscop-C, Siemens, Erlangen, FRG) was used [27]. The left ventricle was opacified with a contrast flow of 12–15 ml/s for 3 s [11]. Images were recorded at 50 frames/s on 35-mm cine film. Only well-opacified ventricular images with clearly defined contours from the first 3–5

* Supported by grant 324-306-003-4 from DAAD (German Academic Exchange Service)

sinus beats after injection were selected for analysis. Extrasystolic or postextrasystolic beats were excluded. All studies were performed by the same experienced observer. Contours from right anterior oblique left ventriculogram were traced at 40 ms intervals (every second frame of the cine film) throughout systole and digitized with a computerized analysis system (AVD, angiographic ventricular dynamics, Siemens) and store d on computer disc for further analysis. The end-diastolic and end-systolic contours were defined as those demonstrating the largest and the smallest ventricular area.

Integrated Analysis Procedure

For wall motion analysis of each frame a radial axis system with a total of 90 radii was used [11]. The midpoint of the long axis between the aortomitral conjunction and the most distant point of the apex was defined as the reference point. The radial distances were measured between the reference point and the edge of each contour, beginning at the aortomitral conjunction with clockwise progression at 4° increments. Radii located on aortic (radii 1–10) and mitral valve (radii 81–90) regions were excluded, leaving 70 myocardium-related radii for further analysis [11]. The anterior wall was defined by radii 11–40, the apical region by radii 41–50, and the inferior wall by radii 51–80. The temporal radial shortening fractions (Yt) were calculated at each 40 ms interval relative to end-diastole as follows:

$$Yt = \frac{\text{end-diastolic radial distance–radial distance at a given time point}}{\text{end-diastolic radial distance}} \times 100\,(\%)$$

The systolic sequential time points (Xt) were expressed as normalized values as a percentage of the holosystole, e.g., at end-diastole, $Xed = 0$, and at end-systole, $Xes = 100\%$. Shortening fractions (Yt) of each radius were then plotted against the corresponding sequential time points (Xt), as shown in Fig. 1. After testing for linearity, the least squares linear regression technique was employed. Starting with the point of ventricular contraction at end-diastole ($Yt = 0$, $Xt = 0$) the intercept (a) of the linear regression line was always defined as $a = 0$ in the present study. That means that the regression equation is written as $Yt = b \cdot Xt$. Linear regression correlation coefficients (r) and regression slopes (b) were calculated for each radius, yielding 70 radial correlation coefficients and regression slopes. Normal values of r and b (mean $\pm$ 1 SD) for each radius were obtained from the 15 normal control subjects. Normal and abnormal radial values were defined as follow:

Normal value: mean $-$ 1 SD $<$ normal value $<$ mean $+$ 1 SD
Borderline value: mean $-$ 1 SD $>$ borderline value $>$ mean $+$ 1 SD
Abnormal value: mean $-$ 2 SD $>$ abnormal value $>$ mean $+$ 2 SD

Normal r values describe normal temporal or homogeneous contraction in a given radius. Significant temporal heterogeneity of contraction is indicated by abnormal r values. The b value describes holosystolic temporally integrated radial shortening. Normal b values describe normokinesis. Abnormal b values

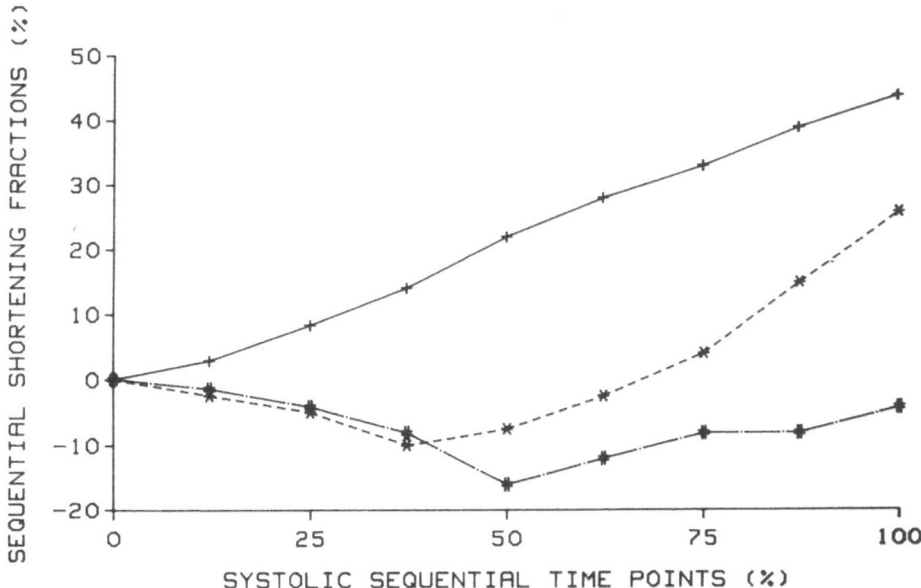

Fig. 1. Correlation between temporal sequential shortening fractions (%) and systolic sequential time points (%). *Solid line with crosses,* radius of normal left ventricle demonstrating approximately linear contraction (end-systolic shortening 45%) resulting in normal high *r* and *b* values. *Dashed line,* radius of borderline hypokinetic left ventricular region (end-systolic shortening 25%) with early systolic dyskinetic motion ("bulging") resulting in wall motion heterogeneity and reduced *r* and *b* values. Dotted line with double crosses: radius of akinetic region (end-systolic shortening < 0%) with midsystolic bulging resulting in motion heterogeneity with low *r* value and low negative *b* value

describe hypokinesis (mean − 2 SD < *b* values > 0), dyskinesis (*b* values < 0) and hyperkinesis (*b* values > means ± 2 SD). A graphic display of normal ranges (mean ± SD) of each radial *r* or *b* value and corresponding observed values from individual subjects allows immediate comparative information (Figs. 2 and 3.). The number of abnormal radii can be counted. The sum of the abnormal *r* or *b* values deviating from mean − 1 SD (or mean ± 1 SD for hyperkinesis) of all abnormal radii can give information about the degree of abnormal wall motion in a given ventricle, expressed in a digital value (Figs. 2, 3).

Variability Study

To determine intraobserver variability, 62 frames of ventriculograms, yielding 4340 radii in three normal subjects and four patients with myocardial infarction, were traced twice by the same examiner. A minimum of three days elapsed between tracings of the same ventriculograms to prevent the memory of the first tracing from influencing the second tracing. Interobserver variability studies

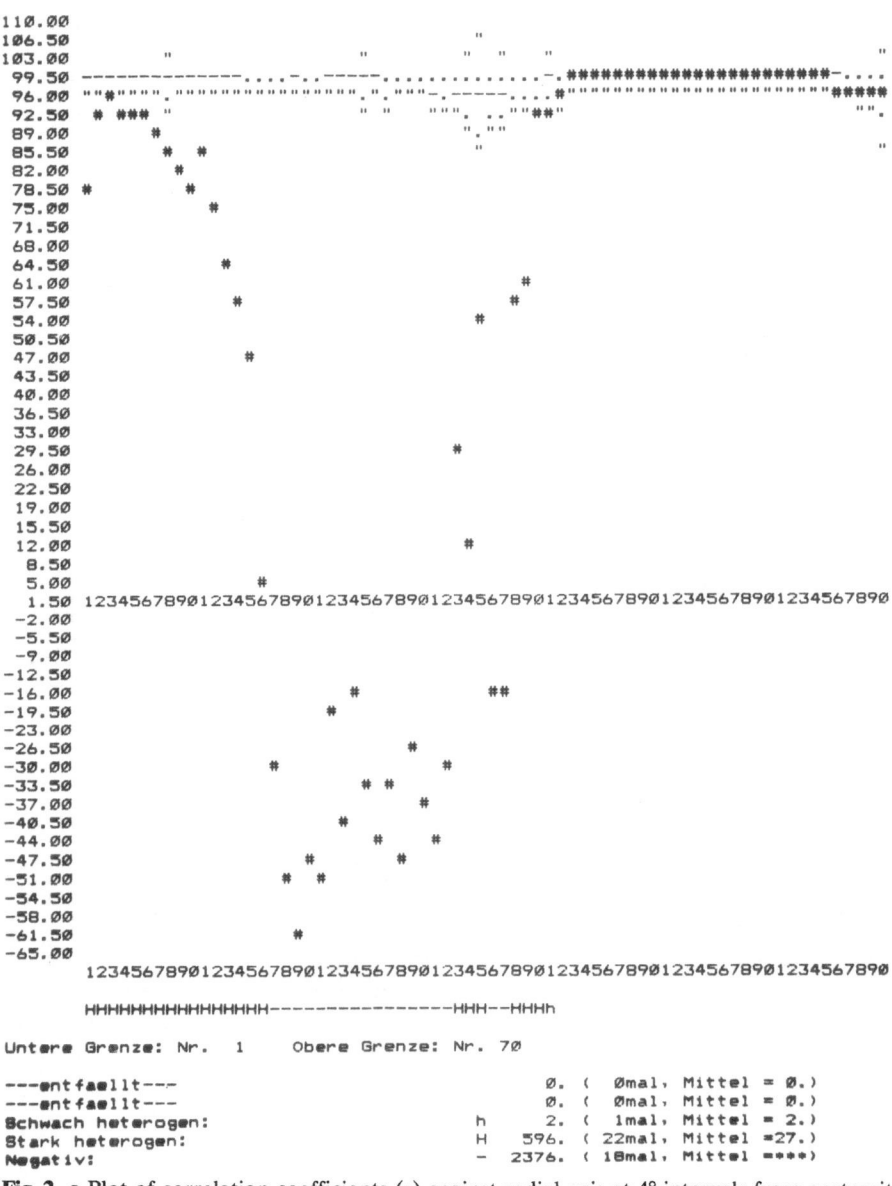

Fig. 2. a Plot of correlation coefficients (*r*) against radial axis at 4° intervals from aortomitral conjunction with clockwise progression around' ventricular contour, excluding aortic and mitral valve regions. Normal values: mean, ----; 1 SD, '''; and 2 SD, """". **b** Simplified graphic display of **a**. Note high *r* values and small standard deviation for normals, suggestive of linear temporally homogeneous inward motion of a given radius. An example of a patient with anterior myocardial infarction showed significant systolic wall motion heterogeneity in the anteroapical region. A total of 40 radii (22 radii had an *r* value < mean ± 2 SD; 18 had a negative *r* value) had significant heterogeneity: the sum of the amplitude of heterogeneity-*r* values of the 40 abnormal radii deviating from mean ± 1 SD was calculated as 29.82

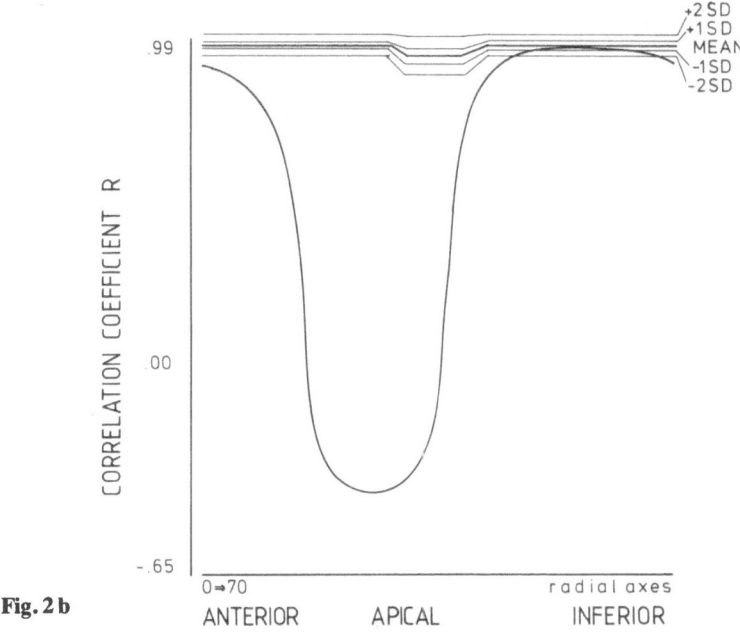

+2 SD
+1 SD
MEAN
-1 SD
-2 SD

.99

CORRELATION COEFFICIENT R

.00

-.65

0→70   radial axes

Fig. 2 b

ANTERIOR   APICAL   INFERIOR

were not performed. The mean intraobserver difference of b values was 0.017 ± 0.012, corresponding to 3.6% of the mean b value, and the correlation of the two studies was high $(r = 0.96)$; the mean intraobserver difference of r values was 0.051 ± 0.042, corresponding to 5.4% of the mean r value, and the r values of the two studies correlated highly $(r = 0.91)$.

Application of the Method in Normal and Infarcted Ventricles

The method described was applied in normal subjects and patients with coronary artery diesease. The total study population consisted of 41 patients with technically high quality angiograms without atrioventricular or intraventricular conduction disturbances. Fifteen patients (age 32–67 years, mean 48 years) were considered as normal control subjects (group 1). These patients had atypical chest pain, but completely normal coronary arteries and cardiac hemodynamic parameters without any history of heart diesease. Twenty-six patients (age 38–72 years, mean 58 years) were considered as group 2. Patients in group 2 had a previous myocardial infarction (MI) between 6 weeks and 2 years before cardiac catheterization and significant coronary artery disease ($>75\%$ stenosis in diameter reduction) in only one major coronary vessel. Nineteen patients of group 2 had left anterior descending coronary artery disease and six patients had right coronary artery disease. Patients with left ventricular aneurysm were excluded.

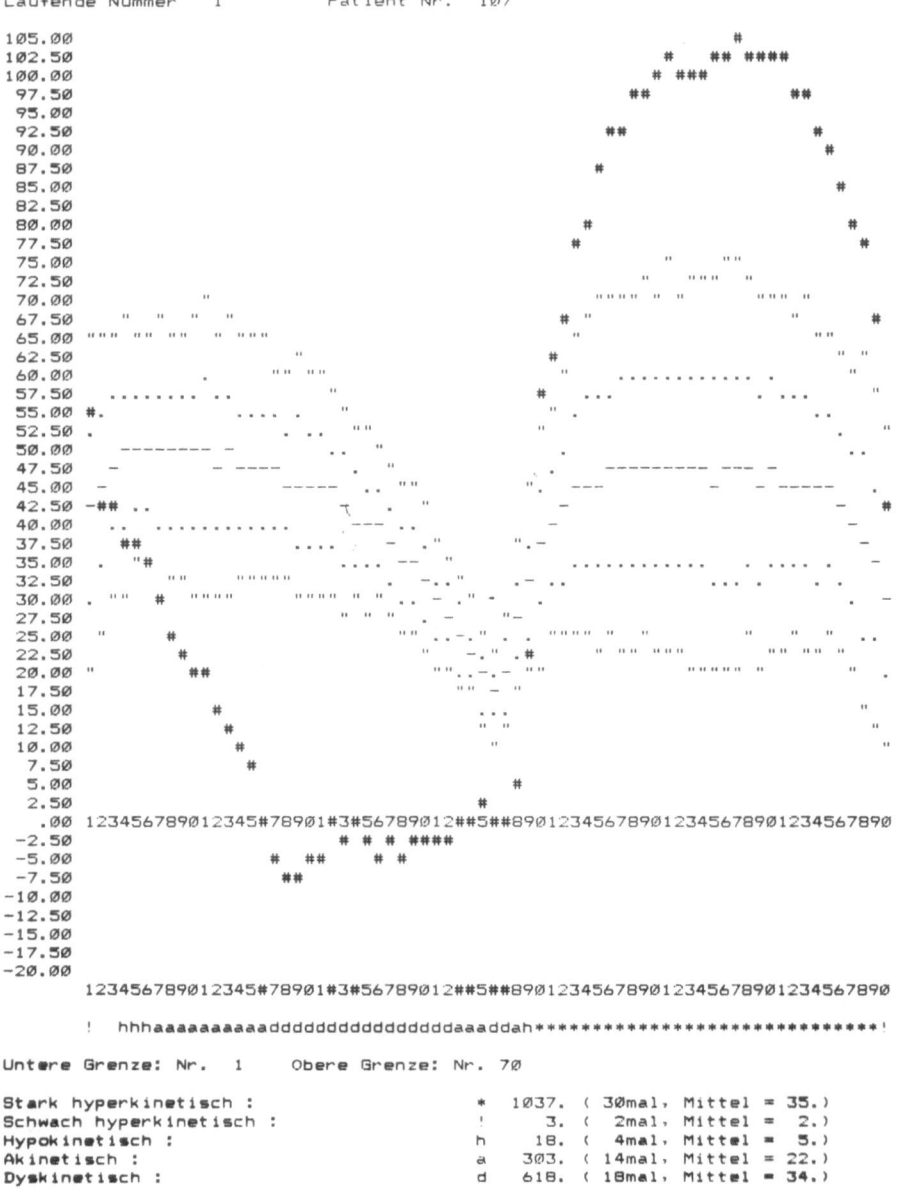

Fig. 3. a Plot of regression slopes (*b*) against radial axis at 4° intervals from aortomitral conjunction with clockwise progression around ventricular contour, excluding aortic and mitral regions. Normal values: mean, ----; 1 SD, ''''; 2 SD, """". **b** Simplified graphic display of **a**. An example of a patient with anterior myocardial infarction showed significantly reduced systolic contraction in anteroapical region. A total of 32 radii had hypokinesis or dyskinesis; the digital value of the abnormal amplitude was 9.12

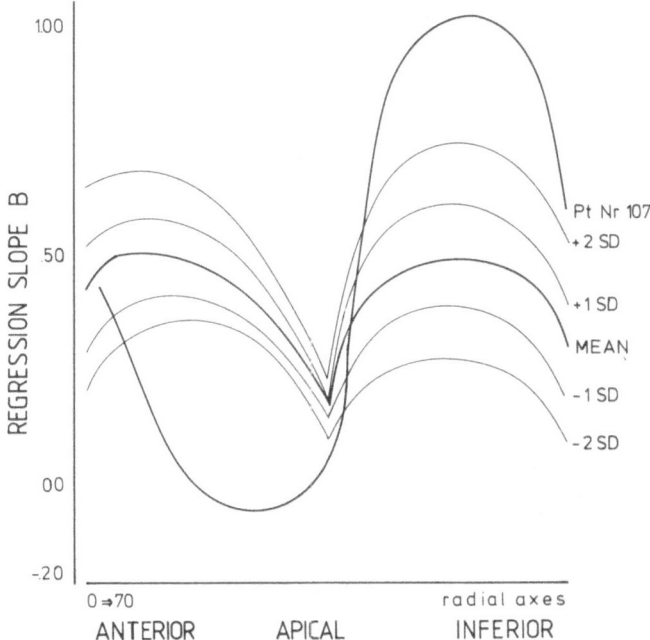

Fig. 3 b

Statistical Analysis

Data were presented as mean values (X) ± standard deviations (SD). The significance of the difference of mean values was tested using Student's t-test, and the significance of radial number differences was tested with the chisquare test. A $P < 0.05$ was considered statistically significant.

Results

Global Left Ventricular Function

Mean global left ventricular ejection fraction (EF) was 69% ± 3% in normal subjects, and 60% ± 8% in patients with myocardial infarction ($P < 0.01$). Six of 26 patients with myocardial infarction had an EF < 55%. The mean heart rate was 72 ± 6 (range 61–89 beats/min) in normal subjects and 70 ± 5 (range 59–86 beats/min) in patients ($P > 0.05$). Left ventricular systolic pressure was 114 ± 12 mmHg in normal subjects and 128 ± 15 mmHg in patients ($P < 0.01$). End-diastolic left ventricular pressure was 7 ± 2 mmHg in normal subjects and 11 ± 5 mmHg in patients ($P < 0.01$), nine of whom had an end-diastolic pressure > 12 mmHg.

Table 1. Comparison of Systolic Integrated Parameters in Groups 1 and 2

	Normals ($n = 15$)	Patients ($n = 26$)	
		MI region	Non-MI region
r	0.972 ± 0.016	0.480 ± 0.304*	0.964 ± 0.018
b	0.449 ± 0.106	0.203 ± 0.211*	0.695 ± 0.213*

* $P < 0.001$, mean ± SD
MI region, infarcted myocardial region; non-MI region, noninfarcted myocardial region; r, radial correlation coefficients; b, radial linear regression slopes

Integrated Parameters of Systolic Wall Motion in Group 1

High r values with small standard deviations in all radii derived from normal ventriculograms proved that a uniform linear segmental contraction pattern without temporal heterogeneity predominates in the normal left ventricle (Table 1 and Fig. 2). When the r values of the radii in the apical region (0.959 ± 0.026) were compared with the r values of the anterior (0.983 ± 0.012) and inferior region (0.983 ± 0.010), only minor, statistically insignificant differences were found ($P > 0.05$).

Radial b values in normal ventriculograms were different in various myocardial regions and showed large standard deviations (Table 1, Fig. 3). In the apical region, b values (26.93 ± 5.64) were significantly lower than those in the inferior (49.73 ± 13.57) or anterior region (46.71 ± 9.91) ($P < 0.01$). The difference between b values in inferior and anterior regions was not significant ($P > 0.05$).

When the above-defined criteria for temporally heterogeneous radial wall motion (reduced r values) and radial hypokinesis or dyskinesis (reduced b values) were applied to normal subjects, none of the latter had more than two temporally heterogeneous adjunctive radii and three hypo- or dyskinetic adjunctive radii.

Integrated Parameters of Systolic Wall Motion in Group 2

First we compared the mean radial r value and b value in myocardial infarct MIregions or non-MIregions with those in the normal ventricles. In case of anterior myocardial infarction, anterior and apical regions were defined as the MIregion; correspondingly, in case of inferior myocardial infarction, inferior and apical regions as the MIregion. In MIregions markedly reduced r values were observed, while r values in non-MIregions were not different from the normal r values (Table 1). The b values of the MIregions were also reduced, demonstrating hypokinesis, whereas b values in the non-MIregions, as compared with the values of normal subjects, were significantly increased (Table 1), indicating hyperkinesis.

When normal values for each radius were used, all patients but one had more than two adjunctive radii, demonstrating temporally heterogeneous radial contraction in the MIregion. Significant temporally heterogeneous contraction in all patients was detected quantitatively in 695 of 1040 radii in MIregions, but only in 10 of 780 radii in non-Miregions ($P < 0.001$). The abnormal radii in non-MIregions were always located in regions closed to the valves, and were observed in no more than two consecutive adjunctive radii. The sum of the reduced r values deviating from mean $\pm$ 1 SD in individual patients was 9.60 $\pm$ 10.46, $n = 25$ in MIregions.

Twenty-three of 26 patients showed hypokinesis or dyskinesis with minimum of abnormal b values in more than three consecutive radii. A total of 571 of 1040 radii of MIregions showed hypokinesis or dyskinesis in all patients. Only 19 of 780 radii in non-MIregions had hypokinesis ($P < 0.001$), and these radii were located almost only in regions closed to the valves and there were no more than three adjunctive radii in any case. The sum of deviations from mean $\pm$ 1 SD was 6.00 $\pm$ 3.40, $n = 23$ in MIregions. In non-MIregions 230 of 690 radii demonstrated a hyperkinetic contraction.

Discussion

Myocardial ischemia is characterized by temporal and spatial patterns of wall motion abnormalities [1–37]. The severity of left ventricular spatial contraction abnormalities has been categorized as akinesis, hypokinesis, and dyskinesis. Much effort has been made to improve detection of these spatial abnormalities [7, 8, 10, 11, 13, 16, 39, 40, 42]. However, conventional qualitative and even quantitative assessment of left ventricular wall motion included only the spatial wall motion at two time points – end-diastole and end-systole. The temporal wall motion, which describes the temporal contraction sequence and pattern throughout systole, has been less investigated [15, 16, 24, 35–37]. In the present study we have described an integrated temporal and spatial systolic wall motion analysis method. This method not only demonstrates a high degree of temporal and spatial resolution, but also has the important advantage of overcoming the large amount of data in wall motion analysis throughout systole. This is achieved by introducing the two simple integrated parameters (r and b) for temporal and spatial information. Furthermore, the graphic plots of r and b values against corresponding radii and the digital sum of abnormal degree in an individual patient allow easy comparisons in various conditions.

Rationale of Temporal Wall Motion Analysis

It is impressive to see that in cineventriculograms the simple measurement of endocardial excursion from end-diastole to end-systole frequently fails to detect systolic wall motion abnormalities, which appear to be obvious by visual interpretation. Such abnormalities may be caused by temporal heterogeneity in wall motion [14–24]. In the earliest efforts to assess temporal wall motion properties, regional wall motion analyses at several given time points in systole, e.g., early, middle, and late systole, were utilized. Some investigators found that early systolic parameters may improve sensitivity in detecting early discrete wall motion abnormalities in coronary artery disease [17–20, 24], while others could not confirm these results [32–34]. The reason for this descrepancy might be related to the difficulty in standardizing the time sequence of contraction due to the wide, individual variability [25, 26, 38]. Another important reason is the temporal characteristics of contraction in ischemic or infarcted myocardium. Wiegner et al. [29] analyzed the isolated muscle preparation and demonstrated that the pattern of shortening during hypoxia becomes polyphasic and heterogeneous. In intact dog hearts, Weyman et al. [16] have observed that during contraction the size of the dyskinetic area within infarct or ischemic zones varies with time. Although a tendency for the maximum of motion abnormalities occurred in the second quartile of the normalized contraction sequence, at most only ⅓ (34%) of all radii showed their maximal motion abnormality within any given decile. This fact suggested that no fixed temporal point in the contraction sequence can be arbitrarily selected that will consistently allow determination of the maximal degree of abnormal motion. Even in normal subjects there is some variability in onset of contraction, in the time sequence, and in spatial regional left ventricular contraction [25, 26]. The underlying mechanism may be complex. It may be related to the variability in electrical activity sequence or the geometric fiber orientation of the ventricle [25]. The ischemic and/or infarcted myocardium is unable to support high stress during early systole. The resulting temporal bulging of the infarcted region has actually an unloading effect for the normal regions of myocardium [28]. Furthermore, the motion of ischemic myocardium is complex and constantly changing because of persistent, polyphasic contractile activity of hypoxic muscle, because of elastic recoil of passive elements within the muscle [29], and because of the passive motion induced by contraction of surrounding areas [16]. All of these mechanisms may contribute to temporal heterogeneity in the infarct regions throughout systole.

Obviously, the human eye has the ability to integrate motion throughout systole. Therefore, an analogous quantitative system that also considers motion at sequential time points in the systolic contraction might provide a more effective means to differentiate ischemic wall motion abnormalities. Such a system is expected to be superior to a system based only on two time points arbitrarily selected [36]. Gillam et al. [36] have demonstrated that the chemohistological infarct size in the dog heart correlated highly with the extent of left ventricular dysfunction evaluated by the integrated method ($r = 0.87$); but only poor correlation was found between chemohistological infarct size and the extent of wall motion abnormalities determined by the conventional method considering motion only from two time points ($r = 0.35$). The same results have also been found in chronic myocardial infarction in the dog model [37]. The fact that failure to consider the entire systolic contraction characteristics may result in misinformation has challenged the precision of the conventional wall motion analysis at two time points (end-diastole and end-systole), especially in the fields of investigation.

Methods Integrating Temporal and Spatial Wall Motion Analysis

Harris et al. [35] were the first to use the integrated method for quantitation of temporal and spatial wall motion heterogeneity from left ventricular cineangiograms in acute myocardial infarction in dogs. More recently, Gillam et al. [36] adapted and modified this method for study of radial wall motion on short-axis echocardiograms in the dog acute myocardial infarction. The principle of the method from Harris et al. and Gillam et al. is to test how well the observed motion can be predicted from composite normal motion in systolic contraction sequence. The normal values of radial shortening fractions were obtained for each systolic sequential time point, which was averaged from all radii of various regions [35, 36]. However, it has been demonstrated that on right anterior oblique left ventricular cineangiograms, the normal onset of contraction and the segmental shortening at a given sequential time point are significantly different in various regions of the left ventricle [11, 23, 24, 38, 41]. If the averaged normal values of temporal shortening fractions are used to correlate observed radial values of temporal shortening fractions in various ventricular regions, large differences of r and b values in various radii should result, inducing large variability of the normal range, as shown in the study by Harris et al. [35] in dog left ventricle. Next, they correlated the observed shortening fractions at given time points to the normal shortening fractions at corresponding time points in systole [35, 36]. Since the ventriculography can only be recorded at limited time intervals (usually 16.7 ms or 20 ms), the correlation can only be taken at approximation or extrapolation of radial shortening at individual sequential time points, which is methodologically complicated and does not allow exact comparison.

To overcome these problems, we designed an essentially different and relatively simple analysis system for integrating temporal and spatial wall motion. The principle of our system is to test whether a linearity in temporal systolic shortening exists in a given radius observed. We simply correlate systolic temporal shortening fractions to corresponding normalized systolic sequential time points for each radius, giving r or b values for each individual radius of observed ventricle.

The correlation coefficient determined by our method describes whether linearity of radial shortening during systole can be observed in the left ventricle. The temporal homogeneous segmental contraction or linearity in sequential systolic radial shortening should have a correlation coefficient equal to 1; otherwise, in the case of temporal heterogeneous contraction the correlation coefficient should significantly deviate from 1.

In the present study, the normal ventricle had a high correlation coefficient with small standard deviation in all myocardial radii, indicating that there is near – linearity in sequential systolic radial shortening. Some deviation of the r value from 1 may be due to the minor temporal heterogeneity of contraction sequence during the preejection phase (60 ms) [26].

In the infarcted region of the human left ventricle, we have demonstrated that the correlation coefficients are low and frequently negative. The poor linear approximation of the motion of infarcted segments indicates significant temporal wall motion heterogeneity. These results agree with the animal experimental findings [35, 36], although the methods used are different.

The slope of the regression line b describes steepness of the systolic radial shortening and gives information about ventricular contractility. A high b value means hyperkinesis, a reduced b value hypokinesis, negative b value dyskinesis. However, in contrast to conventional wall motion analysis of superimposing contours of end-diastolic and end-systolic frames, the slope b describes temporally integrated shortening fractions during systole. Therefore, in cases of obvious radial motion heterogeneity (reduced r) b may yield results significantly different from the conventional two-frame method, as shown in Fig. 1. In the normal ventricle the radial shortening at end-systole relative to end-diastole was nearly equal to that calculated from the temporally integrated systolic shortening parameter of regression slope b (Fig. 1a); however, in the infarcted ventricle the radial shortening at end-systole relative to end-diastole was 44% (in normal range in our laboratory), obviously different from that of 27% (hypokinesis) calculated from b ($Y = b \cdot x$) (Fig. 1b).

Limitations of the Method Presented

The limitations of contrast ventriculography may naturally influence the present analysis. There is no consensus about an optimal reference system for quantitative analysis of segmental wall motion. Although some studies suggest that a radial coordinate system or the centerline method may be better for segmental wall motion analysis, available data do not establish the superiority of any reference system [4–14, 25, 38–42]. The rotation and translation of the heart during systole, as well as endocardial infolding in ventriculograms, cannot be completely overcome by any selected analyzing system. The motion we measured using a radial coordinate system may not correspond to the motion of actual anatomic segments. To make those measurements, the techniques involving endo- or epicardial implantation of radiopaque markers together with biplane fluoroscopy would be required. Fortunately, McDonald [42] compared the measurements obtained using epicardial radiomarkers with those obtained using contrast ventriculography in the same patients and found that in the RAO projection the results of both methods were fairly similar.

A trained observer needs approximately 15 min to trace the contours during systole at 40-ms intervals. This is relatively time-consuming and tedious, and analysis of the data without computer assistance is not practicable. Therefore, widespread application of the integrated method would be difficult. However, development of an efficient automatic edge-detecting system will make this analysis easily available.

Implications of Integrated Wall Motion Analysis

Some investigations suggest that temporal wall motion abnormality may be one of the earliest signs of the myocardial ischemic effects [17–20, 24]. It is expected that integrated wall motion analysis will improve detection of ischemic wall motion abnormalities. For this purpose, in our hospital studies are currently underway to compare sensitivity in detecting ischemic wall motion abnormalities as determined by the integrated method with those determined by the conventional two-frame method. At present, we know little about the significance of temporal wall motion abnormalities [15, 24]. It has been supposed that temporal wall motion heterogeneity makes overall systolic performance of the left ventricle less effective and that temporal region heterogeneous contraction could induce arrhythmia through the mechanical stretching of adjacent muscle cells [15]. The integrated method will make possible further investigation of these unanswered questions. Furthermore, the integrated method is also important for studies of effects of therapeutic interventions on temporal wall motion abnormalities.

Conclusion

In the present study we have described a new method integrating temporal and spatial wall motion of the left ventricle. The method was then used to study normal and infarcted ventricles in human beings. With the integrated method we have demonstrated for the first time that there is an almost temporal homogeneous systolic wall motion pattern of any given radius in the normal human left ventricle. Furthermore, our results agreed with the results of experimental animal studies that there is significant temporal and spatial wall motion heterogeneity in infarcted regions. Using the present method, these abnormalities could be quantitatively assessed with a high degree of temporal and spatial resolution.

References

1. Tennant R, Wiggers CJ (1935) The effect of coronary occlusion on myocardial contraction. Am J Physiol 112:351
2. Herman MV, Heinle RA, Klein MD, Gorlin R (1967) Localized disorders in myocardial contraction. Asynergy and its role in congestive heart failure. N Engl J Med 277:222
3. Heikkila J, Tabakin BS, Hugenholtz PG (1972) Quantification of function in normal and infarct regions of the left ventricle. Cardiovasc Res 6:516
4. Dumesnil JG, Ritman EL, Frye RL, Gan GT, Rutherford BD, Davis GD (1974) Quantitative determination of regional left ventricular wall dynamics by roentgen videometry. Circulation 50:700
5. Leighton RF, Wilt SM, Lewis RP (1974) Detection of hypokinesis by a quantitative analysis of left ventricular cineangiograms. Circulation 50:121
6. Dodge HT (1977) Angiographic evaluation of ventricular function. N Engl J Med 296:551
7. Rickards A, Seabra-Gomes R, Thurston P (1977) The assessment of regional abnormalities of the left ventricle by angiography. Eur J Cardiol 5:167
8. Gelberg HJ, Brundage BH, Glantz S, Parmley WW (1979) Quantitative left ventricular wall motion analysis. A comparison of area, cord, and radial method. Circulation 59:991
9. Ingels NB Jr, Daughters GT, Stinson EB, Alderman EL (1980) Evaluation of methods for quantitating left ventricular segmental wall motion in man using myocardial markers as a standard. Circulation 61:996

10. Sheehan FH, Mathey DG, Schofer J, Krebber H-J, Dodge HT (1983) Effect of interventions in salvaging left ventricular function in acute myocardial infarction: a study of intracoronary streptokinase. Circulation 52:431

11. Bonzel T, Tarnowska R, Wollschlaeger H, Zeiher A, Just H (1986) Quantitative regional wall motion analysis as assessed by biplane hemiaxial isocentric angiocardiography: normal values (submitted for publication. Cardiovascular and Interventional Radiology)

12. Bonzel T, Loellgen H, Just H (1984) Left ventricular wall motion analysis by conventional and hemiaxial biplane left ventricular angiography: choice of views. In: Sigwart U, Heintzen P (eds) Ventricular wall motion. Thieme, Stuttgart, p 43

13. Fuchs M, Behrenbeck W, Hombach V (1984) Die invasive Diagnostik der koronaren Herzkrankheit. In: Hombach V (ed) Kardiologie: Grundlagen – Fortschritte – Klinische Erfahrungen. Schattauer, Stuttgart, p 95

14. Marier DL, Gibson DG (1980) Limitations of two-frame method for displaying regional left ventricular wall motion in man. Br Heart J 44:553

15. Dodge HT, Stewart DK, Frimer M (1978) Implications of shape, stress, and wall dynamics in clinical heart disease. In: Fishman AP (ed) Heart failure. Hemisphere, Washington, p 43

16. Weyman AE, Franklin TD, Hogan RD, Gillam LD, Wiske PS, Newell J, Gibbons EF, Foale RA (1984) Importance of temporal heterogeneity in assessing the contraction abnormalities associated with acute myocardial ischemia. Circulation 70:102

17. Leighton RF, Pollack MEM, Welch TG (1981) Abnormal left ventricular wall motion at mid-ejection in patients with coronary heart diesease. Circulation 52:238

18. Johnson LL, Ellis K, Schmidt O, Weiss MB, Cannon PJ (1975) Volume injected in early systole, a sensitive index of left ventricular performance in coronary artery disease. Circulation 52:378

19. Gibson DG, Doran JH, Traill TA, Brown DJ (1978) Abnormal left ventricular wall movement during early systole in patients with angina pectoris. Br Heart J 40:758

20. Slutsky R, Karliner JS, Battler A, Peterson K, Ross J (1980) Comparison of early systolic and holosystolic ejection phase indexes by contrast ventriculography in patients with coronary artery disease. Circulation 61:1083

21. Hood WB, Covelli VH, Abelmann WH, Norman JC (1969) Persistence of contractile behaviour in acutely ischemic myocardium. Cardiovasc Res 3:249

22. Theroux P, Franklin D, Ross J, Kemper W (1974) Regional myocardial function during acute coronary artery occlusion and its modification by pharmarcologic agent in dog. Circulation 35:896

23. Franklin TD, Weyman AE, Egenes KM (1977) A closed-chest canine model for cross-sectional echocardiographic study. Am J Physiol 233:H417

24. Holman BL, Wynne J, Idoine J, Neill J (1980) Disruption in the temporal sequence of regional ventricular contraction: I. Characteristics and incidence in coronary artery disease. Circulation 61:1075

25. Klausner SC, Blair TJ, Bulawa WF, Jeppson GM, Jensen RL, Clayton PD (1982) Quantitative analysis of segmental wall motion throughout systole and diastole in the normal human left ventricle. Circulation 65:580

26. Clayton PD, Bulawa WF, Klausner SC, Urie PM, Marshall HW, Warner HR (1979) The characteristic sequence for the onset of contraction in the normal human left ventricle. Circulation 59:671

27. Wollschlaeger H, Bonzel T, Loellgen H, Just H (1984) Invasive Diagnostik: Neuere Entwicklungen der Koronarangiographie. Schweiz Med Wochenschr 114 [Suppl 16]: 17–22

28. Lewartowski B, Sedek G (1974) Mechanical performance of the left ventricle at early stage of experimental ischemia. Mechanism of shortening of ejection period. Cardiovasc Res 8:593

29. Wiegner AW, Allen GJ, Bing OHL (1978) Weak and strong myocardium in series; implications for segmental dysfunction. Am J Physiol 235:H776

30. Weisfeldt ML, Armstrong P, Scully HE, Sanders CA, Daggett WM (1974) Incomplete relaxation between beats after myocardial hypoxia and ischemia. J Clin Invest 53:1626

31. Gibson DG, Doran JH, Trail TA, Brown DJ (1978) Regional abnormalities of left ventricular wall motion during isovolumic relaxation in patients with ischemic heart disease. Eur J Cardiol 7:251

32. Jones AA, Goodyer AVN, Cohen LS, Langou RA (1980) Lack of sensitivity of the first third resting ejection fraction for identifying patients with coronary artery disease. Circulation 62 [Suppl III]:78

33. Kemper AJ, Bianco JA, Shulman RM, Folland ED, Parsi AF, Tow DE (1982) The interval ejection fraction: a cineventriculographic and radionuclide study. Circulation 64:1094

34. Sheehan FH, Dodge HT, Bolson EL, Hok-Wai W, Caputo GR, Stewart DK (1983) Value of partial ejection fraction, volume increment, and regional wall motion in identifying patients with clinically significant coronary artery disease. Circulation 68:756

35. Harris LD, Clayton PD, Marshall HW, Warner HR (1974) A technique for the detection of asynergistic motion in the left ventricle. Comput Biomed Res 7:380

36. Gillam LD, Hogan RD, Foale RA, Franklin TD, Newell JB, Guyer DE, Weyman AE (1984) A comparison of quantitative echocardiographic methods for delineating infarct-induced abnormal wall motion. Circulation 70:113

37. Gibbons EF, Hogan RD, Franklin TD, Nolting M, Weyman AE (1985) The natural history of regional dysfunction in a canine preparation of chronic infarction. Circulation 71:394

38. Sheehan FH, Stewart DK, Dodge HT, Mitten S, Bolson EL, Brown BG (1983) Variability in the measurement of regional left ventricular wall motion from contrast angiograms. Circulation 68:550

39. Brower RW, Meester GT (1976) Computer based methods for quantifying regional left ventricular wall motion from cine ventriculogram. Computers in Cardiology, IEEE Computer Society, Long Beach, p 55

40. Urie PM, Jensen RL, Clayton PD, Klausner SC, Marshall HW, Warner HR (1977) Comparison of methods for quantifying segmental wall motion (abstr). Circulation 56 [Suppl III]:III–238

41. Sigel H, Nechwatal W, Stauch M (1981) Quantitative regionale Lävangiographie: Vergleichende Untersuchungen an einem Normalkollektiv. Z Kardiol 70:221

42. McDonald IG (1970) The shape and movements of the human left ventricle during systole: a study by cineangiography and by cineraiography of epicardial markers. Am J Cardiol 26:221

Assessment of Ventricular Muscle Function in Man: The End-Systolic Index

J. F. Spann, B. A. Carabello, B. S. Denenberg, R. M. Donner,
A. K. Gash, A. H. Maurer, J. A. Siegel, and L. S. Malmud

Section of Cardiology, Department of Medicine and Department of Nuclear Medicine,
Temple University Health Sciences Center, Philadelphia, Pennsylvania, USA

Introduction

Accurate assessment of ventricular muscle contractile function is clinically important, but difficult to achieve. Cardiac muscle function before valve replacement [1–7] and before coronary surgery [1, 2, 8–10] is a major determinant of outcome. Selection of appropriate medical therapy for other forms of cardiac disease depends upon knowledge of ventricular muscle contractile function. Full assessment of new cardiac drugs also requires determination of the drugs' effects on cardiac muscle. Unfortunately, accurate assessment of ventricular muscle contractile function in heart disease is impaired by the alterations in afterload, preload, and wall thickness which often accompany disease. Thus, standard ejection phase indices of contractile function which have been used extensively can be misleading. For example, a disease which increases afterload may artificially lower ventricular ejection fraction, while a disease which either lowers afterload or increases preload may artificially elevate the ejection fraction and thus obscure a true reduction of contractile function. The relationship between pressure and volume at end-systole is thought to provide a contractile index which is independent of preload and which accounts for afterload. We have recently used the relationship of end-systolic stress to end-systolic volume index to assess ventricular muscle contractile function in several disease states where preload, afterload, wall thickness, and pump function may be abnormal. This technique of assessing ventricular contractile performance appears clinically useful and it is now possible to acquire the needed measurements of end-systolic pressure, thickness, and volume using several available techniques.

Effects of Loading Conditions on Ejection Phase Indices of Ventricular Muscle Contractile Function

Several intrinsic characteristics of cardiac muscle underlie the alterations of ejection performance by loading conditions. For example, there is an inverse relationship of both velocity and extent of shortening with increasing load [11]. This principle, of course, underlies the well-known force-velocity relationship of isolated papillary muscle. As resting cardiac muscle is lengthened by increasing preload, an increased number of active sites are allowed to interact and length-dependent activation occurs [12–18]. This basic characteristic, of course, dictates an increasing systolic force generated from increased diastolic lengths on the ascending limb of the Frank-Starling relationship. These properties of cardiac muscle extend to the intact ventricle.

Unfortunately, accurate assessment of classic muscle mechanics such as force-velocity or Frank-Starling relationships has been difficult to achieve in the intact ventricle of man. Instead, ejection phase indices, e.g., ejection fraction and Vcf, have been applied in man to assess contractile function. These indices rely upon detection of the extent and velocity of ventricular systolic shortening. Like isolated cardiac muscle, the extent and velocity of systolic shortening of the intact ventricle is dependent on preload and afterload. This may cause inaccurate assessment of contractile function in those diseases where preload and afterload are markedly altered. For example, in mitral regurgitation there is both increased preload and decreased afterload [19]. These altered loading conditions artificially elevate the ejection phase indices and thus obscure a true reduction in cardiac muscle contractile performance [20, 21]. Myocardial wall tension, an expression of afterload, is determined as the product of ventricular pressure and radius. Since mitral regurgitation diminishes ventricular pressure and radius more rapidly than normal during systole as blood flows into the atrium, left ventricular afterload falls more rapidly than normal during systole [19, 22] (Fig. 1). End-diastolic volume, an estimation of preload, is elevated to greater than twice normal in mitral regurgitation [23]. The increased preload and decreased afterload artificially increase ejection fraction. Immediately following mitral valve replacement for regurgitation, ejection fraction declines (Fig. 2). No change in myocardial function is thought to have occured. Instead, afterload suddenly increases (Fig. 3) as the run-off into the low resistance left atrium is abolished. Thus, in this instance, a change in ejection fraction does not reflect a change in contractile function. Further, a normal ejection fraction may conceal depressed muscle function in mitral regurgitation [20].

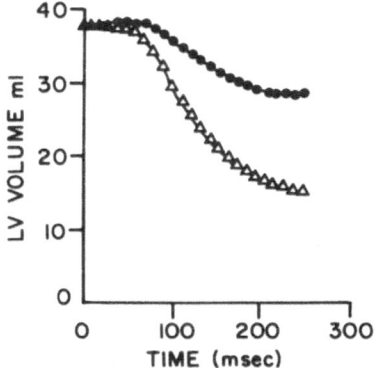

Fig. 1. Effects of acute mitral regurgitation on left ventricular mechanics. The *upper left hand panel* demonstrates that left ventricular pressure is lower throughout the last two-thirds of systole during mitral regurgitation. The *upper right hand panel* demonstrates a similar relationship for left ventricular wall tension or stress. The *bottom panel* demonstrates more complete left ventricular emptying which occurs during mitral regurgitation as a result of lowered afterload. (Modified from [19], with permission)

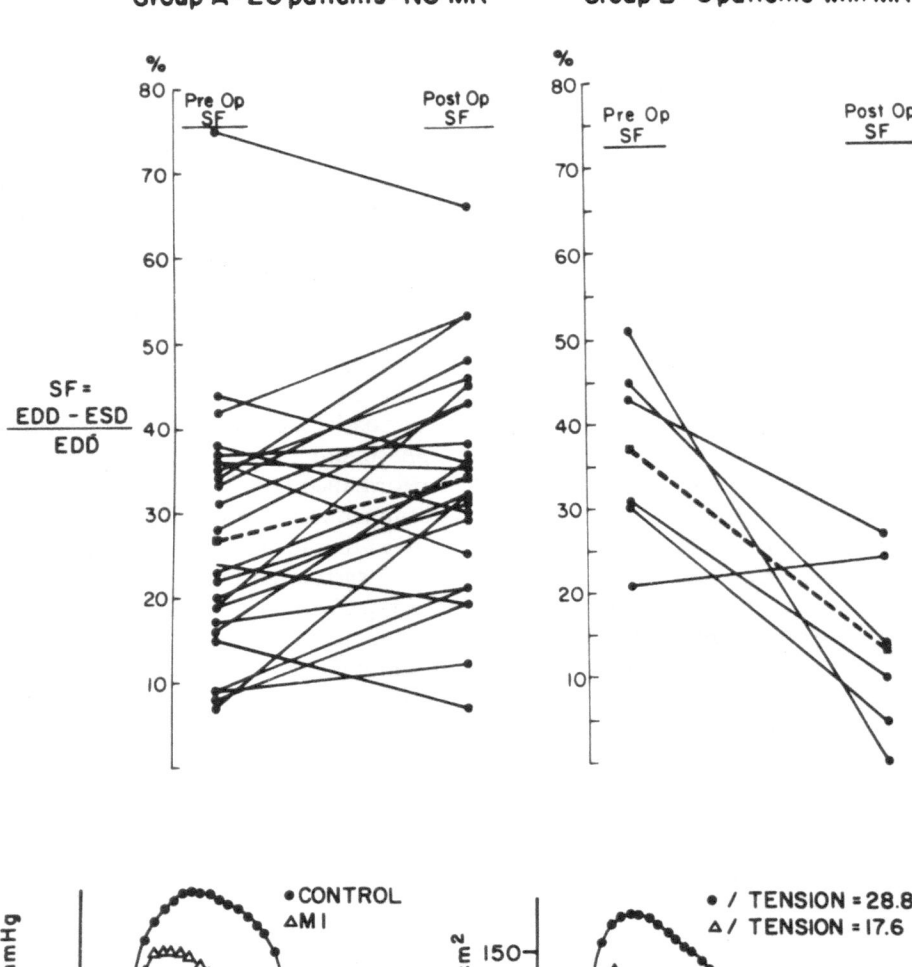

Fig. 2. Effect of surgery on shortening fraction. The *left hand panel* demonstrates that patients without mitral regurgitation had no appreciable change in ejection shortening postoperatively. On the other hand, the *right hand panel* demonstrates that the imposition of a competent mitral valve in patients with mitral regurgitation caused a fall in left ventricular shortening fraction. This occurs as the competent prosthetic mitral valve diminishes left ventricular preload and increases left ventricular afterload from preoperative conditions. (From [21], with permission)

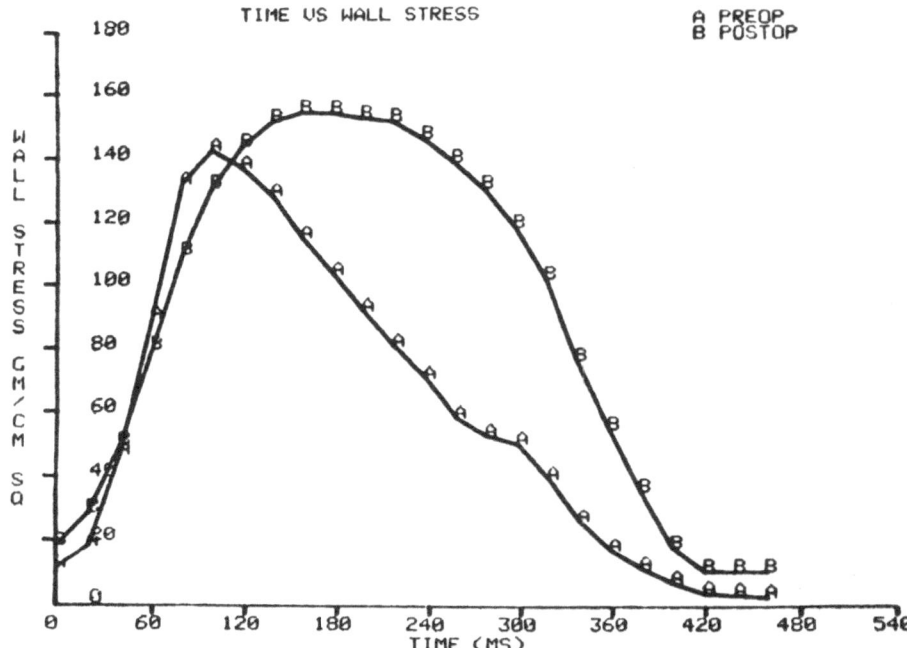

Fig. 3. Systolic wall tension preoperatively (*A*) and postoperatively (*B*) in patients undergoing mitral valve replacement for mitral regurgitations. Note that postoperatively there is a large increase in wall stress of afterload due to the presence of a competent mitral valve which prevents unloading into the left atrium. From [21], with permission)

End-Systolic Stress-Volume Relationships

The recently described relationship between end-systolic ventricular pressure and volume is an index of myocardial contractile function which is independent of preload and is a linear function of afterload [24–32].

This relationship is based on a fundamental property of cardiac muscle. Abbott and Wilkie found that the length tension curves of frog sartorius muscles were identical whether derived from isometric or isotonic studies [33]. From these data it was deduced that the state of the muscle at the end of its contraction was dependent only upon its length and contractile state at the end of contraction. It was not dependent upon its initial length. Wilkie stated "put in more general terms, this means that when the shortening velocity of the contractile component is zero (i. e., when tension rise and shortening have reached their maximum) the tension in the muscle is a function of its length only; it does not depend, for example, on initial conditions or on the route taken to reach final equilibrium" [34]. Working with isolated cardiac muscle, Downing and Sonnenblick reported that all end-systolic force-length points were on a single curve [35]. They concluded that the end systolic force-length relationship was an indication of the contractile state of heart muscle. The force generated at an

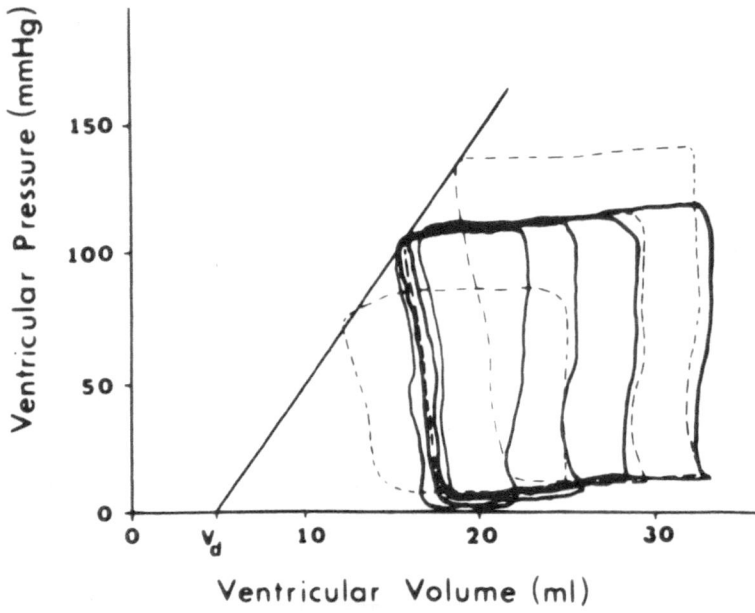

Fig. 4. Pressure-volume relationship of a beating canine ventricle. Note that while left ventricular end-systolic pressure is held constant, end-systolic volume is also constant. Ventricular contractions are initiated from a wide range of end-diastolic volumes which did not effect the end-systolic pressure-volume relationship. From Suga [24], with permission)

instantaneous length of heart muscle is dependent only on that length and the contractile state. It fellows, therefore, that if one knows muscle length and force at end-systole one can deduce the contractile state. This is true in the isolated and intact animal ventricle [24, 28, 30] and in the human ventricle [29, 36].

Figure 4 demonstrates the preload independence of the end-systolic pressure-volume relationship. In these experiments by Suga and Sagawa [24] systolic pressure was held constant while preload was varied. A separate pressure-volume loop is shown for each contraction. Notice that no matter from what end-diastolic volume the beat originates, the same points of ventricular volume and pressure are reached at end-systole. In another set of experiments (Fig. 5) both preload and afterload were varied in ejecting beats [32]. Again, the pressure volume loops are plotted for each of the four contractions. Notice that all points reached by the ventricle at end-systole lie along the same relatively straight line. At higher pressures the ventricle completed its systolic ejection at a higher point along this line. At lower pressures the ventricle was able to eject a greater volume, but again ended its systolic ejection at a point on the line. Thus, neither changes in preload nor afterload changed the slope of this line as long as the contractile state remained constant. The slope of the line is an expression of the contractile state. Thus, when the contractile state was increased by iso-proterenol or norepinephrine (Fig. 6) the slope of this relationship is changed.

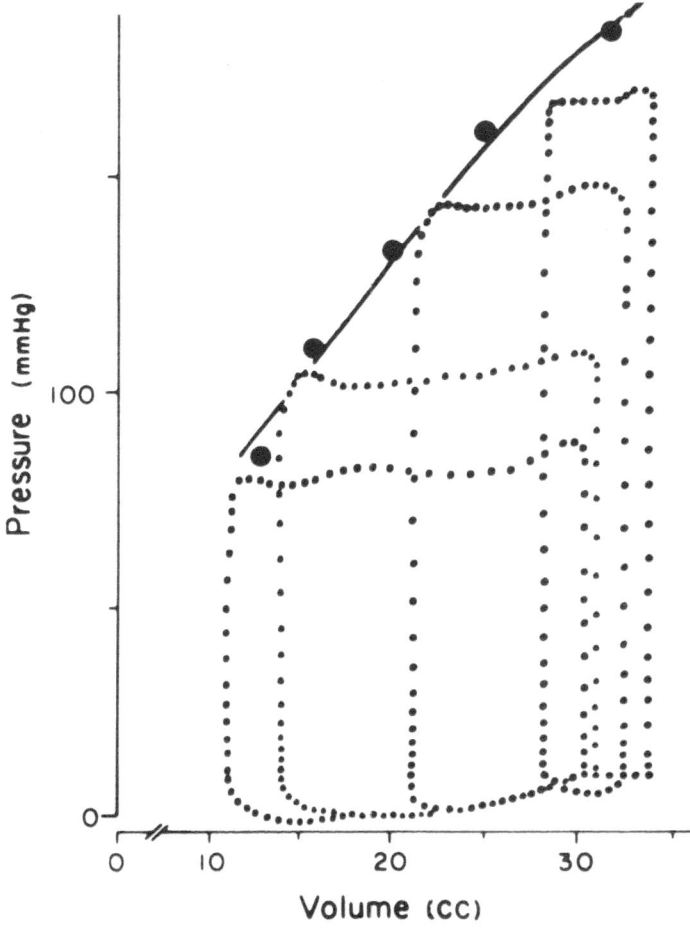

Fig. 5. Pressure-volume relationship of a beating canine ventricle taken at different end-systolic pressures. Note that as end-systolic pressure increases, end-systolic volume increases linearly, as the ventricle shortens progressively less and less against the greater pressure load. The slope of the dark line connecting these end-systolic pressure-volume points is an expression of contractility. (From [32], with permission)

An increase in the slope of the line relating various end-systolic pressures to volume represents an increase in contractile state. At given impedence to emptying (afterload), the ventricle is able to empty more fully and to a smaller volume. One can determine the contractile state of ventricular cardiac muscle by determining the slope of this relationship relating end-systolic pressure to volume. Further, if one assumes that the line goes through or near the zero origin, the slope of the line can be indicated by the simple ratio of end-systolic pressure over end-systolic volume. This ratio could be referred to as the end-systolic index (ESS/ESVI). Wall stress, which takes into account the distribution

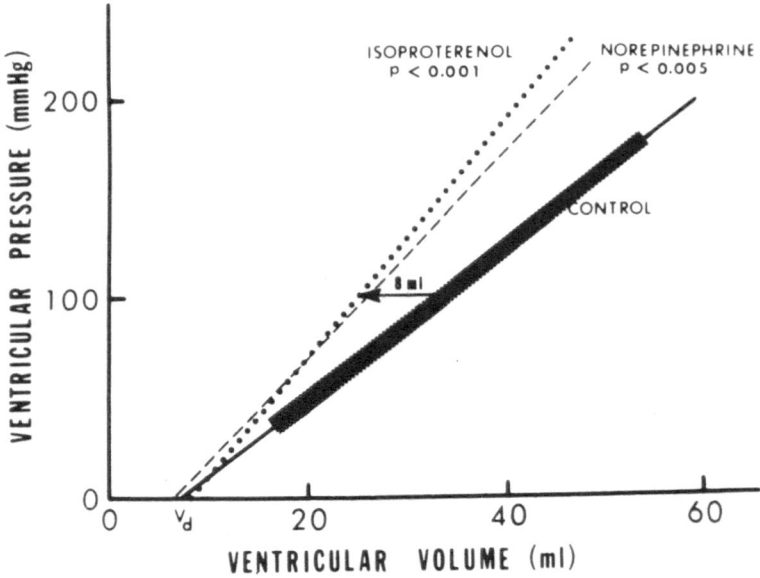

Fig. 6. Pressure-volume relationship in the canine ventricle at rest (*heavy black line*). Note that with the infusion of inotropic agents such as norepinephrine (*dashed line*) or isoproterenol (*dotted line*) the pressure-volume relationship is shifted upward and to the left. The steeper slope obtained with these agents indicates increased contractile function. (From [30], with permission)

of ventricular pressure over the radius and thickness of the ventricle, may be a more precise measure of afterload than is pressure alone. It is substituted by some investigators for pressure in the above-described pressure-volume relationship. According to Mirsky [37]

$$\text{wall stress} = \frac{P \cdot b}{h} \cdot \left\{ 1 - \frac{b}{2h} - \frac{b^2}{2a^2} \right\}$$

where P is the ventricular pressure, b is the ventricular semiminor axis ($\frac{D+h}{2}$), h is the wall thickness, and a is the semimajor axis ($\frac{L+h}{2}$).

Several practical clinical methods are available to obtain the end-systolic stress-end-systolic volume relationship. In order to obtain this relationship, one must obtain left ventricular end-systolic pressure, thickness, and dimension or volume. The four currently available methods for procuring these measurements include angiography, echocardiography, gated blood pool scanning, and digital subtraction angiography. Each has its own specific advantages and disadvantages. Standard angiographic methods can accurately define left ventricular pressure and wall thickness. However, these techniques tend to overestimate volumes and require geometric assumptions in their calculations. Another disadvantage of the standard angiographic approach is that multiple injections of large doses of radiographic contrast used to obtain multiple points at different loading conditions may be clinically hazardous in patients with cardiac problems. Echocardiography, when coupled with sphygmomanometry is a wholly noninvasive way of obtaining the end-systolic index. It also has advantages and limitations. Its noninvasive character is an obvious advantage. Furthermore, multiple measurements at different loading conditions allow one to plot the line relating various end-systolic volumes to various end-systolic pressures or stresses. Real time (2D) echo can also exclude regional wall disease which might produce inaccurate measurement made using M-mode echocardiography. A limitation is that adequate imaging is possible in only 70% of patients. Furthermore, extreme care is required to assure that measurements made at different times are obtained from the same spot in the ventricle. Nuclear methods share the advantage of echocardiography by being noninvasive. A potentially important advantage of the nuclear technique over echocardiography or angiocardiography is that no geometric assumptions are required to make volumetric measurements. Unfortunately, up to now it has not been possible to determine absolute volume using nuclear technique due to inability to account for isotope attenuation.

A new method for determining absolute ventricular volume has been developed by Maurer and colleagues at our institution [38]. An orally administered gelatin capsule containing technetium-99 is used for this purpose. Serial images are obtained in a left anterior oblique projection as the capsule transits the esophagus. An average transmission factor is then determined by dividing the capsule rate count in the region of the left ventricle by the capsule count recorded behind a phantom prior to administration. Thus, experimentally measured transmission factors are directly determined for each patient. The patient is kept in the sampe position and the patient's red blood cells are then labeled by administering an intravenous injection of 16–20 microcuries of technetium-99 sodium pertectnatate after prior administration of stannous pyrophosphate. Routine gated blood pool images are then obtained. Next, a 10-ml venous blood sample is drawn and counted by the same scintillation camera used to obtain the gated blood pool image. The absolute left ventricular volumes are then calculated by dividing the background corrected ventricular count rate by the appropriate transmission factor and the count rate obtained from the venous blood sample:

$$\text{VOLUME} = \frac{\text{net LV counts/s}}{\text{blood counts/cc/s} \times T}$$

where $T = e^{-\mu d}$ = the transmission factor = $\frac{\text{capsule counts in LV}}{\text{capsule counts behind the phantom}}$.

When these absolute end-systolic volumes are compared with angiographic volumes, an excellent correlation was obtained ($r = 0.91$).

Studies in our laboratory have demonstrated that end-systolic pressure can also be determined noninvasively using sphygmomanometry. We have determined the regression equation for the relationship of end-systolic pressure to peak systolic pressure (ESP = 0.66 PSP + 13; $r = 0.88$).

Digital subtraction angiography has certain advantages for measurement of end-systolic volume index. It can be accomplished with a small intraventricular injection of contrast. Thus, multiple 10-cc intraventricular injections providing left ventricular imaging can be accomplished to allow end-systolic pressure volume relationships to be examined with multiple loading conditions. Wall thickness is easily seen with this technique.

Unfortunately, we have little experience with this technique at present. It requires special equipment, depends upon geometric assumptions, and apparently the ventricular volume measurement can be affected by the technique settings used for the subtraction images.

Clinical Use of the End-Systolic Index

We have recently utilized the principles outlined above to study a number of clinical conditions. The techniques have proven useful both in invasive and noninvasive studies. Frequently, assessment of ventricular contractile state with a technique which is independent of preload and afterload has provided new understanding of these diseases. We examined ventricular performance in

a) 11 adult patients with severe aortic stenosis and congestive heart failure symptoms (AS-CHF group),

b) 10 patients with significant aortic stenosis but no heart failure symptoms (AS-C group), and

c) 12 normal subjects [39].

Determination of the end-systolic stress and end-systolic ventricular volume at the naturally occuring variations among the patients in each group provided data for calculation of a linear regression line for each group. These linear regression lines were then used as estimates of the end-systolic stress-volume relationship for each group and is shown as a sloping line in Fig. 7. The groups were compared statistically using nonpaired t-tests where variance of the slope was calculated in a standard fashion. A significant reduction ($P < 0.01$) in the slope of this estimate of the end-systolic index was found in the AS-CHF group (0.9 ± 0.5) compared with both the normal (5.8 ± 1.3) and AS-C groups (3.9 ± 1.3). Although the AS-C group had a lower slope than normal, the difference

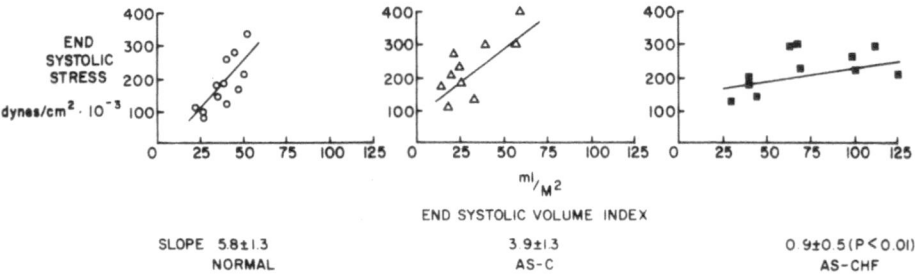

Fig. 7. End-systolic stress-end-systolic volume index relationship of normals (*open circles*), patients with compensated aortic stenosis (*open triangles*), and patients with aortic stenosis and congestive heart failure (*solid squares*). Note that the slope of the end-systolic stress-volume relationship in aortic stenosis patients with congestive heart failure is markedly reduced. This indicates diminished contractility in this group of patients despite the fact that most had normal ejection fractions. (From [38], with permission)

was not statistically significant. Conversely, the average ejection fraction is not significantly altered in AS-C patients (0.67 ± 0.03) or AS-CHF patients (0.53 ± 0.04) compared with normal (0.63 ± 0.03). Ejection fraction was greater than 0.50, the lower limit of normal in our laboratory, in each normal and AS-C patient, and in eight of the eleven AS-CHF patients. This study suggests that contractile function estimated by group end-systolic stress-volume relationships is reduced in patients with severe aortic stenosis and congestive heart failure. Further, contractile function appears relatively normal in patients with significant but less severe aortic stenosis but without heart failure. These techniques also have limitations. Naturally occurring variations in end-systolic stress and end-systolic volume within each group of patients were used to calculate linear regression lines and served as estimates of the end-systolic index lines for each group. These relationships would have been better defined if each heart had been manipulated through a range of volumes and individual curves had been obtained. Such manipulation and the necessary multiple ventriculograms were not considered safe in patients with aortic stenosis.

The ratio of end-systolic wall stress to end-systolic volume index (ESS/ESVI) was recently examined in normal individuals and in 21 patients with symptomatic chronic severe mitral regurgitation [20]. No patient had other valvular disease or coronary artery disease. Various hemodynamic and angiographic determinants were examined to see which might be prognostic of surgical outcome following mitral valve replacement. Sixteen patients were in New York Heart Association functional class I or II postoperatively and formed group A. One patient remained in class 3 postoperatively and four patients died perioperatively; they constitute group B. The end-systolic index (ESS/ESVI) was significantly lower in both groups of patients with mitral regurgitation than in normal persons, suggesting left ventricular dysfunction. The end-systolic index in group B (2.2 ± 0.2) (open circles) was significantly less than in group A

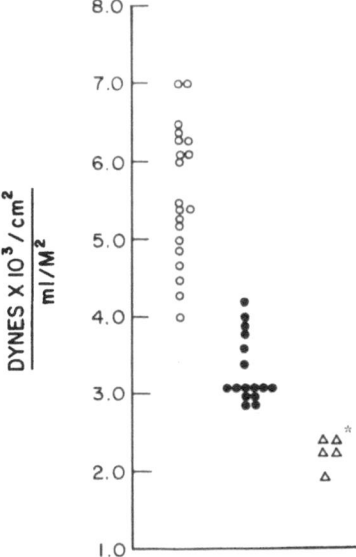

Fig. 8. End-systolic stress-end-systolic volume index for normal patients (*open circles*), patients with mitral regurgitation who had a satisfactory surgical result, group A (*solid circles*), and patients with mitral regurgitation who had an unsatisfactory surgical result, group B (*open triangles*). The end-systolic index in patients with mitral regurgitation and a good result was depressed compared with normals. The end-systolic index was even more depressed in those patients with a poor result. The *asterisk* marks a patient with a poor result who had an ejection fraction of 80% during intraaortic balloon pumping preoperatively. In mitral regurgitation the end-systolic index provided separation of patients with a good and poor surgical result. (From [20], with permission)

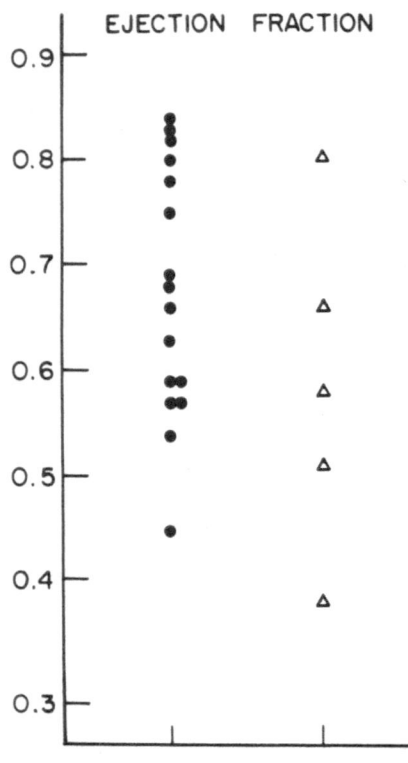

Fig. 9. Ejection fraction in patients with mitral regurgitation who had a good surgical result (*solid circles*) is shown together with patients who had a poor surgical result (*open triangles*). Note that there is great overlap between the two groups. Ejection fraction was normal in most patients who had a poor result as well as most patients who had a good result. (From [20], with permission)

$(3.3 \pm 0.4; P < 0.001)$ (solid circles) (Fig. 8). The variables of age, pulmonary capillary wedge pressure, end-diastolic volume index, end-systolic volume index, ejection fraction, and the end-systolic index (ESS/ESVI) were subjected to stepwise discriminant multivariant analysis to determine if any were independent predictors of outcome. The only independent predictor determined by this method was the end-systolic index (ESS/ESVI) $(P < 0.001)$. One can see in Fig. 9 that there was extensive overlap between the normal and two groups of patients with mitral regurgitation when ejection fractions were compared. Conversely, in Fig. 8, one can see that the end-systolic index overlapped with normal in only two patients with mitral insufficiency. Five patients who either died or had persistent severe symptoms following mitral valve replacement were clearly separated from the patients with mitral regurgitation who had a good result. We conclude that the end-systolic index (ESS/ESVI) may be helpful in evaluating left ventricular function and operative risk in patients with chronic, symptomatic mitral regurgitation. This end-systolic index appeared to be a better predictor of outcome than any of the other hemodynamic findings.

Osbakken and colleagues in our laboratory have recently examined left ventricular muscle and pump performance in 12 normal subjects and 21 patients with aortic regurgitation (10 with minimal symptoms, and 11 with congestive heart failure [40]. Angiographically determined cardiac index was increased in both groups of patients with aortic regurgitation. Ejection fraction was signifi-

AORTIC INSUFFIENCY

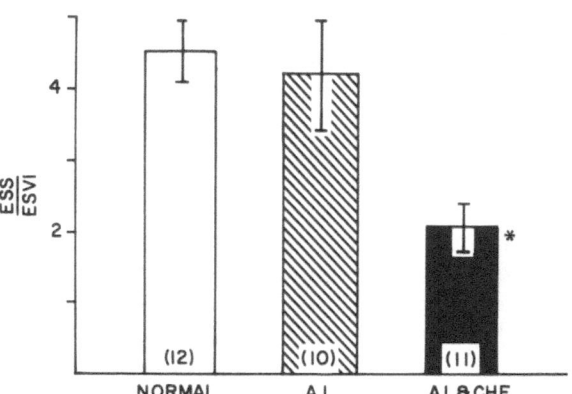

Fig. 10. End-systolic index for normal patients, patients with compensated aortic insufficiency, and patients with aortic insufficiency and congestive heart failure. The depressed end-systolic index in patients with aortic insufficiency and congestive heart failure is indicative of depressed contractile function in this group

cantly decreased in the group with heart failure. Contractile function measured by the end systolic index (ESS/ESVI) was also significantly reduced in patients with aortic insufficiency and congestive heart failure (Fig. 10).

Chakko et al. in our laboratory have very recently utilized the end-systolic stress-volume relationship to examine ventricular contractile function in two groups of patients with systemic hypertension [41]. One group of hypertensives had congestive heart failure, while a second group was free of heart failure. No patient in the study had evidence of coronary artery disease. Arterial pressure and echocardiographic left ventricular volume were measured first in the resting state, then with the legs raised, then during systemic arterial pressure increased by handgrip and then during pressure and volume decrease by amyl nitrate inhalation. End-systolic ventricular wall stress was plotted against end-systolic volume index in each of the four states in each patient. This allowed the determination of the slope of the relationship between left ventricular stress and volume at end-systole for each patient. This end-systolic index was significantly depressed in the patients with systemic hypertension complicated by congestive heart failure, but it was normal in those patients with hypertension but no congestive heart failure. Peak systolic wall stress and ejection fraction were normal in both groups of hypertensive patients. End-diastolic volume was more than doubled when heart failure complicated hypertension. We interpreted these data as indicating that in systemic hypertension, left ventricular function is initially normal. Hypertrophy initially corrects wall stress and pump function is initially maintained without increased preload or heart failure symptoms. However, left ventricular muscle function eventually becomes depressed despite the apparently adequate hypertrophy. Pump function is maintained by increased end-diastolic volume and heart failure symptoms result. Once again, the end-systolic stress-volume relationship provided assessment of ventricular contractile function in a situation where both preload and afterload have been altered by the disease process.

Systolic left ventricular performance in mitral stenosis has been controversial. Potential alterations in preload and afterload in mitral stenosis may have complex effects on left ventricular pump and muscle performance. At the time of cardiac catheterization and left ventriculography, we determined ejection indices consisting of ejection fraction, stroke-work index, and circumferential fiber shortening velocity [42]. We also estimated preload by determining end-diastolic volume index and afterload by measuring end-systolic stress. Muscle contractile function was evaluated by determining the end-systolic index (ESS/ESVI). Nine normal patients and 16 patients with pure mitral stenosis with an average valve area of 0.9 cm^2 who were free of coronary disease were studied. End-diastolic volume index, stroke volume index, circumferential fiber shortening rate, and stroke-work index were higher in normals than in patients with mitral stenosis. The end-systolic index (ESS/ESVI) was 4.87 ± 0.53 in normal individuals and 5.28 ± 0.53 (NS) in the patients with mitral stenosis. Four of five patients with mitral stenosis and an ejection fraction below a limit of normal for our laboratory (0.50) and six of the six patients with mitral stenosis with a reduced circumferential fiber shortening rate had end-systolic indices (ESS/ESVI) within the normal range. Mitral stenosis patients with low ejection fractions and low circumferential fiber shortening rates had a higher end-systolic stress than mitral stenosis patients with normal ejection fractions or circumferential fiber shortening rate. Ventricular thickness was lower in mitral stenosis patients with high end-systolic stress.

We conclude that left ventricular systolic muscle performance is usually normal in mitral stenosis. Reductions in pump function can be explained by low preload and occasionally by high afterload which appears to be due to decreased wall thickness. Once again, utilization of the end-systolic index allowed evaluation of ventricular muscle function in a situation where ejection phase indices indicated abnormal function. However, on further examination, changes in loading conditions had altered the ejection phase indices.

Left ventricular performance has been controversial in patients with atrial septal defects and congestive heart failure. We recently studied 18 patients with large atrial septal defects [43]. Twelve of these patients were asymptomatic (group A), while six had symptoms of left ventricular heart failure (group B). Group B had higher left ventricular end diastolic pressure, mean right atrial pressure, and mean pulmonary artery pressure than group A. There was no significant difference in cardiac index or stroke index between the groups. Two ejection phase indices and the end-systolic index of contractile function are shown in Table 1. No difference in these measures of contractile and pump performance was found. We conclude from this investigation that patients with

Table 1. Two ejection phase indices and the end-systolic index of contractile function

	Normals	Group A	Group B	P
LV ejection fraction	0.74 ± 0.01	0.74 ± 0.02	0.71 ± 0.05	NS
LV-VcF (cps)	1.27 ± 0.04	1.30 ± 0.07	1.38 ± 0.14	NS
LV-ESS/ESVI	5.6 ± 0.19	6.1 ± 0.05	6.0 ± 0.06	NS

large atrial septal defects and congestive heart failure have normal left ventricular systolic function. It can be suggested that impairment of diastolic compliance or effects of the enlarged right ventricle may be responsible for the elevated left ventricular filling pressure seen in this group of patients. In this study, the end-systolic index was concordant with two ejection phase indices of ventricular performance and served to further document normal left ventricular muscle function.

Children with severe aortic stenosis are known to have supranormal ejection performance. This observation has been somewhat puzzling. Parameters of left ventricular function were examined in ten children (average age 10 ± 3.2 years) with severe aortic stenosis and eight normal children [44]. All children were studied at the time of cardiac catheterization with left ventricular contrast injection. The average peak left ventricular aortic gradient was 89 ± 33 mmHg in the children with aortic stenosis. Ejection fraction was greater in children with aortic stenosis and averaged 0.78 ± 0.04 compared with the normal value of 0.62 ± 0.05 ($P < 0.01$). The velocity of fiber shortening was significantly increased in the children with aortic stenosis averaging 1.8 ± 0.22 cps compared with the value of normal children of 1.09 ± 0.13 ($P < 0.001$).

End-systolic volume index was less in aortic stenosis, averaging 14.9 ml/m^2 compared with the normal value of 31 ± 7 ($P < 0.001$). End-systolic wall stress was less in aortic stenosis averaging $60 \pm 25 \times 10^3$ dynes/cm^2 than the value in normal children, which averaged 125 ± 40 ($P < 0.01$). The end-systolic index (ESS/ESVI) was similar in the children with aortic stenosis where it averaged 4.7 ± 1.4 to the normal value which was 4.0 ± 0.8. We conclude that in children with severe aortic stenosis, the increased wall thickness, produced lower than normal wall stress. This combined with normal cardiac muscle function to produce the lower than normal end-systolic volume and supranormal ejection performance observed in our studies and by others in these children. This study once again represents an example of alteration in loading conditions which altered ejection phase indices. In this case they gave a false impression of supranormal ventricular contractile function. The end-systolic index, however, showed normal muscle function and the extreme reduction in ventricular systolic loading provided the explanation for increased ejection performance.

Ventricular dysfunction has been suspected to underlie congestive heart failure in sickle cell anemia. However, ejection indices of left ventricular pump performance have been demonstrated to be normal in the past [45]. The increased preload and decreased afterload of sickle cell anemia would be expected to increase the ejection phase indices and might obscure true left ventricular dysfunction. Therefore, we compared the preload and afterload independent end-systolic index of left ventricular contractile function in six adults (average age 31 ± 7 years) with sickle cell anemia without other disease and in seven normals [46]. Similar measurements were made in five children (average age 12 ± 4 years) with sickle cell anemia and in four normal children. All sickle cell anemia patients had pulmonary venous congestion, three had overt congestive heart failure, and one had pulmonary edema. End-systolic pressure and echocardiographic left ventricular dimensions were determined during rest, leg raise, hand-grip, and amyl nitrate inhalation. End-systolic ventricular wall stress was plotted against end-systolic volume index in each of the four states in each patient. This allowed determination of the slope of the relationship between left ventricular stress and volume at end systole in each patient. Cardiac index was significantly increased to a value of 70% above normal in the patients with sickle cell anemia. The ejection fraction was normal in sickle cell anemia patients. There were striking changes in ventricular loading conditions. Afterload as measured by systemic vascular resistance was reduced significantly to 60% of normal in the sickle cell anemia patients. Preload was increased in sickle cell anemia patients who had an end-diastolic volume index which was significantly increased to 140% of normal in sickle cell anemia patients. Ventricular contractile function was severely depressed in sickle cell anemia patients. The end-systolic index was significantly reduced to 55% of normal in sickle cell anemia patients. The slope of the relationship between end-systolic stress and end-systolic volume index was also significantly depressed to a value of approximately one-half of normal in the sickle cell anemia patients. The decreased slope of the end-systolic stress volume relationship and the decreased end-systolic index demonstrates the left ventricular dysfunction present in sickle cell anemia.

We conclude that intrinsic left ventricular muscle contractile performance is severely depressed in sickle cell anemia. Increased preload and decreased afterload compensate for the left ventricular dysfunction and maintain a normal ejection fraction and a high cardiac output. These compensations account for the previous misconception that the heart muscle is normal in sickle cell anemia.

Summary and Conclusion

We conclude that determination of the slope of the line relating end-systolic stress and end-systolic volume index and determination of the end-systolic index (ESS/ESVI) are effective new techniques which allow assessment of ventricular contractile performance in diseases where preload, afterload, and wall thickness are abnormal and thus confound other measurements of ventricular contractile performance. This more accurate assessment of contractile function has proved useful in advancing our understanding of the effects of various desease states on cardiac muscle. The ability to obtain this index easily and from a variety of different imaging techniques should make it a clinically useful tool. It should have efficacy in evaluating patients for surgery, assessing prognosis, and in determining the effects of various therapeutic modalities on pump and muscle function.

Acknowledgement. The authors would like to express their appreciation to Maxine Blob for typing the manuscript.

References

1. Cohn PF, Gorlin R, Cohn LH, et al. (1974) Left ventricular ejection fraction as a prognostic indicator guide in surgical treatment of coronary and valvular heart disease. Am J Cardiol 34:136–141
2. Singh R, Green W, McGuire LB (1974) Left ventricular ejection fraction and results of cardiac surgery. Cardiology 59:342–349
3. Kennedy JW, Doces JG, Stewart DK (1979) Left ventricular function before and following surgical treatment of mitral valve disease. Am Heart J 97:592–598
4. Carabello BA, Green LH, Grossmann W, Cohn LH, Koster JK, Collins JJ Jr (1980) Hemodynamic determinants of prognosis of aortic valve replacement in critical aortic stenosis and advanced congestive heart failure. Circulation 62:42–48
5. Huber D, Grimm J, Koch R, Krayenbuehl HP (1981) Determinants of ejection performance in aortic stenosis. Circulation 64:126–134
6. Henry WL, Bonow RO, Borer JS et al. (1980) Observations on the optimum time for operative intervention for aortic regurgitation. I. Evaluation of the results of aortic valve replacement in symptomatic patients. Circulation 61:471–482
7. Henry WL, Bonow RO, Rosing DR, Epstein SE (1980) Observations on the optimum time for operative intervention for aortic regurgitation. II. Serial echocardiographic evaluation of asymptomatic patients. Circulation 61:484–492
8. Hammermeister KE, Kennedy JW (1974) Predictors of surgical mortality in patients undergoing direct myocardial revascularization. Circulation [Supp II]:112–115
9. Moraski RE, Russell RO Jr, Smith M, Rackley CE (1975) Left ventricular function in patients with and without myocardial infarction and one, two or three vessel coronary artery disease. Am J Cardiol 30:1–10
10. Cohn PF, Gorlin R, Herman MV et al. (1975) Relationship between contractile reserve and prognosis in patients with coronary artery disease and a depressed ejection fraction. Circulation 51:414–420
11. Sonnenblick EH (1962) Force-velocity relations in mammalian heart muscle. Am J Physiol 202:931–939
12. Frank O (1959) On the dynamics of cardiac muscle. Am Heart J 58:282–317, 467–478
13. Starling EH (1918) Linacre Lecture on the Law of the Heart (1915). Longmans, Green, London
14. Sonnenblick EH, Spiro D, Cottrell JS (1963) Fine structural changes in heart muscle in relation to the length-tension curve. Proc Nat Acad Sci USA 49:193–200
15. Grimm AF, Katele KV, Kubota R, Whitehorn WV (1970) Relation of sarcomere length and muscle length in resting myocardium. Am J Physiol 218:1412–1416
16. Pollack GH, Huntsman LL (1974) Sarcomere length-active force relations in living mammalian heart muscle. Am J Physiol 227:383–389
17. Sonnenblick EH, Skelton CL, Spotnitz WD, Feldman D (1973) Redefinition of the ultrastructural basis of cardiac length-tension relations. Circulation 48 [Suppl 4]:65–70
18. Pollack GH (1974) Discussion of light diffraction of cardiac muscle. In: The Physiological Basis of Starling's Law of the Heart. Elsevier, New York, p 90 (Ciba Foundation Symposium 24, New Series)
19. Urschel CW, Covell JW, Sonnenblick EH, Ross J Jr, Braunwald E (1968) Myocardial mechanics in aortic and mitral valvular regurgitation. The concept of instantaneous impedenace as a determinant of the performance of the intact heart. J Clin Invest 47:867–883
20. Carabello BA, Nolan SP, Maguire LB (1981) Assessment of left ventricular function in patients with mitral regurgitation: value of the end-systolic wall stress-end-systolic volume ratio. Circulation 64:1212–1217
21. Wong CYH, Spotnitz HM (1981) Systolic and diastolic properties of the human left ventricle during valve replacement for chronic mitral stenosis Am J Cardiol 47:51–55
22. Eckberg DL, Gault JH, Bouchard RL, Karliner JS, Ross J Jr, Braunwald E (1973) Mechanics of left ventricular contraction in chronic severe mitral regurgitation. Circultion 47:1252–1259

23. Vokonas PS, Gorlin R, Cohn PF, Herman MV, Sonnenblick EH (1973) Dynamic geometry of the l44 left ventricle in mitral regurgitation. Circulation 48:786–796
24. Suga H, Sagawa K, Shoukas AA (1973) Load independence of the instanteous pressure-volume ratio of the canine left ventricle and effect of epinephrine and heart rate on the ratio. Circ Res 32:314–322
25. Marsh JD, Green LH, Wynne J, Cohn PF, Grossman W (1979) Left ventricular end-systolic pressure-dimension and stress-length relations in normal human subjects. Am J Cardiol 44:1311–1317
26. Imperial ES, Levy MN, Sieske H Jr (1961) Outflow resistance as an independent determinant of cardiac performance. Circ Res 9:1148–1153
27. Weber KT, Janicki JS (1977) Instantaneous force-velocity-length relations: experimental findings and clinical correlates. Am J Cardiol 40:740–747
28. Sagawa K, Suga H, Shoukas AA, Bakalar KM (1977) End-systolic pressure/volume ratio: a new index of ventricular contractility. Am J Cardiol 40:748–753
29. Grossman W, Braunwald E, Mann T, McLaurin LP, Green LH (1977) Contractile state of the left ventricle in man as evaluated from endsystolic stress pressure-volume relations. Circulation 56:845–852
30. Suga H, Sagawa K (1974) Instantaneous pressure-volume relationships and their ratio in the excised supported canine left ventricle. Circ Res 35:117–126
31. Mahler F, Covell JW, Ross J Jr (1975) Systolic pressure-diameter relations in the normal conscious dog. Cardiovasc Res 9:447–455
32. Weber KT, Janicki JS, Hefner LL (1976) Left ventricular force-length relations of isovolumic and ejection contractions. Am J Physiol 213:337–343
33. Abbott BC, Wilkie DR (1953) The relation between velocity of shortening and the tension-length curve of skeletal muscle. J Physiol (Lond) 120:214–220
34. Wilkie DR (1956) The mechanical properties of muscle. Br Med Bull 12:177–183
35. Downing SE, Sonnenblock EH (1964) Cardiac muscle mechanics and ventricular performance: force and time parameters. Am J Physiol 207:705–715
36. Mehmel HC, Stockins B, Ruffmank, Olhausen K, Schuler G, Kubler W (1981) The linearity of the end-systolic pressure-volume relationship in man and its sensitivity for assessment of left ventricular function. Circulation 63:1216–1222
37. Mirsky I (1969) Left ventricular stress in the intact human heart. Biophys J 9:189–208
38. Maurer AH, Siegel JA, Denenberg B, Robbins PS, Malmud LS (1982) Absolute left ventricular volume from gated blood pool imaging using an esophageal transmission measurement. [Abstr] J Nucl Med 23:70
39. Spann JF, Bove AA, Natarjan G, Kreulen T (1980) Ventricular performance, pump function and compensatory mechanisms in patients with aortic stenosis. Circulation 62:576–582
40. Osbakken M, Bove A, Spann JF (1981) Left ventricular function in chronic aortic regurgitation with reference to end-systolic pressure, volume and stress relations. Am J Cardiol 47:193–198
41. Chakko S, Troy A, Gash A, Bove AA, Spann JF (1982) Decreased ventricular contractile function, normal pump function and compensatory mechanisms in patients with systemic hypertension. [Abstr] Am J Cardiol 49:978
42. Cepin D, Gash A, Carabello BA, Spann JF (1982) Normal left ventricular systolic muscle function in patients with mitral stenosis. (Abst) Am J Cardiol 49:990
43. Carabello BA, Gash A, Mayer D, Spann JF (1982) Normal left ventricular systolic function in adults with atrial septal defect and left heart failure. [Abstr] Am J Cardiol 49:978
44. Donner RM, Carabello BA, Black I, Spann JF (1982) Diminished wall stress, normal muscle function and supranormal pump function in children with aortic stenosis. (Abstr) Am J Cardiol 49:978
45. Gerry JL, Baird MG, Fortuin (1976) Evaluation of left ventricular function in patients with sickle cell anemia. Am J Med 60:968–972
46. Denenberg BS, Criner G, Jones R, Troy A, Spann JF (1982) Impaired left ventricular contractile function sickle cell anemia. (Abstr) Am Fed Clin Res

Evaluation of Myocardial Function Using Power Indices*

P. Spiller, R. Unterberg, J. Jehle, R. Körfer, B. Pölitz, and F. K. Schmiel

Medizinische Klinik und Poliklinik der Universität Düsseldorf

Introduction

The assessment of myocardial performance in the intact heart is usually based upon the concept of an inverse relationship between force and velocity. Since Sonnenblick showed that the velocity of the contractile element V_{CE} is proportional to the relative rate of pressure rise during the isovolumic phase, this scheme has been applied to several experimental and clinical studies [3–7, 9, 14, 15]. Although controversy still exists as to the proper choice of the muscle model and as to the comparability of V_{max} from different subjects, there is general agreement that the rate of pressure rise cannot be interpreted in the case of valvular insufficiency [1, 10, 13]. The parameters of the ejection phase, too, are dependent on the loading conditions of the ventricle. An acute increase of the afterload, for instance, combined with no change of contractility results in a reduction of the ejection fraction and of the velocity of fiber shortening [8, 12].

To analyze myocardial performance independently of the loading conditions, a parameter has to be established which takes pre- and afterload into account. Afterload is included in left ventricular systolic power, a parameter which is calculated from instantaneous pressure and volume or wall stress and fiber length. Preload can be described by end-diastolic parameters, e. g., end-diastolic wall stress. Relating systolic power to the volume of the myocardial wall and to end-diastolic wall stress, a myocardial power index results which is hypothetically independent of pre- and afterload.

This paper has the following three main objectives:
1. To validate the proposed index of myocardial performance by demonstrating its load independence
2. To prove the superiority of the power index for analysis of myocardial performance compared with other parameters
3. To simplify the power index in order to be able to determine it from routinely measured pressures and dimensions

Independence with regard to the ventricular loading conditions can only be proved if a parameter remains nearly unaltered in spite of considerable changes of pre- and afterload. During routine heart catheterization, ventricular load can

---

* Supported by Deutsche Forschungsgemeinschaft (SFB 30)

only be changed to a limited extent and contractility may be influenced during this intervention by reflex mechanisms. Our experiments were therefore performed during cardiac surgery, where extreme changes of the loading conditions are achieved routinely by the extracorporeal circulation.

Materials and Methods

Two cineventriculographies with simultaneous pressure recordings were conducted in 12 patients after coronary revascularization and aortic valve replacement. For assessment of the control conditions the first ventriculogram was recorded with ejecting nonbypassed left ventricle. Six min later, on average, the second ventriculogram was performed with ejecting left ventricle during partial cardiopulmonary bypass, i.e., during reduced volume loading. Mean arterial pressure was held constant by the extracorporeal circulation. The angiograms were recorded using a single-plane C-arm unit with 50 frames/s in right anterior oblique (RAO) projection. The contrast medium – 30 ml amidotrizoate, on the average – was injected manually via the vent catheter, which was introduced into the left ventricle through the mitral valve. Left ventricular pressure was recorded by a 5F catheter tip manometer introduced through the lumen of the vent catheter. Arterial pressure was measured using a fluid-filled catheter connected to an external pressure transducer.

In six groups of patients (normal left ventricle, $n = 13$; aortic stenosis, $n = 9$; coarctation of the aorta, $n = 9$; aortic insufficiency, $n = 10$; congestive cardiomyopathy, $n = 10$; and mitral insufficiency, $n = 9$) biplane cineangiograms of the left ventricle with simultaneous pressure recordings (catheter tip manometer) were performed during routine heart catheterization.

Left ventricular volumes were determined according to the area-length method of Dodge et al. [2]. Wall volumes were calculated according to Rackley et al. [11] and wall stresses were determined using the formula of Wong and Rautaharju [16].

Results and Discussion

In Fig. 1 the pressure parameters under control conditions and under partial unloading are plotted. As intended, mean arterial pressure remains unchanged. Compared with peak systolic pressure the decrease of end-diastolic pressure is more pronounced, i.e., primarily left ventricular preload is changed. This becomes evident, too, from the volume parameters, depicted in Fig. 2. End-diastolic and stroke volumes are markedly reduced, whereas end-systolic volumes reflect only a small, but significant decrease.

In Fig. 3 the usual parameters of myocardial function – ejection fraction, mean circumferential fiber shortening rate, and the relative rate of pressure rise – are compiled. Additionally, myocardial power per wall volume is depicted; it is calculated from the pressure volume loop by dividing the stroke work through the ejection time and the myocardial volume. As this parameter is

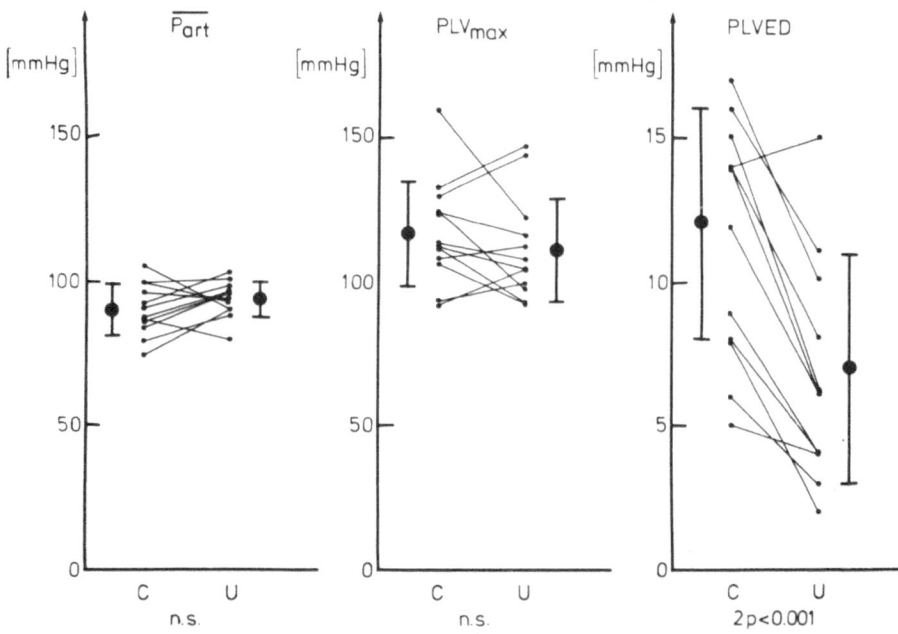

Fig. 1. Mean arterial pressure (P_{art}), left ventricular systolic (PLV_{max}) and end-diastolic pressure (*PLVED*) during control (*C*) and unloading (*U*) in 12 patients. Mean arterial pressure remains unchanged. End-diastolic pressure decreases considerably more than systolic pressure

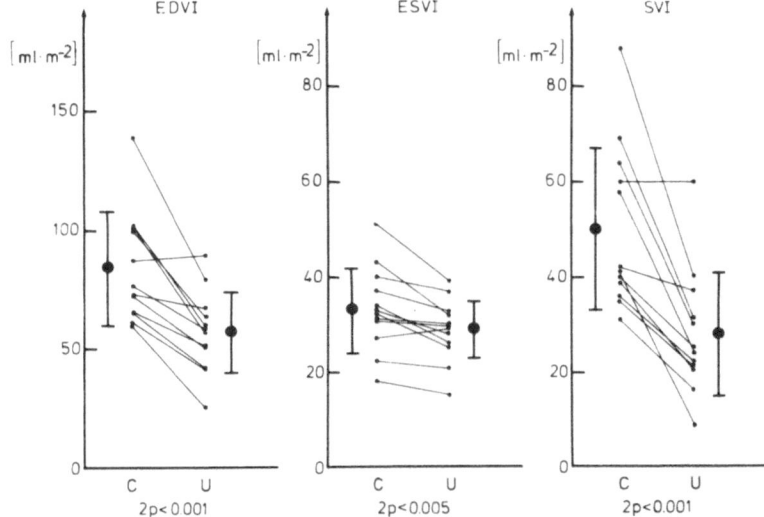

Fig. 2. End-diastolic (*EDVI*), end-systolic (*ESVI*), and stroke volumes (*SVI*) during control (*C*) and unloading (*U*) in 12 patients. Left ventricular volumes and stroke volume decrease significantly

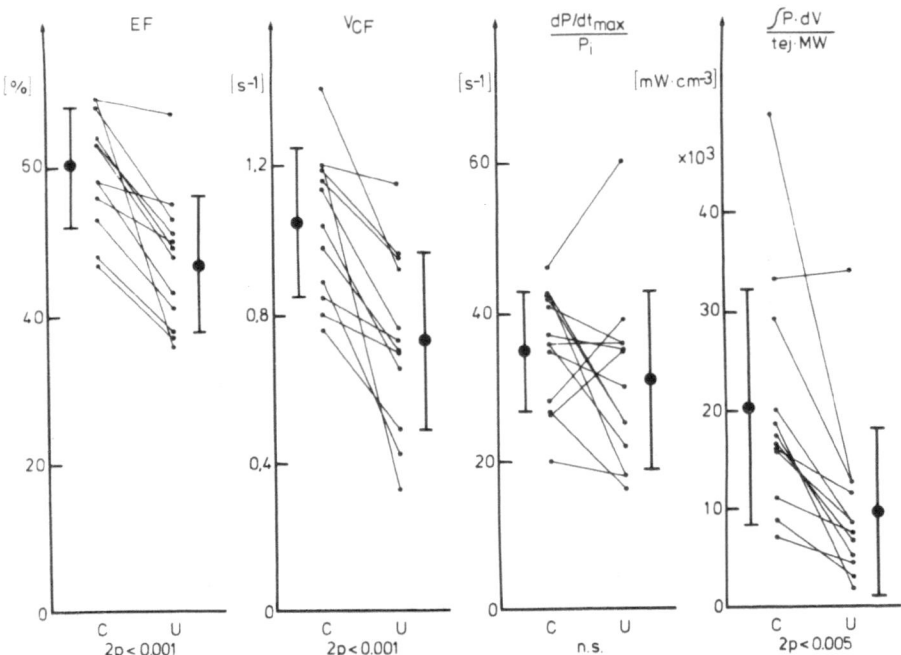

Fig. 3. Ejection fraction (*EF*), mean circumferential fiber shortening rate (*V$_{CF}$*), relative rate of pressure rise (dp/dt_{max}/P_I) and systolic myocardial power per wall volume ($\int PdV/t_{ej} \cdot MV$) during control (*C*) and unloading (*U*) in 12 patients. All parameters except (dp/dt_{max}/P_I) decrease significantly

a function of systolic pressure and ejected volume, it can be used as a measure of myocardial performance, which takes the afterload into account.

All ejection phase parameters decrease significantly, although no change of contractility can be supposed. The changes of dp/dt max divided by the instantaneous pressure are pronounced, but not uniform, probably in part due to mitral regurgitation caused by the vent catheter. Myocardial power per wall volume decreases about 50%. Thus, all these parameters of ventricular and myocardial function are considerably altered by the loading conditions of the left ventricle.

Since myocardial power takes the afterload into account, its decrease must be explained by the changes of myocardial preload. To demonstrate the relationship between power and preload, in Fig. 4 myocardial power per wall volume is plotted vs end-diastolic wall stress. Prolonging the straight lines which reflect the changes of both parameters for each single patient, to the left, it becomes evident that the intercepts of the axes are all near the origin. Thus, for each single patient the ratio of myocardial power per wall volume and end-diastolic wall stress remains constant when the preload is reduced. The constancy of this ratio – the so-called myocardial power index – is confirmed by the mean values corresponding to control and unloading (right panel).

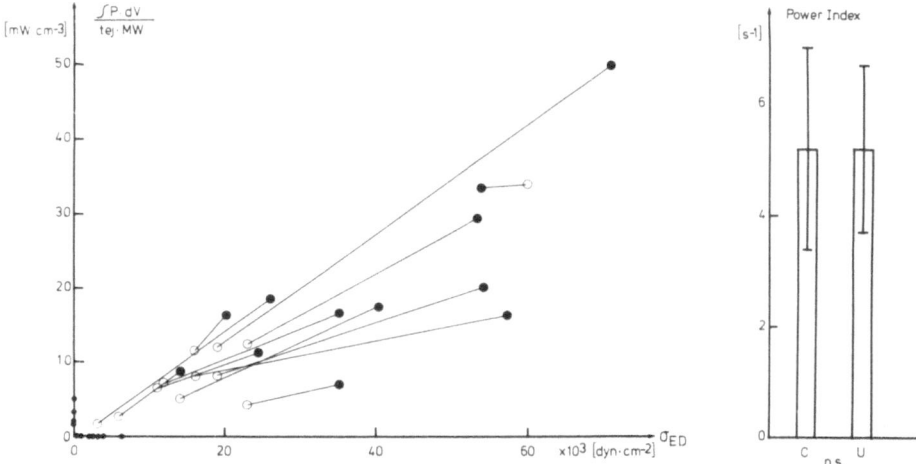

Fig. 4. Correlation between myocardial power per wall volume ($\varsigma PdV/t_{ej} \cdot MV$, *ordinate*) and end-diastolic wall stress (σ_{ED}, *abscissa*) during control (*points*) and unloading (*circles*) in 12 patients. The *columns* represent the mean value and the standard deviation of the power index (ratio of myocardial power per wall volume and end-diastolic wall stress)

The validity of this power index to describe myocardial performance taking pre- and afterload into account was proved in six patient groups. In Fig. 5 the values of the power index of ventricles with aortic stenosis, coarctation of the aorta, aortic insufficiency, mitral insufficiency, and congestive cardiomyopathy, are compared with those of normal ventricles. The five patient groups are significantly separated from the group with normal ventricles. Most of the values of the ventricles with pathologic loading conditions and with congestive cardiomyopathy are below the lowest normal value. Only few patients have normal power indices indicating an unaltered myocardial performance. As expected, the lowest mean value is found in congestive cardiomyopathy.

Figure 6 demonstrates the ejection fraction of the six patient groups. This parameter, indeed, separates the groups with abnormal from those with normal myocardial function. Regarding the individual cases, however, it becomes evident that the power index permits an essentially more selective separation. Compared with ejection fraction, mean velocity of circumferential fiber shortening and parameters of the isovolumic contraction phase reveal a similar pattern.

Since, for the evaluation of parameters derived from instantaneous pressures and dimensions, a frame by frame analysis of the angiograms is necessary, we considered substituting the power index by a less sophisticated parameter. Therefore, 15 usual parameters of systolic function and 20 parameters of preload obtained from both ventriculographies were combined to calculate 300 power indices. In Fig. 7 that simplified index which is nearly identical under both conditions, as proved by the paired *t*-test, is correlated with the original power index.

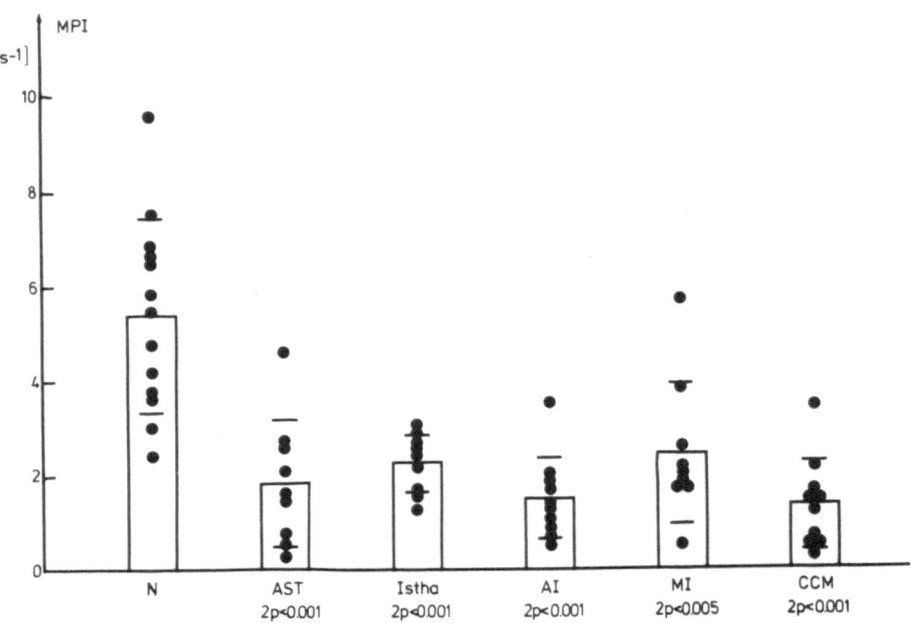

Fig. 5. Myocardial power index (*MPI*) of six patient groups (*N*, normal left ventricle; *AST*, aortic stenosis; *Istha*, coarctation of the aorta; *AI*, aortic insufficiency; *MI*, mitral insufficiency; *CCM*, congestive cardiomyopathy). Most of the values of the ventricles with pathologic loading conditions and with *CCM* are below the lowest normal value

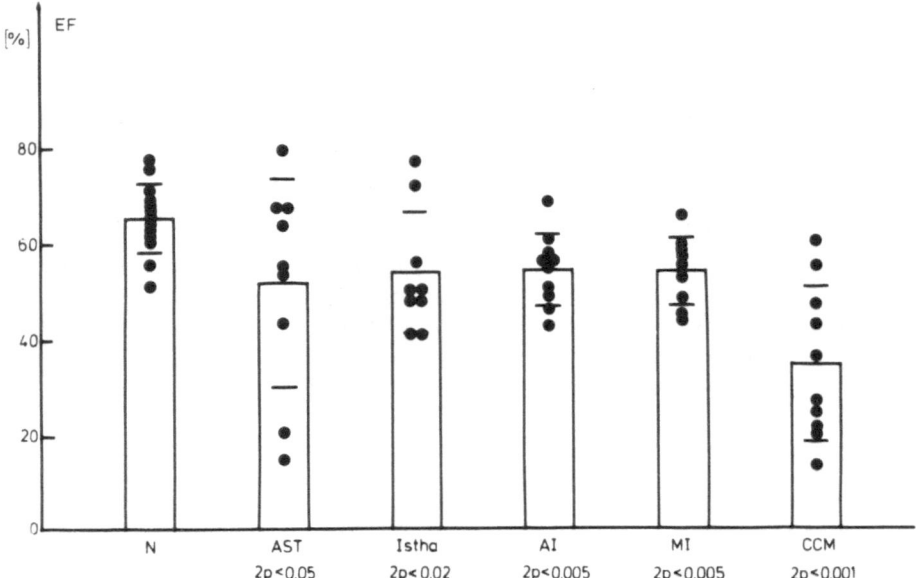

Fig. 6. Ejection fraction (*EF*) of the six patient groups (see Fig. 5). Compared with the myocardial power index the ejection fraction permits only a poor separation of abnormal from normal ventricles

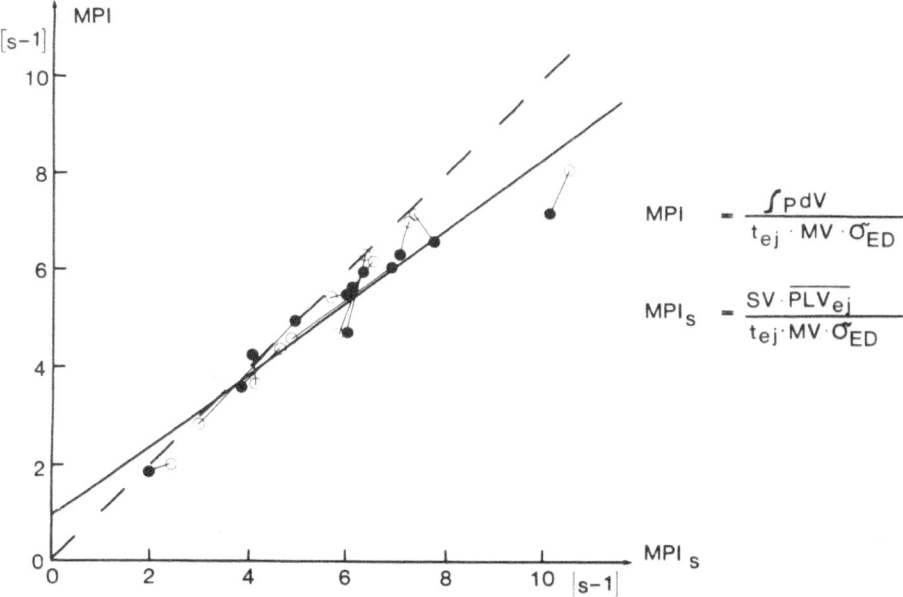

Fig. 7. Correlation of the myocardial power index (*MPI*) and a simplified index (*MPI*$_s$) during control (*points*) and unloading (*circles*) in 12 patients. Both parameters are closely correlated

In this index MPI$_s$, one part of the term systolic power, the integral PdV, is approximated by the product of stroke volume and mean systolic pressure. Preload is again described by end-diastolic wall stress. It is evident that this simplified index MPI$_s$ is closely correlated to the power index MPI which is calculated from instantaneously determined data.

Summarizing, one can conclude:

1. The ratio of myocardial power per wall volume and end-diastolic wall stress is independent of the loading conditions of the myocardium.
2. This power index permits a clear separation of patients with abnormal left ventricular function from those with a normal left ventricle on an individual basis.
3. A simplified index which describes myocardial function with the same accuracy can be calculated from usually derived pressure and dimension parameters.

References

1. Van Den Bos GC, Elzinga G, Westerhof N, Noble MIM (1973) Problems in the use of indices of myocardial contractility. Cardiovasc Res 7:834
2. Dodge HT, Kennedy JW, Petersen JL (1973) Quantitative angiocardiographic methods in the evaluation of valvular heart disease. Progr Cardiovasc Dis 16:1
3. Gunther S, Grossman W (1979) Determinants of ventricular function in pressure-overload hypertrophy in man. Circulation 59:679

182   P. Spiller, R. Unterberg, J. Jehle, R. Körfer, B. Pölitz, and F. K. Schmiel

4. Huber D, Grimm J, Koch R, Krayenbuehl HP (1981) Determinants of ejection performance in aortic stenosis. Circulation 64:126
5. Kochhäuser M, Jehle J, Neuhaus KL, Spiller P (1978) Systolische und diastolische
Myokardfunktion bei druckbelastetem linken Ventrikel. Z Kardiol 67:583
6. Krayenbuehl HP, Rutishauser W, Amende I, Mehmel H (1973) High-fidelity left ventricular pressure measurements for the assessment of cardiac contractility in man. Am J
Cardiol 31:415
7. Levine HJ (1967) Muscle mechanics in the in situ heart. In: Tanz RD, Kavaler F, Roberts
J (eds) Factors influencing myocardial contractility. Academic, New York
8. Mahler F, Ross J, O'Rourke RA, Covell JW (1975) Effects of changes in preload,
afterload, and inotropic state on ejection and isovolumic phase measures of contractility
in the conscious dog. Am J Cardiol 35:626
9. Mason DT, Spann JF, Zelis R (1970) Quantification of the contractile state of the intact
human heart. Am J Cardiol 26:248
10. Pollack GH, Huntsmann LL, Verdugo P (1972) Cardiac muscle models. Circ Res 31:569
11. Rackley CR, Dodge HT, Coble YD, Hay RE (1964) A method for determining left
ventricular mass in man. Circulation 29:666
12. Rönsberg D, Benn M, Karsch KR, Kreuzer H, Neuhaus KL, Spiller P (1978) Der Einfluß
der Nachbelastung auf normales und ischämisches Myokard beim Hund. Z Kardiol 67:595
13. Sonnenblick EH (1974) Contractility in the intact heart: progress and problems. Eur J
Cardiol 1:319
14. Spann JF, Bove AA, Natarajan G, Kreulen T (1980) Ventricular performance, pump
function and compensatory mechanisms in patients with aortic stenosis. Circulation
62:576
15. Weber KT, Janicki JS (1977) Instantaneous force-length-relations: experimental findings
and clinical correlates. Am J Cardiol 40:740
16. Wong AYK, Rautaharju PM (1968) Stress distribution within the left ventricular wall
approximated as an elipsoidal shell. Am Heart J 75:649

Angiographic Analysis of Left Ventricular Diastolic Function

J. Jehle, H. Rose, F. K. Schmiel, P. Spiller, and L. J. Ulbricht

Medizinische Klinik und Poliklinik B, University of Düsseldorf, Düsseldorf, FRG

The elastic properties of the left ventricle are described by the pressure-volume relationship during the passive filling phase in diastole [2, 5, 7, 8]. In experimental studies Diamond and Forrester found this relationship to be "almost perfectly exponential" [1]. The measured pressures and volumes could be fitted best to the function:

$$p = b_1 * e^{a_1 * V} + c_1$$

Diamond and Forrester concluded from their investigations that the constant a_1 reflects the elastic properties of the left ventricle. An even more simplified expression of the original equation with the constant c equal to zero is usually used [2,5,7]:

$$p = b_2 * e^{a_2 * V}$$

It is the purpose of the following study to demonstrate the problems of evaluation of the diastolic pressure-volume relationship using these two equations and angiographically determined left ventricular volumes.

Five patients with reduced ventricular function and an abnormal ventricular geometry as well as three anaesthetized mongrel dogs with normal ventricular geometry were investigated. Quantitative high-speed left ventriculograms were performed with simultaneous pressure recordings by means of catheter-tip manometers. In the patients two and in the dogs three consecutive heart cycles without any interventions were analysed. The measured diastolic pressures and volumes were fitted – by means of a computer program – to the exponential functions mentioned above [8].

Using the equation of Diamond and Forrester, the analysis of two or three consecutive beats shows that the calculated pressure-volume curves are significantly different (Fig. 1).

In nearly all patients all parameters b_1, a_1 and c_1 of the first and second cycle are significantly different. Similar results were found in the three consecutive beats of the experimental studies. This means that the elastic properties of the ventricle seem to have changed from beat to beat. This is unlikely. In contrast to these results, the beat-to-beat reproducibility of the pressure-volume relationship can be improved using the simplified formula (Fig. 2). In contrast to the results obtained by the formula with three parameters, no statistical differences were found in the same patients as well as in the experimental studies.

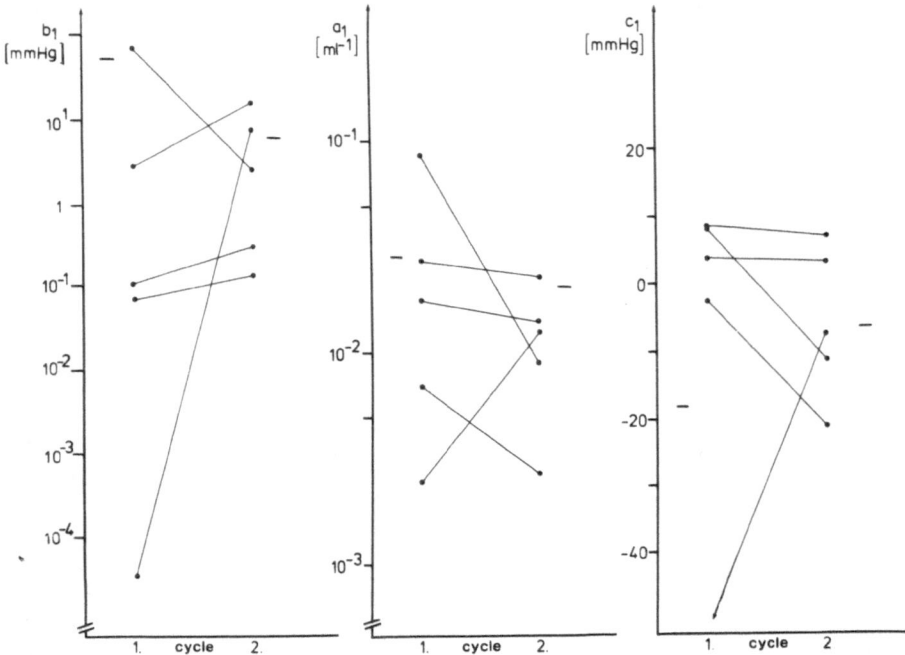

Fig. 1. Parameters a_1, b_1, and c_1 of the pressure-volume relationship using Diamond and Forrester's formula (two consecutive cycles in five patients). Nearly all parameters of the first and second cycle are significantly different

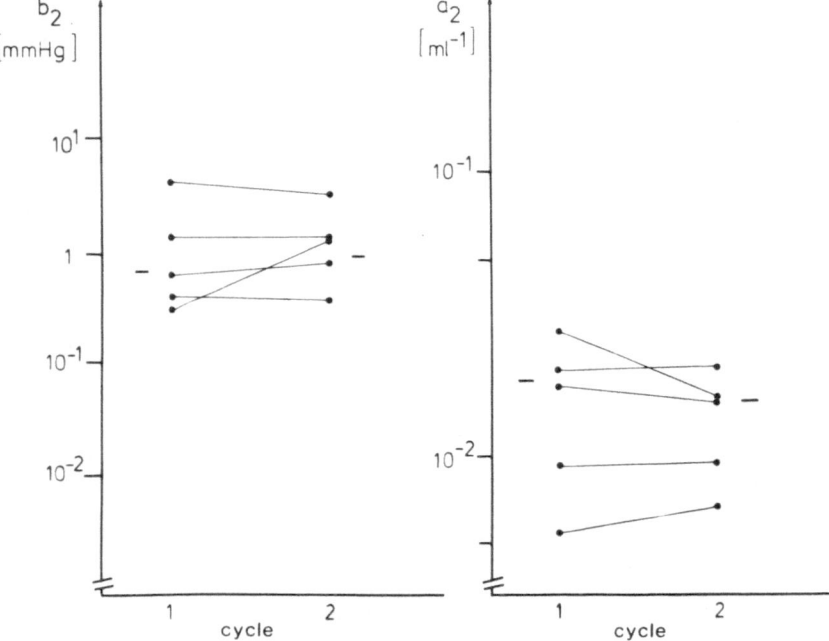

Fig. 2. Parameters a_2 and b_2 of the pressure-volume relationship using the simplified formula (two consecutive cycles in five patients). The parameters of the first and second cycle are not significantly different

Although these results are reproducible, the application of this formula for the determination of diastolic function is not suitable, for the following reasons:

1. Two pressure-volume curves with identical slopes but a different operating pressure level cannot be described exactly, because the computed slope is influenced by shifts of the operating pressure level.
2. Using the simplified formula implies that the ventricular pressure cannot reach the value of zero.
3. Using the constant $c_1 = 0$ for all ventricles, the residual sums of squares of the approximation applying the formula with three parameters were about 8% less (on the average) than those of the formula with two parameters. That means that the pressures and volumes measured were less exactly fitted by the simplified formula.

A combination of the good approximation properties of Diamond and Forrester's formula with the good beat-to-beat reproducibility of the simplified formula can be achieved by predefining the additive constant c for each individual ventricle. This can be done by taking the isovolumic relaxation period into account (Fig. 3). The solid line represents the measured pressure from dp/dt_{min} to end-diastole; the dots, the measured volumes. The pressure-volume relationship is usually calculated between the two vertical lines. Relaxation is evaluated

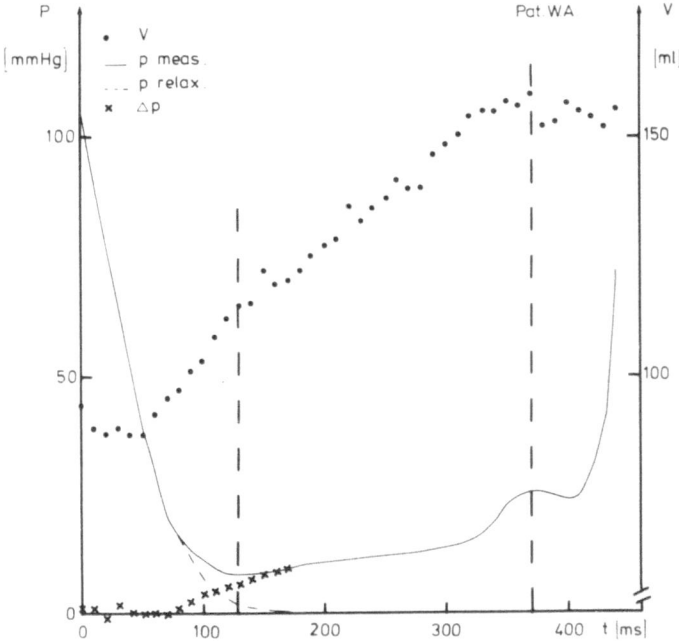

Fig. 3. Diastolic pressure-time curve (*solid line*) and volume-time curve (*dots*) of a patient. The pressure-volume relationship is usually calculated between the two vertical lines. The pressure decline is computed during the isovolumic relaxation period and extrapolated in diastole (*dashed line*). The difference between measured and extrapolated pressure is drawn in as *crosses*. This difference should represent the pressure increase caused by the passive inflow of volume

according to a formula used in our working group [4]. By this method the pressure decline is calculated during the isovolumic phase and extrapolated into the early filling phase; the extrapolated pressures are drawn in as the dashed line. The crosses represent the differences between the extrapolated relaxation curve and the measured pressures in the early filling phase, which should represent the increase of left ventricular pressure caused by the passive inflow of volume after mitral valve opening. The time when the pressure equals zero corresponds well with the time of the end-systolic volume, here called V_o [4].

Introducing this V_o into Diamond and Forrester's formula, the following equation will result. According to our definition, V equals V_o if the pressure p equals zero. Finally, a last equation results; a formula fulfilling our demands mentioned above:

$$p = b_1 * e^{a_1 * V} + c_1$$
$$p = b_3 * e^{a_3 * (V - V_o)} + c_3$$
$$\text{if } p = 0 \text{ then } V = V_o$$

therefore
$$p = b_3 * (e^{a_3 * (V - V_o)} - 1)$$

Extending the "conventional" pressure-volume relationship in the manner described, the parameters of the approximation do not differ significantly when obtained from two or three consecutive cycles. An example is shown in Fig. 4. The conventionally determined pressure-volume relationship is drawn in as dots. Extending this conventional relationship (dots) in the manner described

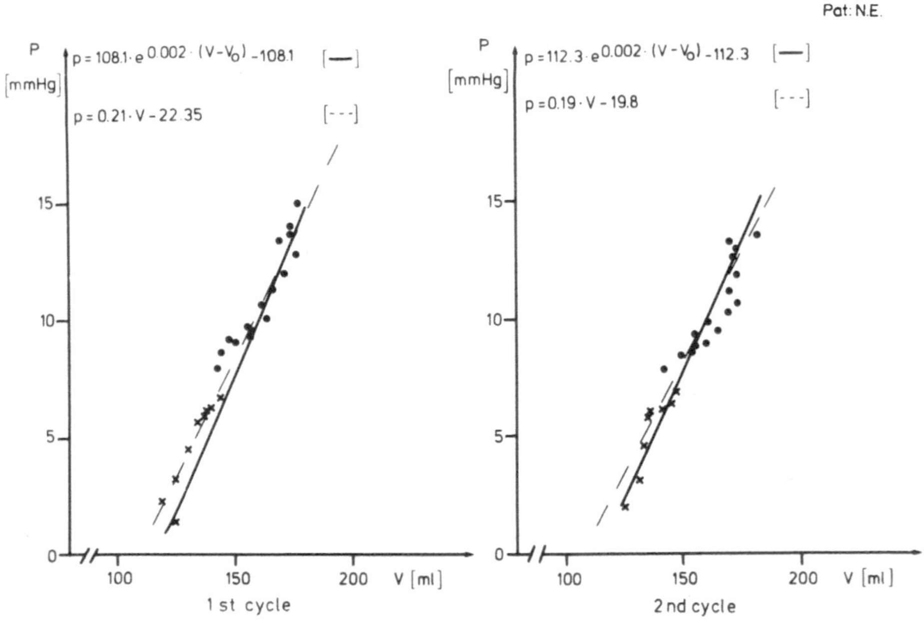

Fig. 4. Conventionally determined (*dots*) and extended (*crosses*) pressure-volume relationship of a patient in two consecutive cycles. The approximation using the modified exponential function (*solid line*) and the linear function (*dashed line*) shows good reproducibility. From this perspective both pressure-volume relationships seem to be linear

(crosses), the parameters of the modified exponential function (solid line) do not differ, when obtained from two or three consecutive cycles.

From this perspective, this curve and all other pressure-volume relationships analysed could be fitted to a linear function as well (dashed line), given as:

$$p = a_4 * V + b_4$$

The parameters of this function do not differ significantly. The value of V_o computed by the linear function corresponds well with the angiographically determined end-systolic volume in both cycles. Even from theoretical considerations, the extended pressure-volume relationships cannot be fitted to an exponential function, if the stress-strain relationship is an exponential function which could be shown in several experimental studies [3, 6].

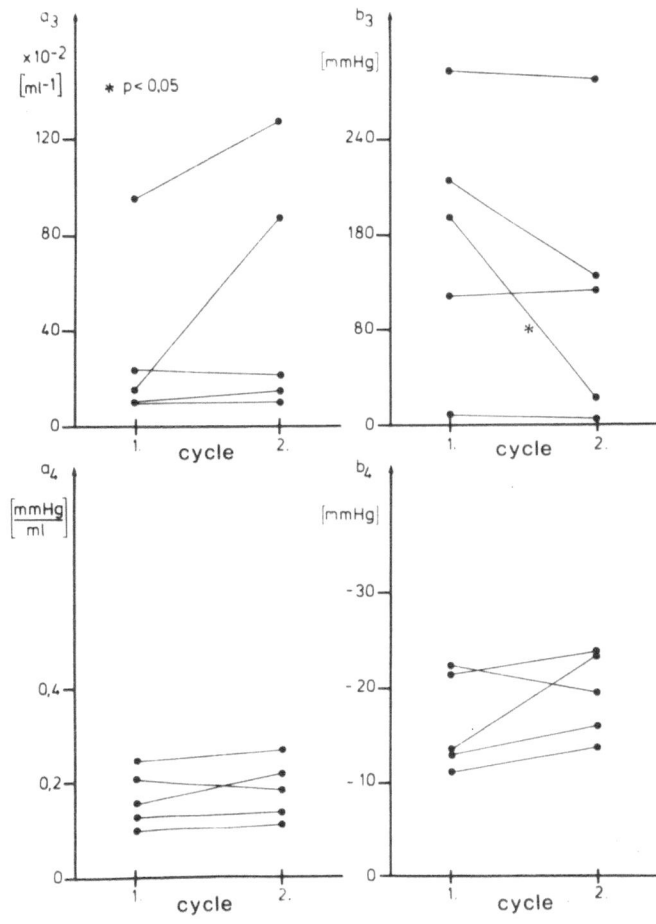

Fig. 5. Parameters a_3 and b_3 of the modified exponential function and a_4 and b_4 of the linear function in the two consecutive heart cycles of five patients. Regarding the scatter of the parameters (not drawn in), both approximations reveal a good reproducibility from beat to beat

Our extended pressure-volume relationships were therefore analysed using both the modified exponential and the linear equation. The computed values of the residual mean squares do not differ significantly when the exponential and the linear approximation are compared. That means that under these conditions both methods seem to be equivalent. The parameters of the corrected exponential equation b_3 and a_3 and of the linear equation b_4 and a_4 reveal a similarly good reproducibility from beat to beat in the normally as well as in the abnormally shaped ventricle, but the scatter of the parameters (not shown in Fig. 5) of the corrected exponential function is much greater than the scatter of the parameters of the linear function (Fig. 5). Therefore, using angiographically determined volumes, the elastic properties of the left ventricle should be described by a linear function with a constant passive elastic modulus for each ventricle.

Using this approach, a simple parameter for the description of elastic ventricular properties can be derived using haemodynamic parameters like end-diastolic and end-systolic volumes as well as end-diastolic pressure (Fig. 6). As the slope of the linear function equals the quotient of end-diastolic pressure and stroke volume, a frame by frame analysis of diastole is not necessary. Regarding the different sizes of the ventricles in various heart diseases, the stroke volume must be divided by the resting volume, which is about equal to the end-systolic volume. Thus, the stiffness index of the ventricle E'_v results. In several experimental studies it could be shown that this simplified parameter reflects the known effects of certain interventions on the elastic properties of the ventricle.

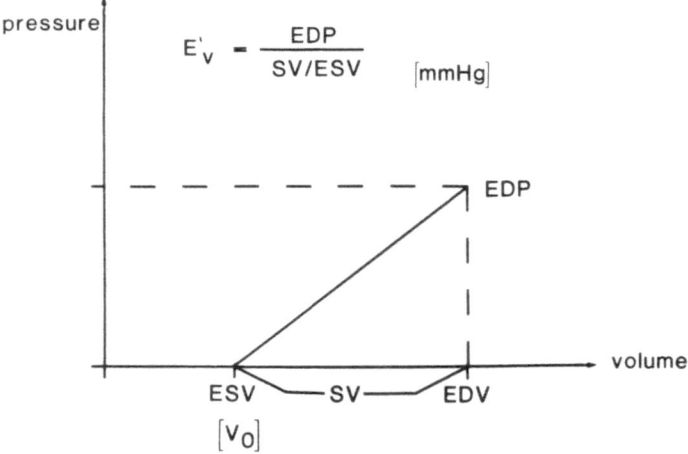

Fig. 6. Calculation of the stiffness index E'_v derived from the linear function to describe the elastic properties of the left ventricle. This index can be calculated by means of the usual haemodynamic parameters end-diastolic pressure (*EDP*), end-diastolic volume (*EDV*), end-systolic volume (*ESV*) and stroke volume (*SV*)

In summary

1. The diastolic pressure-volume relationship cannot be described exactly by using the formula of Diamond and Forrester or the commonly used, simplified one, when angiographically determined volumes are used.
2. Regarding relaxation, an extended pressure-volume relationship can be determined. This relationship can be described by a linear function.
3. Using this approach, a simple expression of usual haemodynamic parameters can be derived to describe the elastic properties of the ventricle.

References

1. Diamond G, Forrester JS, Hargis J, Parmley WW, Danzig R, Swan HJC (1977) Diastolic pressure-volume relationship in the canine left ventricle. Circ Res 29:267
2. Gaasch WH, Levine HJ, Quinones MA, Alexander JK (1976) Left ventricular compliance: mechanisms and clinical implications. Am J Cardiol 38:645
3. Holubarsch C, Jacob R (1979) Evaluation of elastic properties of myocardium. Z Kardiol 68:123
4. Jehle J, Körfer R, Schmiel FK, Spiller P (1981) A new approach to description of left ventricular relaxation. 2nd Joint Meeting of the Working Groups of the European Society of Cardiology, Pavia, 1981
5. Mehmel HC, Stockins B, Ick A, Olshausen von K, Kübler W (1979) Diastolische Druck-Volumen-Beziehung des linken Ventrikels bei Koronarkrankheit unter Belastung und im postextrasystolischen Schlag (abstr.) Z Kardiol 68:287
6. Mirsky I (1976) Assessment of passive elastic stiffness of cardiac muscle: mathematical concepts, physiologic and clinical considerations, directions of future research. Progr Cardiovasc Dis 18:277
7. Neuhaus KL, Tebbe U, Kreuzer H (1979) Der Einfluß körperlicher Belastung auf die diastolische Druck-Volumen-Beziehung des linken Ventrikels. Z Kardiol 68:791
8. Ulbricht L, Jehle J, Schmiel FK, Spiller P (1981) Untersuchungen zur angiographischen Bestimmung der diastolischen Druck-Volumen-Beziehung des linken Ventrikels. Basic Res Cardiol 76:224

Evaluation of Left Ventricular Function Using Biplane Quantitative Ventriculography with Supine Leg Exercise

U. Gleichmann, G. Trieb, D. Fassbender, and H. Mannebach

Gollwitzer-Meier-Institute, D-4970 Bad Oeynhausen, FRG

Despite the fact that most coronary patients develop problems during exertion, many cardiologists are not used to exercising the patient in the catheter laboratory. So in many cases the functional significance of a coronary stenosis remains a matter of speculation needing further evaluation in a second test, most often using radionuclide scintigraphy or angiography.

Stenosis of less than 50% is generally accepted as insignificant at rest and with exercise, while stenosis of more than 90% is critical [13, 17]. At this point all compensatory mechanisms are exhausted at rest [9].

Problems arise in the interpretation of the functional significance of moderate stenosis between 50%–75% (Fig. 1). From experimental data [9] we know that this degree of stenosis could be partially compensated by a reduction of peripheral coronary resistance which is in series with a proximal stenosis [13]. On the other hand, an increase in oxygen demand of the myocardium, or a small increase in stenosis percentage due to coronary artery spasm or thrombosis, may suddenly decrease coronary artery flow in this type of moderate stenosis.

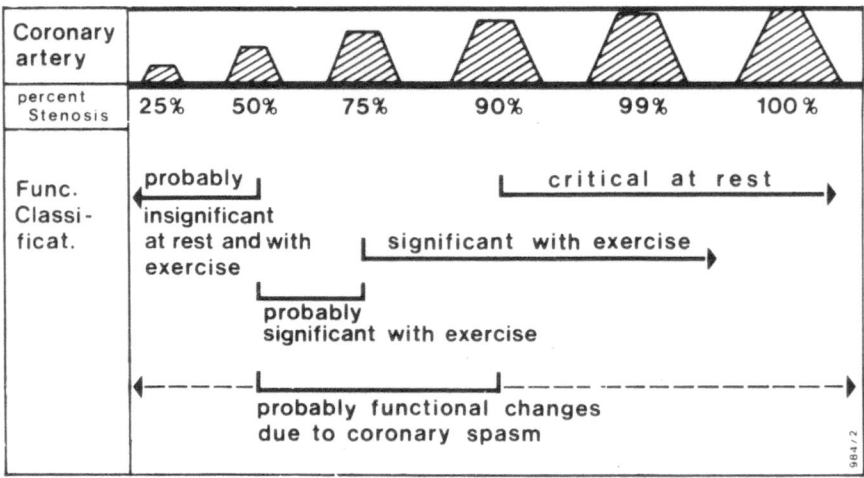

Fig. 1. Grading system of coronary stenosis in percent diameter reduction and significance of coronary stenosis in coronary heart disease

Furthermore, the functional significance of this moderate stenosis depends on the area and thickness of the perfused muscle and is influenced by perfusion pressure, the determinants of myocardial oxygen consumption, and collateral flow to this area or from this area to other parts of the ventricle.

With these variables in mind, one must conclude that the critical lumen diameter reduction lies somewhere between 50%–90% stenosis, and that for any individual patient it must be impossible to define a sharp borderline between significant and insignificant stenosis. A higher angiographic resolution would not resolve this problem. The intercorrelation of these parameters for an individual patient and the prediction of the extent of myocardium in jeopardy in a given patient prior to myocardial infarction could only be tested experimentally with exercise and by analyzing global left ventricular (LV) function and local wall motion using exercise angiography [5, 6, 14–16, 18, 19] or perfusion scintigraphy [1, 11].

In our experience, LV angiography during exercise is a safe and effective method for improving diagnostic accuracy in coronary patients. In some patients with angina pectoris in the absence of coronary heart disease exercise, ventriculography may also give further information of LV function and prognosis. This is true, for instance, in patients with syndrome X. Results in this group were published by our group earlier [8]. Therefore, here we will give some technical remarks regarding the method and present some results of the correlation of LV function with various degrees and locations of coronary stenosis.

Material and Methods

During a 7-year period (1974–1980) LV exercise angiograms were performed in 896 patients out of a total group of more than 4000 (Table 1). The diagnoses of these patients are given in Table 1. There were 89 really normal subjects, 223 coronary patients without scar and with normal ventricles at rest, and 273 coronary patients with scar due to prior myocardial infarction. In a group of 152 coronary patients LV function was evaluated after heart surgery. The remaining 159 patients suffered from other diseases like syndrome X, hypertension, cardiomyopathy, and aortic regurgitation.

Catheters were introduced in most cases using Judkins technique; in a small group (3%), using Sones's technique. Introduction through the right or left groin does not interfere with bicycle exercise in any way. Before exercise, measurements of pressure and cardiac output (using the thermodilution technique), and a biplane left ventriculogram at rest were performed. The resting LV angiogram was obtained with power injections of approximately 0.5–0.6 ml/ kg body wt. Urografin 76 with a flow rate of 12 ml/s. For the exercise LV angiogram, a slightly higher quantity of 0.6–0.7 ml/kg body wt. with a higher flow rate of 14–16 ml/s was chosen. For the exercise ventriculogram the patient was asked to continue the effort on the electrically braked bicycle ergometer in the supine position. Mild inspiration was assured during injection. Cineangiograms employing a 40° right anterior oblique projection an a 50° left anterior oblique projection were obtained simultaneously at a film speed of 50 frames/s.

Table 1. Clinical diagnosis in 896 patients with LV exercise angiography (1974–1980)

		n
1. Normal subjects		89
2. CHD without scar		223
1-Vessel disease	77	
2-Vessel disease	111	
3-Vessel disease	35	
3. CHD with scar		273
4. CHD after heart surgery		152
After bypass grafting	34	
After aneurysmectomy	118	
5. Other diagnosis		159
Syndrome X	18	
Cardiomyopathy	33	
Hypertensive heart disease	91	
Aortic regurgitation	17	
Total		896

CHD, coronary heart disease

Selective coronary angiography was performed in 8–10 min after cessation of exercise. Thus, the time for the whole catheterization procedure amounts to 40–45 min. With the experience of some 750 exercise ventriculographies behind us, we now prefer to perform coronary angiography before ventriculography, the main advantage being that then we can know exactly the patient's coronary state. In this way maximal exercise could be achieved more often. There were 12% extrasystoles at rest and 11% with exercise.

Angiography during exercise was performed either

a) symptom limited, when the patient evaluated angina pectoris, ST depression of more than 3 mm, or an end-diastolic pressure of more than 40 mmHg, or

b) heart-rate limited, when heart rate increased to more than 115 beats per min.

On this basis, in many patients exercise level was submaximal. The work load used depended upon the patient's history and preceding noninvasive or semi-invasive studies using ECG at rest and with exercise, echocardiography, and pulmonary artery pressure measurements with a floating catheter. Mean work load was 55 watts with a range between 25–100 watts, mean exercise duration was 3 min with a range of 2–5 min.

There were no complications at the catheter entrance or due to constrast injections involved with this procedure. For the evaluation of the results, coronary stenosis was graded according to Gensini [7, 10, 12], analysis of the ventriculogram was performed according to the biplane area-length method of Dodge [2, 3, 4] (using a videometric device and a calibration ball exactly positioned at the side of the left ventricular cavity). Written informed consent was obtained by all patients.

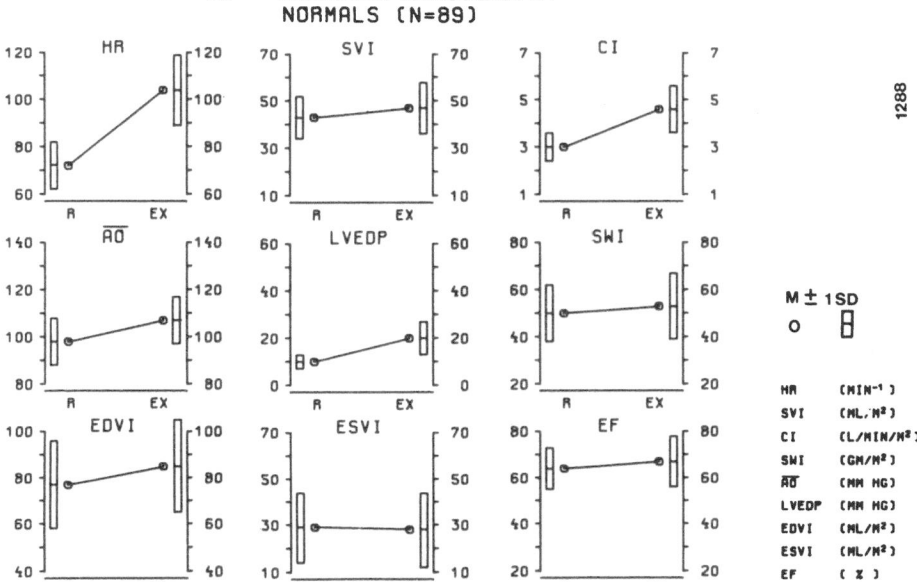

Fig. 2. LV volume and pressure changes in 89 patients without significant heart disease (normal subjects)

Results

Only some of our results in normals and in patients with coronary heart disease without myocardial infarction should be used as a basis for drawing general conclusions. First, with regard to the normal reaction: A group of 89 subjects turned out to be normal (Fig. 2). That means no coronary heart disease, no evidence of cardiomyopathy and no history of hypertension could be detected. In this group the resting heart rate (HR) increased from 71.9 ± 10.9 to 104 ± 15.6 beats/min, LV end-diastolic pressure (LVEDP) increased from 9.6 ± 3.0 to 20.1 ± 7.3 mmHg, end-diastolic volume index (EDVI) increased from 77.1 ± 18.9 to 84.6 ± 22.4 with unchanged end-systolic volume index (ESVI) and a small increase in ejection fraction (EF) from 64.8 ± 9.1 to 67.2 ± 10.9%. Cardiac index (CI) increased from 3.0 ± 0.6 to 4.6 ± 1.0 l/min/m².

With regard to single left circumflex (CX) or right coronary artery (RCA) stenosis, there is nearly the same increase in heart rate, systolic pressure (LVSP), EDVI, and CI, with unchanged ESVI and EF, but an abnormal increase of the LVEDP from 12 to 26.6 mmHg (Table 2). Thus, pump function remains unchanged with a higher filling pressure. The diminished contraction of the posterior wall is compensated by an increased contraction pattern of the normally perfused anterior wall.

Table 2. Hemodynamic parameters at rest and during exercise (mean and SD) in isolated stenosis of right coronary artery or circumflex branch of left coronary artery ($n = 10$)

Parameters	Rest	Exercise	Δ
HR (beats/min)	66.5 ± 13	94.5 ± 15	+ 28.0
LVSP (mmHg)	131.7 ± 9	156.3 ± 23	+ 24.6
LVEDP (mmHg)	12.4 ± 6	26.6 ± 5	+ 14.2
EDVI (ml/m²)	73.7 ± 12	81.0 ± 12	+ 7.3
ESVI (ml/m²)	28.2 ± 12	28.1 ± 17	− 0.1
EF (%)	64.3 ± 8	64.9 ± 8	+ 0.6
CI (l/min/m²)	3.02 ± 0.6	4.45 ± 1.1	+ 1.43

Of particular interest are the findings in single left anterior descending (LAD) stenosis of 50% compared with 75% stenosis with and without angina pectoris during exercise (Fig. 3). Compared with normal subjects, in 50% LAD stenosis there is a slight increase in LVEDP and mean pulmonary artery pressure (PAP), but a normal increase in CI and EDVI, and a slight decrease in ESVI, so that ejection fraction increases as in normal subjects. Thus, in isolated 50% LAD stenosis all volume parameters under exercise behave not significantly differently from normal subjects, with a small increase in filling pressure. Perhaps with more sophisticated methods it would also be possible to demonstrate segmental wall motion disorders in 50% stenosis. This is true for the 75% stenosis without angina pectoris in which EDVI and ESVI increased to the same amount, so that EF does not increase but remains unchanged. In 75% LAD stenosis with angina pectoris during exercise there is the greatest increase of LVEDP, EDVI and ESVI, resulting in a drop in the ejection fraction. But in spite of this decreased ejection fraction, cardiac index remains increased, although on a somewhat lower level compared with the other groups.

More recently we have observed a couple of patients with isolated 75% LAD stenosis and decreasing ejection fraction during exercise without angina pectoris. Thus, absence of angina does not mean normal ejection fraction during exercise. An example is shown in Fig. 4. In this case, with exercise-induced anterior wall and septal hypokinesia and normal function at rest, thallium myocardial scintigraphy showed only a minor redistribution after exercise and a septal scar. With exercise the ejection fraction decreased from 68% to 38%; LVEDP increased from 8 mmHg at rest to 47 mmHg with exercise.

In two- or three-vessel disease including the LAD, most often patients developed changes similar to or more pronounced than those in 75% LAD

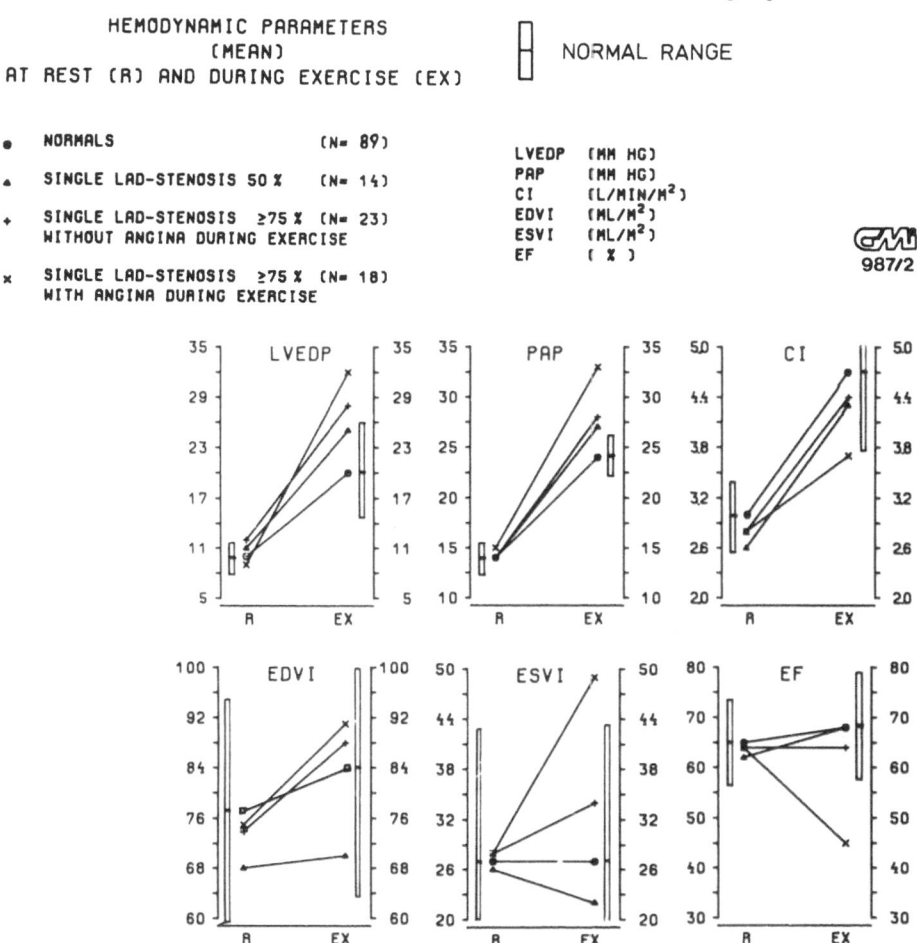

Fig. 3. LV volume and pressure changes in different degrees of left anterior descending (LAD) stenosis

stenosis with exercise angina (Table 3). This was true for patients with multivessel disease and no exercise angina.

According to our protocol, only some 25% of exercise was symptom limited and in most cases limited by a heart rate of about 110 beats/min to get a better opacification of exercise angiography. Thus, we are able to analyze the time course of hemodynamic parameters from the results of many tests (Fig. 5).

During the first phase of ischemia there is an increase of filling pressure without significant changes of volume parameters. End-diastolic volume and end-systolic volume increase up to the same degree, so that ejection fraction remains constant. With angina pectoris there is a sudden drop of ejection fraction, but cardiac index remains unchanged up to this point. However, with a further increase of ischemia a further decrease of ejection fraction and finally of cardiac index was also observed.

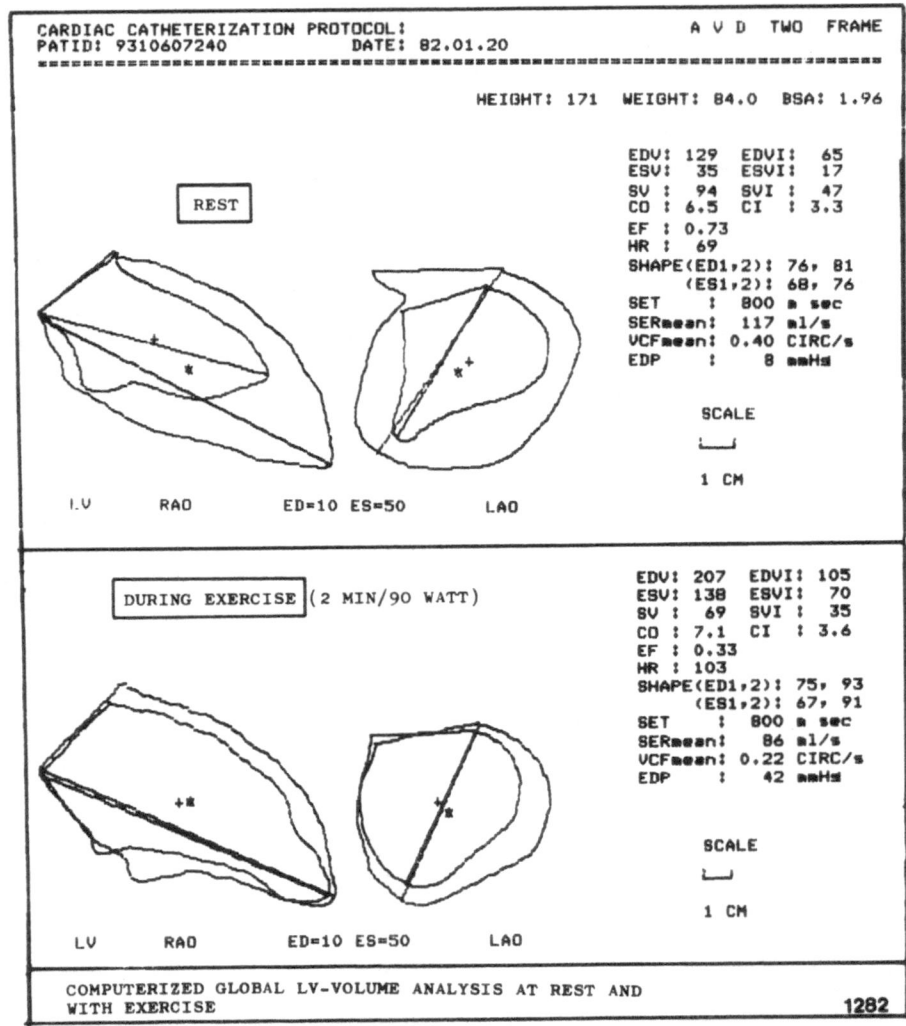

Fig. 4. a Global (*left*) and segmental (*right*) changes in LV function during exercise in a patient with 75% LAD stenosis and no angina during exercise. **b** Myocardial imaging with thallium-201 (*left*) and ECG at rest and with exercise (*right*)

Not only the extent of stenosis but the extent and the position of the ischemic segment during exercise influence LV pump function to various degrees (Fig. 6). From our results we can summarize as follows. The first level of ischemia appears to cause only compliance disturbances, as was shown in Fig. 5. At this level, the overall contractile behavior might still be unchanged. But there are first ST-T changes. A second level of ischemia would seem to cause contractile disturbances starting with regional wall motion disorders such as retarded con-

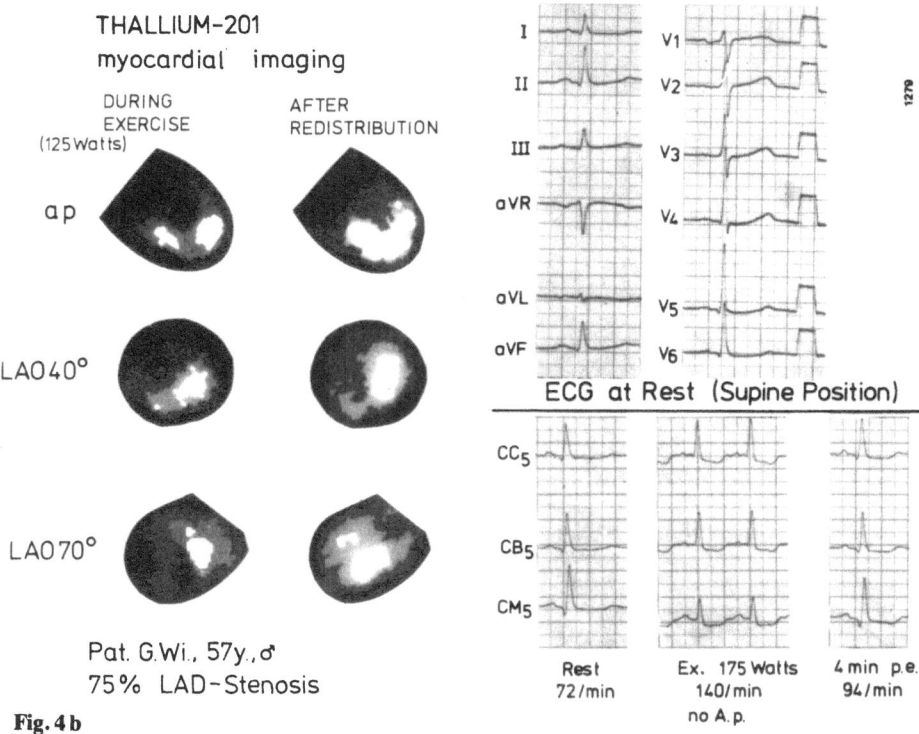

THALLIUM-201
myocardial imaging

DURING
EXERCISE
(125 Watts)

AFTER
REDISTRIBUTION

ap

LAO 40°

LAO 70°

Pat. G.Wi., 57y., ♂
75% LAD-Stenosis

Fig. 4 b

ECG at Rest (Supine Position)

Rest
72/min

Ex. 175 Watts
140/min
no A.p.

4 min p.e.
94/min

Table 3. Hemodynamic parameters (mean and SD) at rest and during exercise in three-vessel disease or left main stenosis ($n = 19$)

Parameters	Rest	Exercise	Δ
HR (beats/min)	70.4 ± 10	103.2 ± 14	+ 32.8
LVSP (mmHg)	138.8 ± 16	152.9 ± 20	+ 14.1
LVEDP. (mmHg)	10.8 ± 3	31.1 ± 9	+ 20.3
EDVI (ml/m²)	73.5 ± 20	83.4 ± 24	+ 9.9
ESVI (ml/m²)	27.8 ± 11	39.8 ± 20	+ 12.0
EF (%)	61.9 ± 10	54.3 ± 14	− 7.6
CI (l/min/m²)	2.59 ± 0.5	4.12 ± 1.2	+ 1.53

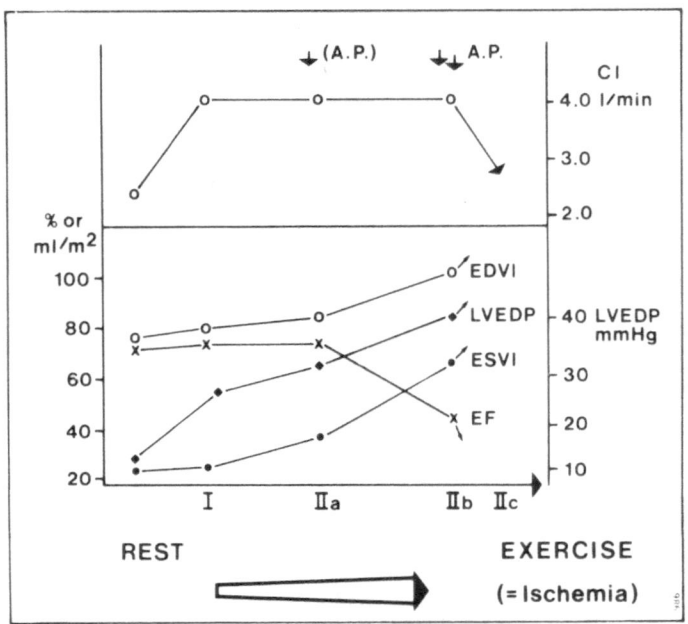

Fig. 5. Time course of volume and pressure changes during exercise in patients with coronary heart disease

traction of one or two segments (Fig. 6). If the ischemic segment is 20%–30% and positioned in the posterior wall of the left ventricle, there is only a slight increase in EDVI with normal ejection fraction due to better contraction of the anterior wall. This ist true also for an ischemic posterior segment of about 40%, where EDVI increases somewhat more but without decrease of ejection fraction. In sharp contrast to this, an ischemic segment of 45% or more in or including the anterior wall could not be compensated by better contraction of the posterior wall, so ejection fraction and CI decrease.

In summary, there are some correlations between coronary anatomy and pathophysiology in coronary heart disease. In cases with normal LV function at rest, the correlation could be best seen during exercise ventriculography, which has been shown to be a safe and effective method that could be used routinely, and which has proved in our experience more sensitive than thallium scintigraphy. The most important is the correlation in LAD stenosis, provided there ist a normal or dominant and not a diminutive LAD. In dominant LAD coronary, stenosis of 50%–60% should be classified as significant. This ist not true for circumflex and RCA stenosis, where 75% or more may be significant, but in absence of LAD stenosis could be well compensated by an increased contraction of the anterior wall. Thus we see that the main applications (Table 4) of exercise LV angiography in patients with angina pectoris and normal LV function at rest are, first, in evaluation of the functional significance of isolated LAD stenosis or one- or two-vessel disease and, second, in complex hemodynamic analysis of

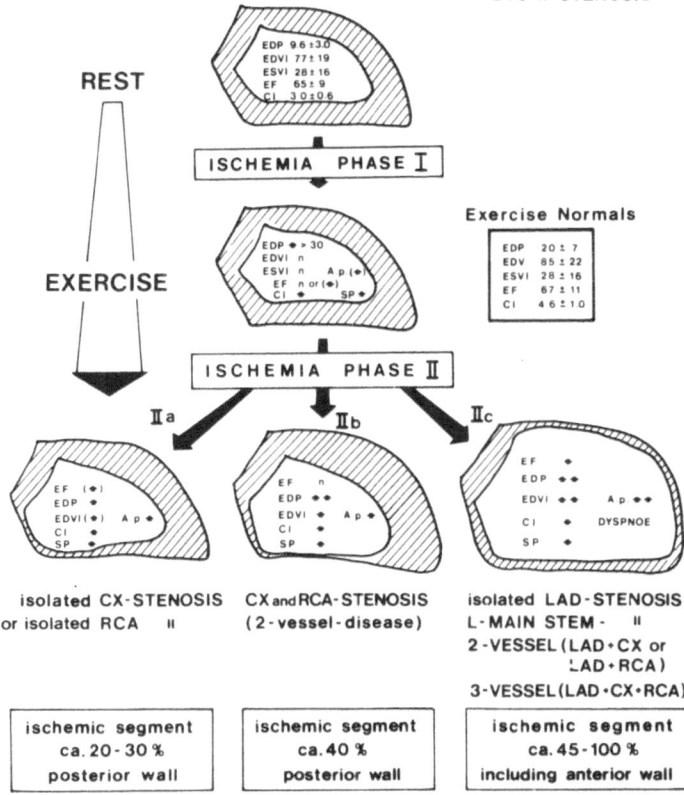

LV-PRESSURE AND VOLUME CHANGES DURING DYNAMIC EXERCISE
IN PATIENTS WITH CHD, NORMAL LV-FUNCTION AT REST AND
≥ 75 % STENOSIS

Fig. 6. Time course of hemodynamic changes with exercise in relation to location and extent of the ischemic segment in coronary heart disease

Table 4. Summary of main indications for LV exercise angiography

1. Coronary heart disease:
   Detection of ischemia in normal or nearly normal wall motion at rest:
   LAD stenosis 50%–75%
   LAD stenosis 75% with:
   - Local hypokinesis
     (nontransmural infarction)
   - Small apical scar
     (small apical infarction)

   Indication for aneurysmectomy:
   - Exercise EF of rest ventricle > 50%
   - Resting EDVI > 60 ml/m^2

2. Complex hemodynamic analysis in patients with:
   - Syndrome X
   - Cardiomyopathy
   - Aortic insufficiency
   - Hypertensive heart disease

patients with syndrome X, cardiomyopathy, hypertensive heart disease, or other unknown causes of ST-T changes at rest or exercise. A third group consists of patients with aortic insufficiency or anterior wall aneurysm, where the aim is to predict prognosis (indications for surgery and postoperative pump function) [18]. Especially in cases with proximal LAD stenosis of 50%–75% and normal or borderline normal LV function at rest, and history of small transmural infarction or no infarction at all, we complete catheterization with LV exercise angiography, which proves to be more helpful in decision making for either drug treatment or percutaneous transluminal coronary angioplasty or bypass surgery.

The real advantages of the method are that it is a rapid and safe test for analyzing global and local LV function in the catheter laboratory during routine LV angiography, thus avoiding further tests with possibly lower specificity and sensitivity.

References

1. Borer JS, Bacharach SL, Green MV, Kent KM, Epstein SE, Johnson GS (1977) Realtime radionuclide cineangiography in the noninvasive evaluation of global and regional left ventricular function at rest and with exercise in patients with coronary heart disease. N Engl J Med 296:839
2. Chapmann CB, Baker O, Reynolds H, Bonke FJ (1958) Use of biplane cinefluorography for measurement of ventricular volume. Circulation 18:1105
3. Davis K, Kennedy JW, Kemp HG, Judkins P, Gosselin A, Killip T (1979) Complications of coronary arteriography from the collaborative study of coronary artery surgery (CASS). Circulation 59:1105
4. Dodge HT, Sandler H, Baxley WH, Hawley RR (1966) Usefulness and limitations of radiographic methods for determing left ventricular volume. Am J Cardiol 18:10
5. Eubanks DE, Tsakiris AG, Davis GD, Wallace RB, Frye RL (1970) Left ventricular volumes during exercise induced angina in patients with coronary artery disease. Circulation [Suppl] 41–42/III:151
6. Frischknecht J, Steele P, Kirch D, Jensen D, Vogel R (1979) Effect of exercise on left ventricular ejection fraction in men with coronary artery disease. Am Heart 97:494
7. Gensini G (1975) Coronary-arteriography. Futura, New York
8. Gleichmann U, Ohlmeier H, Mannebach H, Faßbender D (1981) Hemodynamics and prognosis of patients with angina pectoris without coronary heart disease (Syndrome X). Cardiology 68 [Suppl II]:108
9. Gould L, Lipscomb K, Hamilton G (1974) Physiologic basis for assessing critical coronary stenosis. Am J Cardiol 33:87
10. Iskandrian S, Segal BL (1979) Structure and function of the coronary arteries: how are they related? Cathet Cardiovasc Diagn 5:101–105
11. Leong K, Joner RH (1982) Influence of the location of left anterior descending coronary artery stenosis on left ventricular function during exercise. Circulation 65:109
12. Lichtlen P (1979) Koronarangiographie. Strunke, Erlangen
13. Paulin S (1979) Grading and measuring coronary artery stenosis. Cathet Cardiovasc Diagn 5:213–218
14. Sharma B, Goodwin JF, Raphael MJ, Steiner RE, Rainbow RG, Taylor SH (1976) Left ventricular angiography on exercise: a new method of assessing left ventricular function in ischemic heart disease. Br Heart J 38:59
15. Sigwart U, Schmidt H, Bonzel T, Mertens HM, Gleichmann U (1975) Biplane cineangiographic evaluation of left ventricular contraction in ischemic heart disease at rest and during bicycle exercise. Circulation 51 [Suppl II]:37

16. Sigwart U, Schmidt H, Steiner J, Mertens HM, Gleichmann U (1975) Linksventrikuläre Geometrie und Volumina in Ruhe und während Ergometerbelastung bei koronarer Herzkrankheit. Verh Dtsch Ges Kreislaufforsch 41:193
17. Swan HJ (1979) Mechanical function of the heart and its alteration during myocardial ischemia and infarction. Circulation, 60/7:1587.
18. Trieb G, Mannebach H, Faßbender D, Müller A, Merte HM, Mertens HM, Gleichmann U (1980) The effect of left ventricular aneurys-mectomy on left ventricular function at rest and during exercise: a retrospective study of 350 patients. In: Bircks W, Ostermeyer J, Schulte HD (eds) Cardiovascular Surgery. Springer, Berlin Heidelberg New York, pp 410–414
19. Trieb G, Sigwart U, Mannebach H, Mertens HM, Gleichmann U (1979) Evaluation of left ventricular dysfunction in coronary heart disease by pressure, flow, and volume parameters during stress. Kardiol 68(4):260

Computer Assisted Angiographic Evaluation of Left Ventricular Function

J. Meyer*, K. Hagemann, R. Erbel*, W. Krebs, P. Schweizer, P. Jensch, W. Ameling, and S. Effert

* Present adress: II. Medizinische Klinik und Poliklinik der Univ. Mainz, Langenbeckstr. 1, D-6500 Mainz, FRG

Department of Internal Medicine I and Department of Electronic Data Processing Systems, Klinikum der RWTH, Goethestr. 27, D-5100 Aachen, FRG

Left ventricular (LV) dynamics can be described in terms of pressure, volume, and time. Modern techniques of computer analysis facilitate on-line analysis of pressure signals. In scientific studies LV and aortic pressure measurements are taken via tip micromanometers and analyzed using computer systems [1, 2]. The computer results are displayed within seconds, together with the analog curves, on the video screen or sheets produced by a printer (Fig. 1). The computer indicates with small vertical marks the exact points within the curves where the measurements were taken. In this way, visual quality control of the computer's performance is made possible [3]. Numerical pressure values are simultaneously displayed in the same frame (Fig. 1).

Furthermore, numerous derived pressure parameters are additionally calculated by the computer. Using a sampling rate of 400 Hz and an adequate smoothing procedure (smoothing over 11 points, differentation over seven

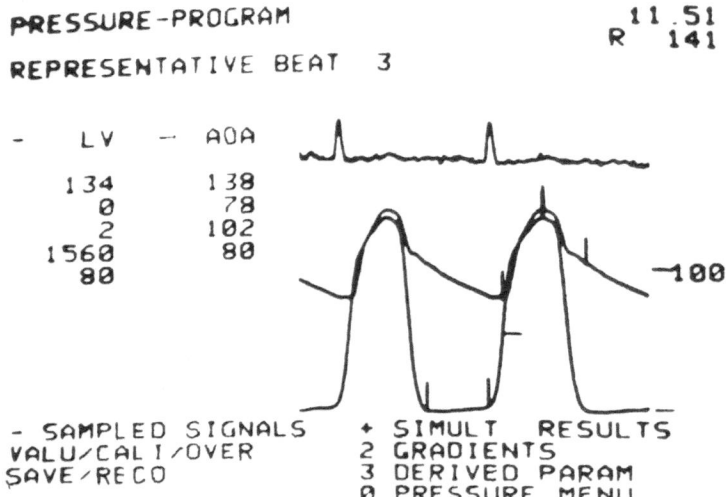

Fig. 1. Original video display of the computer measurements of left ventricular (*LV*) and aortic pressure (*AOA*). Representative beat of a sampling period, computer marks of the measurement points within the curves. Numerical values of *LV* pressure: systolic, begin- and end-diastolic, maximum d*p*/d*t*, heart rate; aortic pressure: systolic, end diastolic, mean pressure, heart rate

points) contractility parameters like dp/dt and V_{CE} can be calculated with a high level of reliability [4] (Fig. 2). The complete V_{CE} loop of the individual cardiac cycle can be displayed on the screen and then edited by the X-Yplotter. With the sampling rate of 400 Hz the individual points of the V_{CE} loop are available in steps of 2.5 ms. V_{pm}, the maximum value of the V_{CE} curve, is calculated as well as V_{max}. Since, because of simultaneous pressure recordings, the time of the aortic valve opening is also marked within the V_{CE} loop, one can easily check

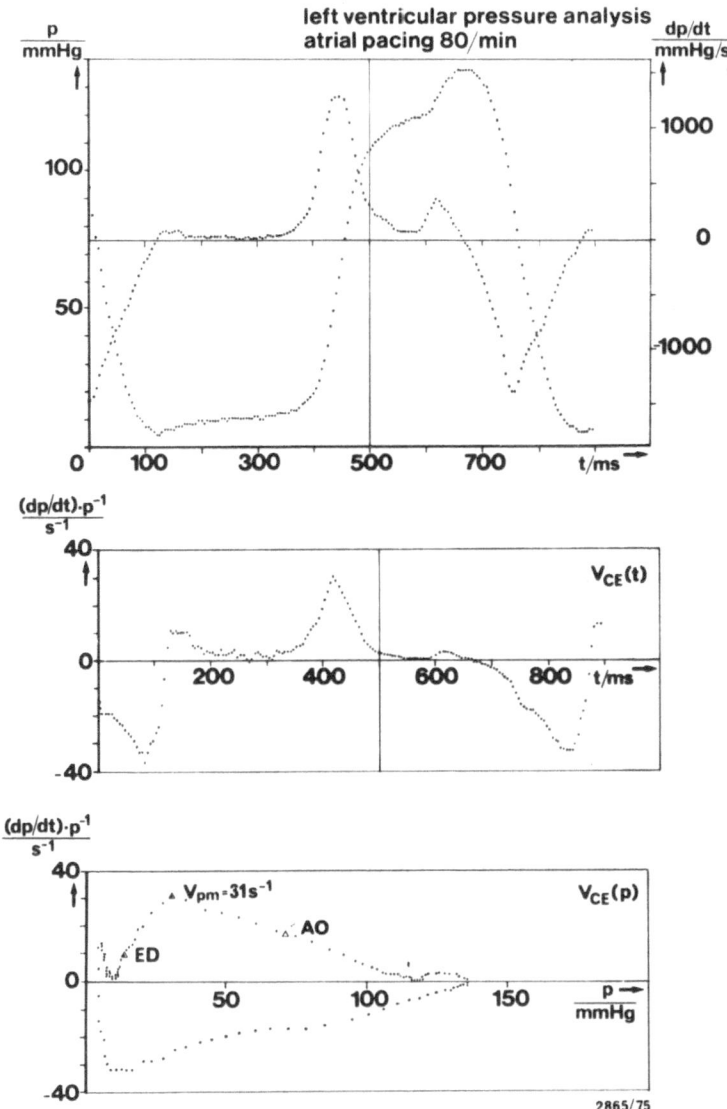

Fig. 2. Computer analysis of LV pressure with simultaneous display of the curves of dp/dt, dp/dt/p ($V_{CE}(t)$), and the V_{CE}loop ($V_{CE}(p)$). Identification of V_{pm} and aortic valve opening (AO). Heart rate 80 beats/min using atrial pacing

whether the contractility parameters are really taken within the isovolumic phase (Fig. 2).

These sophisticated parameters of the force-velocity-length relation [5,6], however, have lost some of their importance during the past years. Modern techniques of videometric and digital image analysis have improved quantitative angiocardiography [7–21]. Combined with computer analysis, it is now possible to carry out a truly simultaneous and continuous study of pressure, volume, and time. To ensure identical heart rates, right atrial pacing is performed routinely. LV angiography is performed by injection of 60–70 ml contrast medium into the pulmonary artery (Fig. 3). With this technique premature ventricular contractions can be avoided. The ventriculograms obtained are of adequate quality for quantitative analysis using computerized videometry. Only the earliest cycles providing good opacification of the LV cavity are analyzed.

Biplane cineangiography is performed employing the 30° RAO projection, at a camera speed of 50 frames/s. Frame-by-frame analysis of the angiograms is performed by projecting the cinefilms onto a video screen and outlining the ventricular contours by hand with a light-pen. By this means the ventricular angiogram is cut into 100–256 slices. Each slice is determined by the height of the video lines.

Besides volume analysis, the function and morphology of the heart valves and the contraction pattern of the wall areas can be analyzed. The information is transmitted from the video screen directly to the computer. The thickness of the LV wall is determined from the free wall of the ventricle in 30° RAO projection by taking the average difference of epicardial and endocardial positions. We use the single-plane method of Trenouth et al. [22] to calculate muscle mass with its correction in the valvular and the apical region. This method produces slight underestimation of LV mass. Because of irregularities in trabecular and

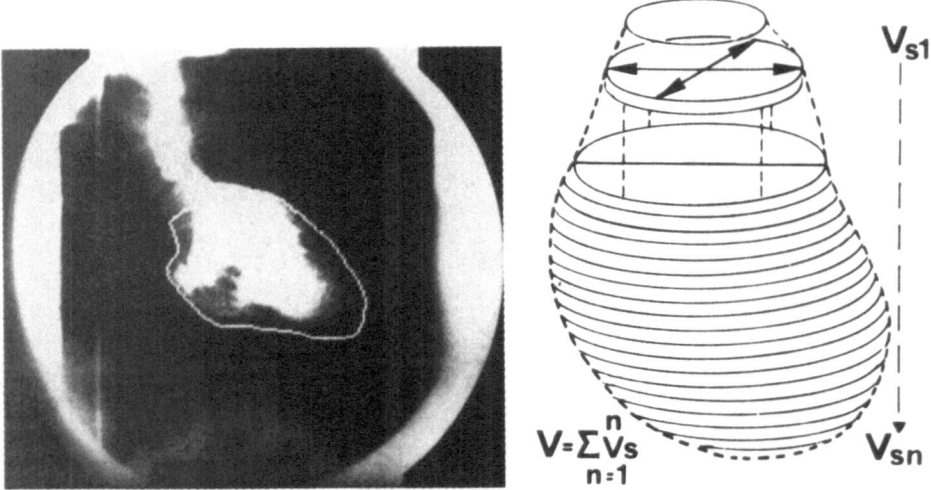

Fig. 3. LV angiography with outlining of contours by light-pen. Calculation of ventricular volume using the Simpson method. Separation of the ventricle into numerous slices of known height according to the television lines

papillary structures, and because of scars, some uncertainty arises even in angiograms with good opacification. The LV volume is calculated using Simpson's rule. No regression equation for correction of volumes is used. Smoothing and differentation of the pressure and volume curve is performed as described by Savitzky and Golay [23].

The volume analysis can be correlated with the instantaneous pressure value by a synchronization signal to both the angiographic and the pressure recordings (Fig. 4). In this way, simultaneous pressure-volume analysis is possible [17, 20, 21, 24]. The pressure and volume curves of the whole cardiac cycle are both plotted by the computer using a common time scale. The number of curve-points is determined by the speed of the cine cameras and the pictures/s (in our institution 50 frames/s). Using a linear interpolation procedure between two

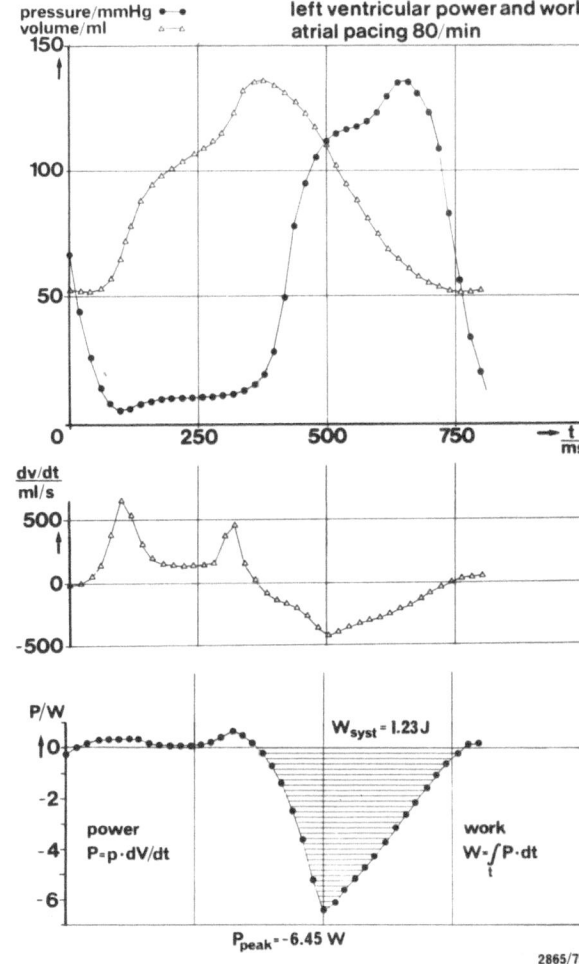

Fig. 4. Simultaneous pressure and volume curves of the left ventricle (pacing rate 80 beats/min). First derivative (dV/dt) of LV volume and continuous power curve. LV work corresponds to the area of the power curve. Sampling points according to the camera speed (see text)

points of the volume curve, calculations can be made automatically at 10-ms intervals [23]. Knowing LV pressure, wall thickness, and the interior ventricular diameter, the maximal systolic wall stress can be calculated by the computer according to the method of Sandler and Dodge [25, 26]. The meridional wall stress is calculated by

$$\delta = \frac{pD}{4\,W\,(1 + W/D)}$$

where p is the left ventricular pressure, D ist the maximum interior LV diameter, and W is the wall thickness.

Corresponding to the first derivative of the LV pressure dp/dt, the volume change dV/dt can also be analyzed continuously (Fig. 4). The systolic peak of this curve is negative corresponding to the systolic decrease of LV volume. From this curve the rate of volume change and thus the speed of volume ejection at any moment of the systole can be measured. It can be defined whether the moment of the maximal volume change max dV/dt lies in the first, second, or third part of the systole [12, 18, 21, 22, 27].

The parameter "left ventricular power" combines the time-dependent changes of ventricular pressure and volume [12, 17, 19, 23, 28]. This has been shown to be a useful index of cardiac performance under various hemodynamic conditions. By plotting power against time a continuous systolic-diastolic power curve (Fig. 4) is obtained. LV power during the ejection period is calculated according to the equation

$$P = p \times dV/dt$$

where P is power, p is instantaneous LV pressure, and dV/dt is the instantaneous ejection blood flow. According to the common time scale of pressure and volume changes, LV power can be determined at any moment of the cardiac cycle. The analog power-curve is plotted, while the individual numeric values are edited by the line printer. We mostly take the values of peak power and the mean value throughout systole.

LV systolic work [10, 18–21, 24, 28] can be represented by

$$W = \int p \times dt$$

and is calculated automatically from the area under the power curve. This is equivalent to the area under the pressure-volume diagram.

The systolic parameters maximum power, mean power, and work are analyzed alone and also standardized with respect to the individual LV end-diastolic volume and muscle mass [10, 17, 20, 21, 24, 29]. Thus, the amount of power and work per gram of LV muscle mass can be calculated. This gives some information on the work load and the performance of the individual ventricle.

In intervention studies using pharmaceutical drugs, in pre- and postoperative comparative studies after valve replacement, exact intra- and interindividual measurements can be made [17, 20, 21, 24, 30–32]. Some results of such combined pressure-volume analysis may be demonstrated: Fig. 5 shows the end-diastolic volume index (EDV/BSA) and the LV muscle mass index (MM/BSA)

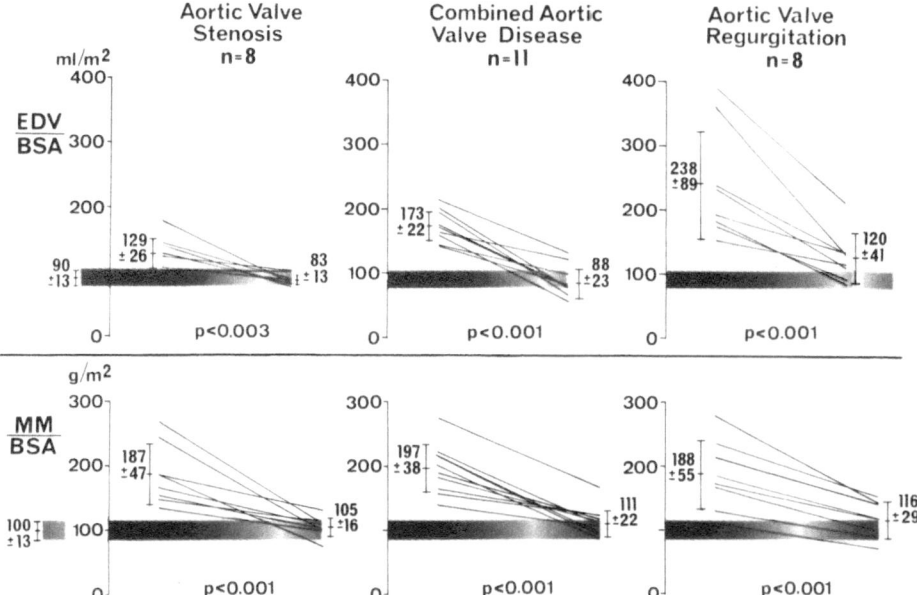

Fig. 5. End-diastolic volume (*EDV/BSA*) and muscle mass index (*MM/BSA*) before and after valve replacement in aortic valve replacement in aortic valve diseases. *Hatched zone,* normal range

before and at 9 ± 3 months after valve replacement by a Björk-Shiley prosthesis in eight patients with pure aortic valve stenosis (regurgitation fraction less than 25%), in eight patients with pure valve regurgitation (valve gradient less than 10 mmHg), and in 11 patients with combined valve disease [20, 21, 31]. Since the pressure-volume parameters are rate-dependent, identical heart rates in the individual patient were achieved by atrial pacing. Preoperatively EDV/BSA was slightly elevated in aortic stenosis (normal range indicated). With rising degree of aortic regurgitation, the end-diastolic volume index rose, reaching up to $390 \, ml/m^2$. One year after operation this parameter normalized quite remarkably in all patients with a greater tendency to aortic stenosis. Even very large ventricles in aortic regurgitation showed a regression of at least 50%.

LV muscle mass was augmented much more uniformly in all three categories. Despite maximal values of up to $300 \, g/m^2$, threefold the value of normal hearts, muscle mass had nearly always normalized within the first 10–15 months after operation.

LV wall stress (Fig. 6) in patients with prevailing valve stenosis showed a significant regression. In patients with aortic regurgitation and large ventricles, however, this parameter was not that informative. LV wall stress and muscle mass were increased approximately equally in both pressure and volume overload [11, 18, 26, 31–33].

There was a substantial increase in wall thickness in the pressure overloaded ventricles, but only a mild increase in the volume overloaded ones. The latter

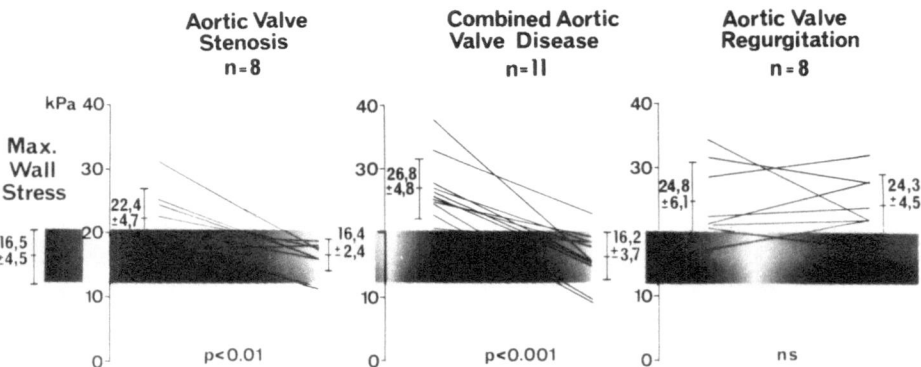

Fig. 6. Maximum wall stress before and after valve replacement

was just sufficient to counterbalance the increased radius. By this means the ratio of wall thickness to radius remained normal in volume overload. By contrast, in pressure overloaded ventricles this ratio was augmented because of the thickening of the ventricular wall.

If pressure overload is the primary stimulus, wall thickening and concentric hypertrophy result, in order to balance systolic stress. In volume overloaded ventricles, increased diastolic wal stress leads to fiber elongation and ventricular enlargement. This then induces wall thickening to return systolic stress to normal. Thus, in both cases the variations in ventricular geometry and wall thickness lead to a normalization of wall stress. In case of decompensation the values of wall stress rise.

After valve replacement, ventricular hypertrophy in aortic stenosis shows much steeper regression than LV volume in aortic regurgitation. Consequently systolic wall stress declined in all instances of aortic stenosis postoperatively, while this parameter was inconsistent in patients with aortic regurgitation.

The functioning of the human heart can broadly be compared to a hydraulic pump. The data needed for the determination of the pump power are pressure, volume, and time. Studies of LV power have been reported by several groups [12, 17, 19, 24, 28]. Measurements, however, can only be compared if the heart rate is kept constant [17].

Systolic mean power (Fig. 7) was elevated preoperatively in all cases with mean values twice the normal. This parameter also showed a remarkable decline postoperatively. In some patients, however, it failed to normalize. Two patients with aortic stenosis and one with aortic regurgitation with an unexpected rise of mean power after operation also suffered from coronary artery disease. Despite good functional results of the artificial valves and a significant reduction of LV volume and muscle mass, their ventricles did not impove in performance. Thus, the positive influences of valve replacement on LV volume and muscle mass and the negative influences of the coronary artery disease can be separated [34].

LV systolic work (Fig. 8) was especially elevated in patients with predominant valve insufficiency [12, 18–20, 21, 24, 34]. In all patients less systolic work was

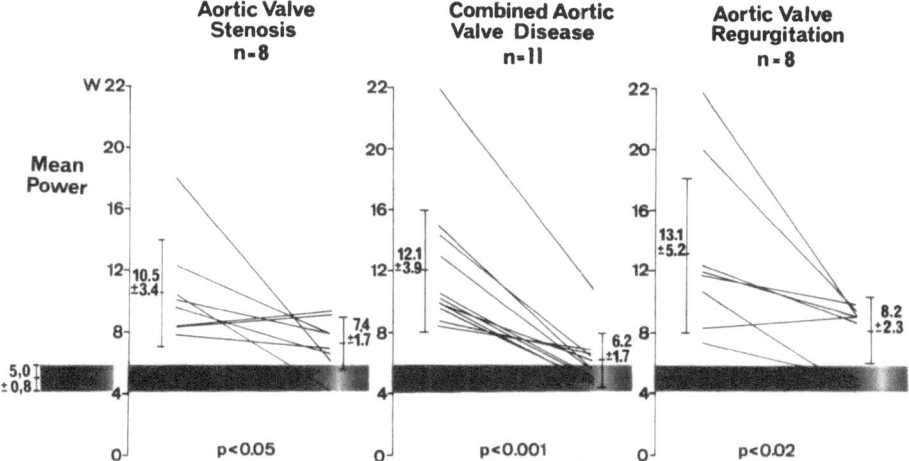

Fig. 7. Mean power before and after valve replacement

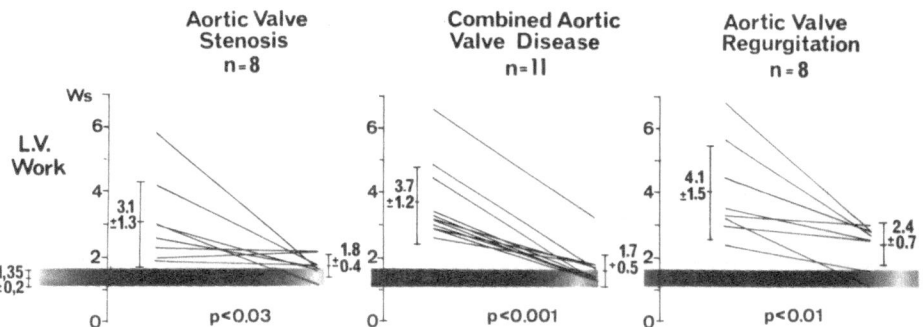

Fig. 8. LV systolic work before and after valve replacement

needed postoperatively. In pure valve regurgitation the values were still above the upper normal level. LV systolic power and work normalized for muscle mass are good parameters of myocardial performance [10, 24, 29–35]. As long as the ventricle is sufficient, the ratio remains constant. Declining power and work per gram of muscle mass, however, are sensitive indicators of myocardial insufficiency. As was also described by Dodge [10, 29], LV work is a better indicator of myocardial performance when related to muscle mass than when related to end-diastolic volume.

Figure 9 shows the application of the pressure-volume analysis to an intervention study [35]. Ten patients with proven coronary artery disease were given 4 mg molsidomine. In order to reach comparable results, atrial pacing (80 beats/min) was performed before and after treatment. After 45 min, systolic wall stress, maximum and mean power, and systolic work in the individual patient showed a significant decline. This demonstrates the amount of the immediate unloading of the left ventricle by this vasodilator. It also demonstrates the fact

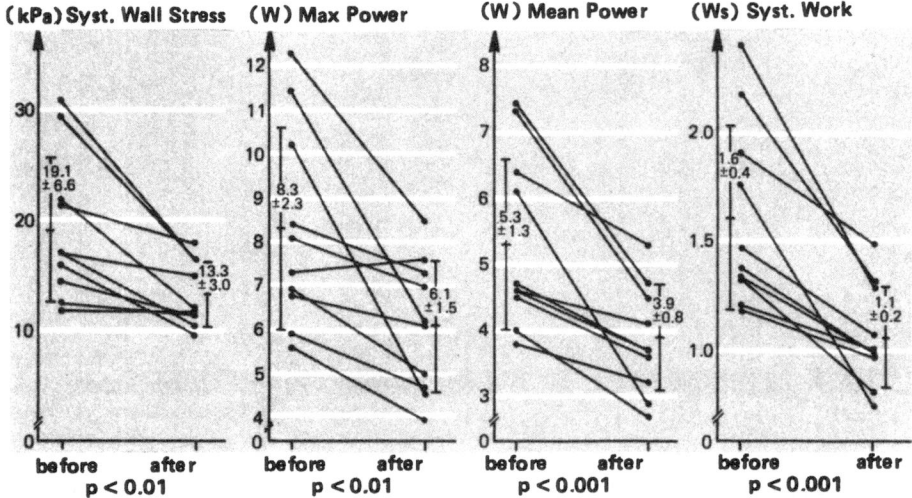

Fig. 9. Analysis of systolic wall stress, maximum power, mean power, and systolic work in patients ($n = 10$) with coronary artery disease before and 45 min after 4 mg molsidomine [35]

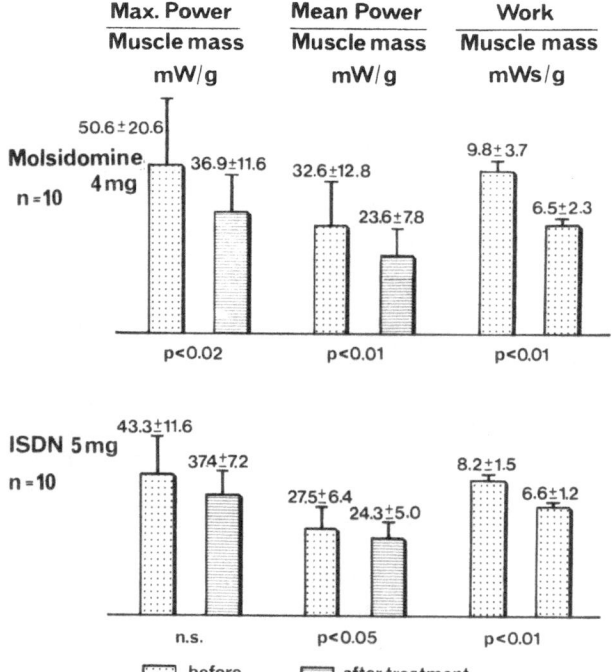

Fig. 10. Changes of maximum power, mean power, and work of the left ventricle related to the individual LV muscle mass before and after molsidomine (4 mg) and isosorbide dinitrate (*ISDN*; 5 mg). No significant differences between both groups ($n = 10$ patients each) [30]

that even 4 mg molsidomine is quite sufficient to induce a remarkable and significant unloading of the left ventricle in the acute intervention.

In comparative studies (Fig. 10), these parameters may also be used to evaluate the qualitative effects of different drugs [30]. Even if the acute effects of molsidomine (4 mg) and isosorbide dinitrate (5 mg) in two different groups of patients ($n = 10$) cannot be compared quantitatively, the qualitative improvements can be demonstrated. Both vasodilators led to a remakable reduction of maximum and mean power and of work per gram of LV muscle mass showing the unloading of the diseased heart and the improvement of LV function.

Thus, computer-assisted pressure-volume analysis provides a precise and detailed analysis of LV function. In the individual patient these indices help in the estimation of operative risk and to compare pre- and postoperative findings. In intervention studies, such analyses give exact information on work load and improvement of ventricular performance.

Although, because of the expense involved, this type of detailed study may not be suitable for routine clinical use, it does allow better quantification, definition, and understanding of the pathophysiological changes of the left ventricle.

References

1. Meyer J, Jensch P, Ameling W, Effert S (1974) A new program for the automatic analysis of cardiac catheterization data. First World Conference on Medical Informatics (Medinfo), Stockholm. North-Holland, Amsterdam, p 677
2. Jensch P, Meyer J, Ameling W, Effert S (1976) Ein Prozeßrechnersystem für Herzkatheterlabors und Hämodynamikmeßplätze. Z Kardiol 65:850
3. Meyer J, Jensch P, Zimmer K, Braun PC, Hagemann K, Platte G, Ameling W, Effert S (1978) Computersystem für die automatische Analyse von Herzkatheterdaten – Zuverlässigkeit der Kurvenerkennung und Vermessung. Klin Wochenschr 56:81
4. Meyer J, Hagemann K, Jensch P, Platte G, Ruppert G, Effert S, Ameling W (1976) Umfassende On-line-Berechnung von Kontraktilitätsparametern mit einem Computersystem – Möglichkeiten und Grenzen. 42. Verh Dtsch Ges. Kreislaufforschg, Bad Nauheim. Steinkopff, Darmstadt, p 271
5. Brutsaert DL, Sonnenblick EH (1973) Cardiac muscle mechanics in the evaluation of myocardial contractility and pump function: problems, concepts and directions. Prog Cardiovasc Dis 16:337
6. Sonnenblick EH, Strobeck JE (1977) Derived indexes of ventricular and myocardial function. N Engl J Med 296:978
7. Rackley CE, Dodge HT, Coble YD, Hay RE (1964) A method for determining left ventricular mass in man. Circulation 29:666
8. Kennedy JW, Baxley WA, Figley MM, Dodge HT, Blackmon JR (1966) Quantitative angiocardiography. I. The normal left ventricle in man. Circulation 34:272
9. Kennedy JW, Twiss RD, Blackmon JR, Dodge HT (1968) Quantitative angiography. III. Relationship of left ventricular pressure, volume, and mass in aortic valve disease. Circulation 38:838
10. Dodge HT, Kennedy JW, Petersen JT (1973) Quantitative angiographic methods in the evaluation of valvular heart disease. Prog Cardiovasc Dis 16:1
11. Rackley CE (1976) Quantitative evaluation of left ventricular function by radiographic techniques. Circulation 54:862
12. Spiller P (1978) Quantitative Lävokardiographie. Urban & Schwarzenberg, Munich, p 103
13. Heintzen PH, Malerczyk V, Pilarczyk J, Scheel KW (1971) On-line processing of the videoimage for left ventricular volume determination. Comput Biomed Res 4:474

14. Lange PE, Onnasch DGW, Farr FL, Malerczyk V, Heintzen PH (1978) Analysis of left and right ventricular size and shape as determined from human casts. Description of the method and its validation. Eur J Cardiol 8:431
15. Alderman EL, Sandler H, Booker JZ, Sanders WJ, Simpson C, Harrison DC (1973) Light-pen computer processing of videoimage for the determination of left ventricular volume. Circulation 47:309
16. Brower RW, Meester GT, Hugenholtz PG (1975) Quantification of ventricular performance: a computer-based system for the analysis of angiographic data. Cathet Cardiovasc Diagn 1:133
17. Hagemann K, Meyer J, von Essen R, Krebs W, Effert S (1979) Left ventricular ejection power in coronary artery disease during atrial pacing. Br Heart J 41:231
18. Bove AA, Kreulen TH, Spann JF (1978) Computer analysis of left ventricular dynamic geometry in man. Am J Cardiol 41:1239
19. Snell RE, Luchsinger PC (1965) Determination of external work and power of the left ventricle in intact man. Am Heart J 69:529
20. Meyer J, Krebs W, Hagemann K, Verstraeten K, Jensch P, Effert S, Ameling W (1978) Computergestützte, simultane Druck-Volumen-Zeitanalyse des linken Ventrikels. I. Untersuchungen bei der Druckhypertrophie durch reine valvuläre Aortenklappenstenose. Z Kardiol 67:809
21. Meyer J, Krebs W, Hagemann K, Verstraeten K, Jensch P, Effert S, Ameling W (1978) Computergestützte simultane Druck-Volumen-Zeitanalyse des linken Ventrikels. II. Untersuchungen bei der Volumenhypertrophie durch reine valvuläre Aortenklappeninsuffizienz. Z Kardiol 67:818
22. Trenouth RS, Phelps NC, Neill WA (1976) Determinants of left ventricular hypertrophy and oxygen supply in chronic aortic valve disease. Circulation 53:644
23. Savitzky A, Golay ME (1964) Smoothing and differentiation of data by simplified least squares procedures. Anal Chem 36:1627
24. Meyer J, Krebs W, Hagemann K, Erbel R, Verstraeten K, Jensch P, Ameling W, Effert S (1980) Computerized simultaneous pressure-volume analysis in aortic valve disease. Eur Heart J 4:171
25. Sandler H, Dodge HT (1963) Left ventricular tension and stress in man. Circulation Res 13:91
26. Grossmann W, Jones D, Laurin LP (1975) Wall stress and patterns of hypertrophy in the human left ventricle. J Clin Invest 56:56
27. Mathes P, Delius W, Sebening H, Blömer H (1978) Initiale systolische Austreibungsgeschwindigkeit als Maß der Ventrikelfunktion bei Herzklappenerkrankungen. Z Kardiol 67:233
28. Russel PO, Porter CM, Frimer M, Dodge HT (1971) Left ventricular power in man. Am Heart J 81:799
29. Dodge HT, Baxley WA (1969) Left ventricular volume and mass and their significance in heart disease. Am J Cardiol 23:528
30. Meyer J, Erbel R, Schweizer P, Effert S (1982) Kombinierte Druck-Volumen-Analyse vor und nach der Gabe verschiedener Vasodilatatoren. 2. Molsidomin-Workshop, Rottach-Egern, Thieme, Stuttgart
31. Rackley CE, Hood WP Jr (1973) Quantitative angiographic evaluation and pathophysiologic mechanisms of valvular heart disease. Prog Cardiovasc Dis 15:427
32. Pantley G, Morton M, Rahimtoola SH (1978) Effects of successful, uncomplicated valve replacement on ventricular hypertrophy, volume and performance in aortic stenosis and in aortic incompetence. J Thorac Cardiovasc Surg 75:383
33 Hood WP Jr, Rackley CE, Rolett EL (1968) Wall stress in the normal and hypertrophied left ventricle. Am J Cardiol 22:550
34. Meyer J, Josephs W, Krebs W, Braun PC, Hagemann K, Bardos P, Messmer BJ, Effert S (1981) Normalisation von Muskelhypertrophie und Pumpfunktion des linken Ventrikels nach Klappenersatz bei schweren Aortenklappenerkrankungen. Thorac Cardiovasc Surg 29:41
35. Meyer J, Sprauer R, Krebs W, Erbel R, Schweizer P, Effert S (1980) Wirkung von Molsidomin auf die Belastung des linken Ventrikels bei koronarer Herzkrankheit. Dtsch Med Wochenschr 105:1210

Use of Endocardial Landmarks in the Evaluation of Left Ventricular Function:
Advantages and Limitations of Automated Analysis of the Ventriculogram

C. J. Slager, T. E. H. Hooghoudt, J. H. C. Reiber, J. C. H. Schuurbiers, and P. D. Verdouw

Thoraxcenter, Erasmus University Ee 2322, P.O. Box 1738, 3000 DR Rotterdam, The Netherlands

Introduction

In this study a method to assess left ventricular wall motion, relying on the pathways of anatomical landmarks recognizable on the endocardial border, is described and evaluated. Although contrast angiography provides detailed information on left ventricular contours, quantitative manual analysis of ventriculograms has not been able to reveal the actual pathways of specific sites on the endocardium. Previously described methods [1–5] to assess left ventricular wall motion are based on preconceived notions about the motion pattern of the left ventricular wall and lack any actual anatomical base. In animals these pathways can easily be followed with endocardially implanted metal clips [6, 7, 8] and roentgen cinematography. For obvious reasons this approach was never performed in humans, although midwall motion [9] and epicardial motion [10–13] have been studied in humans with surgically implanted markers. However, due to wall thickening, major differences exist in extent and direction between the motions of neighbouring endocardial, midwall and epicardial sites [6, 14]. Therefore none of these methods can specifically provide an outline of endocardial movement.

In an attempt to track the endocardium in humans a new-high resolution automated outlining system [15] was employed. This revealed small landmarks at the left ventricular contrast border, which can be followed throughout the cardiac cycle by analysis of consecutive frames of the cineangiogram. The hypothesis that these landmarks actually represent specific anatomical sites has been tested, so that the mean systolic pathways of these anatomical landmarks in normal individuals could be used to define a method for the assessment of human left ventricular wall motion.

Materials and Methods

The first study group consisted of eight anaesthetized pigs with a mean weight of 24 kg ± 3 kg (mean + SD). Left ventricular pressures were obtained from catheters with a micromanometer at the tip (7F Millar, Millar Instruments,

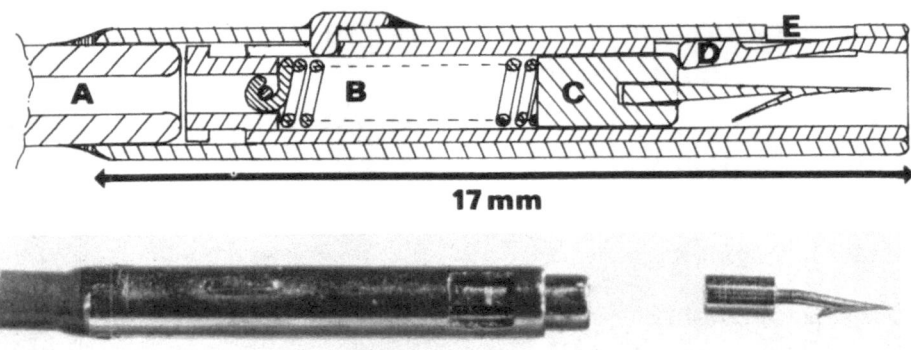

Fig. 1. Schematic drawing and photograph of spring-loaded metal marker insertion device attached to the tip of a 7F catheter. The inner tube, including trigger lever *D* is advanced by manual injection of saline into the catheter *A*, thus releasing metal marker *C*

Houston). A 7F Gorlin pacing catheter was introduced into the coronary sinus. A fixed heart rate of 10 bpm above resting heart rate was chosen and maintained during the study.

A left ventriculogram was made during injection auf 0.75 ml/kg body wt. Urografin 76 (Schering, Berlin) through an 8F angiocatheter at a rate of 12 ml/s. The opacified ventricles were filmed from the left lateral projection at a rate of 50 frames/s. During angiography artificial respiration was stopped to exclude extracardiac motion.

After the acquisition of a technically satisfactory cine angiogram, specific sites of the endocardial wall were marked with small metal darts. For this purpose a spring-loaded insertion device (Fig. 1) attached to the tip of a flexible catheter (USCI Muller Guide System and Variflex 7F catheter) with tip-steering facilities was used. The combination of a sharp barbed hook and a blunt body guarantees both an excellent fixation of the marker with minimal damage of the myocardium and an accurate delineation of the endocardium.

In each pig five markers were inserted along the anterior and infero-posterior margins of the left ventricle in a pattern outlining the ventricular cavity as seen in the left lateral projection (Fig. 2). Care was taken to insert the marker in the outermost position. In order to detect possible myocardial injury due to the insertion procedure, the ECG and left ventricular pressure were monitored continuously. Once marker insertion was completed a second left ventricular angiogram was made with identical X-ray geometry and with the respirator turned off. A centimetre grid was filmed for calibration purposes. An interval of at least 30 min was observed between consecutive angiograms.

The second study group consisted of 23 individuals, submitted to a diagnostic heart catheterization because of suspected heart disease, who appeared to have no haemodynamic or angiographic abnormality. Patients were studied after an overnight fast without premedication; all drugs which might influence left ven-

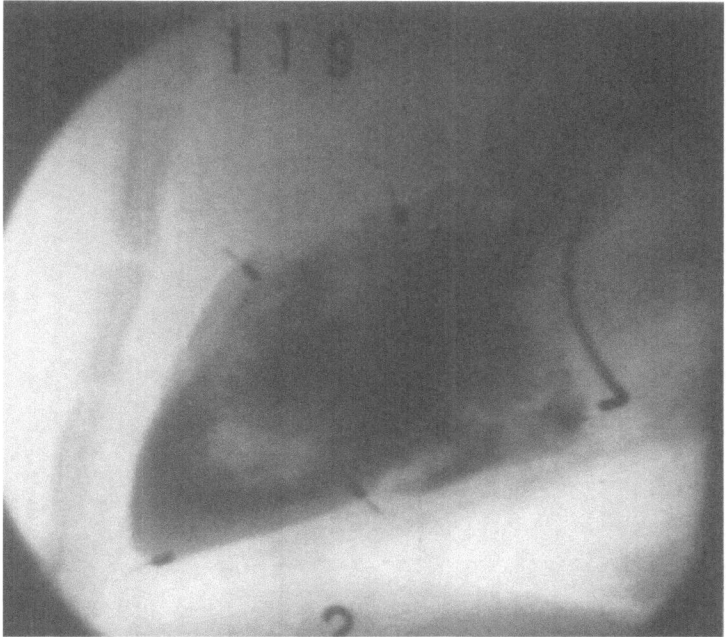

Fig. 2. End-diastolic frame from pig left ventricular angiogram with metal markers outlining the left ventricular cavity as seen in the left lateral projection

tricular contractile function were stopped at least 24 h prior to the study. Left ventricular cineangiograms were made at resting heart rate, during injection of 0.75 mg/kg Urografin 76 at a rate of 16–18 ml/s with a 7F or 8F angiographic catheter. The 30° RAO projection of the opacified ventricle was filmed at a rate of 40–80 (typically 50) frames/s with a 35-mm Arriflex cine camera (Arnold and Richter, Munich). During angiography care was taken to maintain the patients' position with regard to the X-ray equipment unchanged, while respiratory motion was prevented by sustained respiration. For calibration purposes a centimetre grid was filmed at midthoracic level.

The endocardial outlines of all ventriculograms in this study were determined frame by frame with an automated contour detection system, the "Contouromat" [15]. In each frame, left ventricular volume was determined according to Simpson's rule [16]. End-diastole and end-systole were defined as the moment of maximal and minimal left ventricular volume, respectively. The detected contours of all frames of the systolic period were displayed on a video monitor and were recorded on a single 8.3 × 10.8 cm Polaroid photograph. As the contours were displayed according to a fixed external reference system [1] no procedures such as translation and rotation were employed. One such set of superimposed contours is shown in Fig. 3a. Small landmarks at the left ventricular contrast border can be followed through the systolic period; however, the information is partially obscured by the overlap of the successive contours.

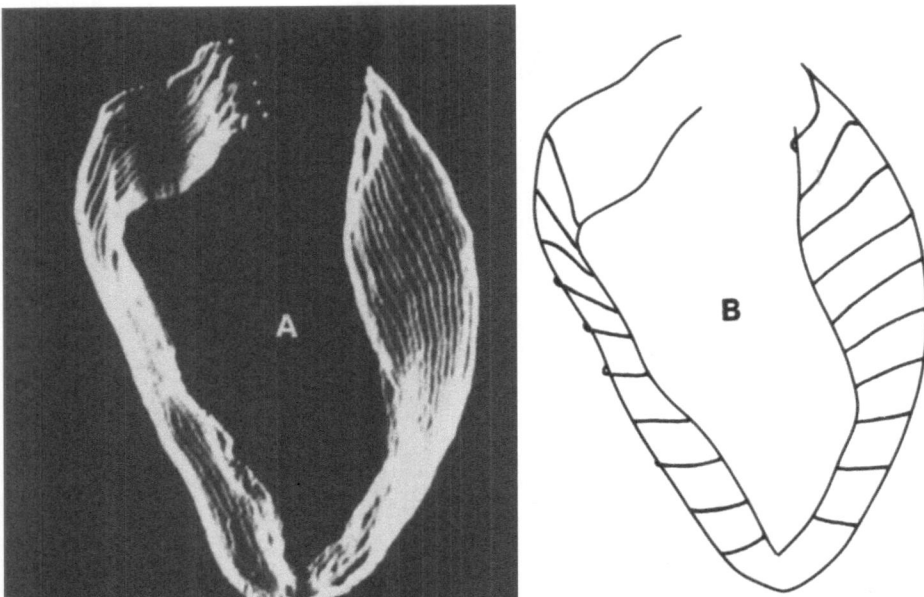

Fig. 3a. Result of automated frame by frame analysis of the endocardial contours in the systolic period from a left ventricular cine angiocardiogram. **b** Pathways of small irregularities at the left ventricular contrast border were analyzed, resulting in a pattern of sytolic trajectories

Therefore a "shift" procedure [17] was applied, which avoids superimposition of these landmarks. After enlargement of the photographs the systolic pathways of these landmarks were drawn manually. Subsequent correction for the previously added shift yielded the actual systolic trajectories with respect to the original frame of reference (Fig. 3b). For further calculations the curved systolic trajectories were represented by straight vectors leading from the end-diastolic to the end-systolic landmark positions.

For each ventricle a non-indexed rectangular coordinate system was defined with its origin coinciding with the end-diastolic apex, the point at maximal distance from the superior aspect of the aortic valve [18]. A basal transverse axis, which extends from the mitral valve fornix to a point on the opposite anterior wall, was constructed, so that an isosceles triangle with its vertex at the ventricular apex was the result (Fig. 4). The ventricular long axis was defined as the median of this triangle through the vertex; the y-axis of the coordinate system coincides with this line.

To be able to compare the pathways of the landmarks of ventricles with different shapes and sizes, a normalization procedure was performed. From base to apex, twenty points were defined by the intersections of the end-diastolic contour and ten equidistant lines perpendicular to the y-axis (Fig. 4). These points were taken to be the end-diastolic starting points for the assessment of pathways of the previously mentioned landmarks at the endocardial

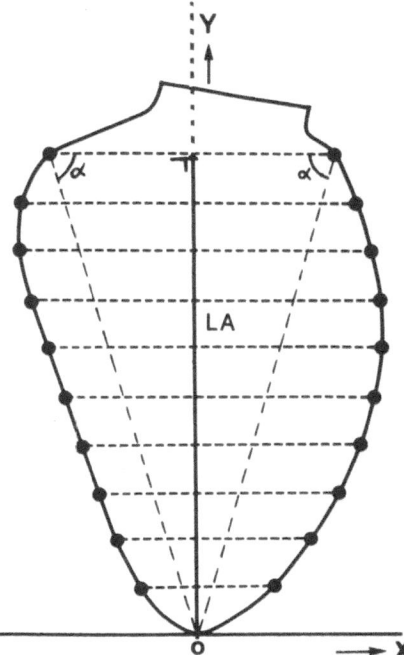

Fig. 4. The median of an isosceles triangle with its vertex at the ventricular apex and its base extending from the mitral valve fornix defines the y-axis of the applied rectangular coordinate system. Left ventricular long axis length (*LA*) is definded as the distance from base to apex. At equidistant y-levels 20 end-diastolic starting points are defined for the assessment of pathways of the endocardial landmarks

border. For both the human and pig ventricles, left ventricular dimensions were normalized such that for each study group the end-diastolic long axis lengths became equal to the mean value. After this procedure, corresponding starting points had equal y-coordinates, but still different x-coordinates (Fig. 5a). For this reason the (normalized) systolic trajectories with corresponding starting points were shifted parallel to the x-axis, such that the starting points coincided at the x-coordinate equal to the mean x-value (Fig. 5b). After decomposing the

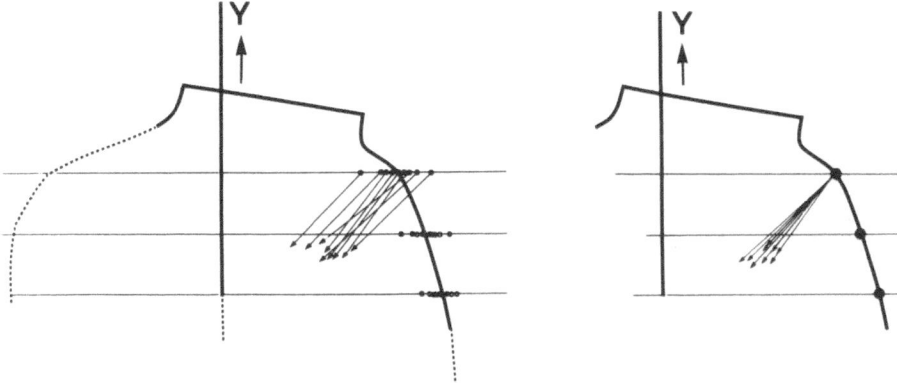

Fig. 5. After normalization of the ventriculograms for long axis length, corresponding starting points were shifted along the x-axis such that they coincide and have an x-coordinate equal to the mean x-value

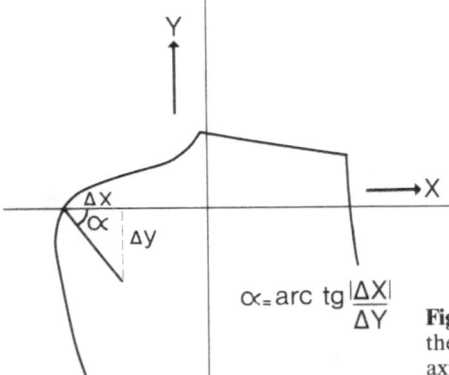

Fig. 6. The direction of the pathways is defined as the acute angle between the pathway and the x-axis

trajectory vectors originating from a common starting point, the mean value and the standard deviation of their x- and y-components were calculated.

From the projected contrast angiogram the end-diastolic and end-systolic contours and the respective positions of the implanted metal markers were drawn on a sheet of paper. Again a non-indexed rectangular coordinate system was defined as described above. With reference to this coordinate system the calibrated x- and y-coordinates of the end-diastolic and end-systolic marker positions were computed, thus defining the systolic marker pathways.

With respect to the coordinate system, the individual pathways were decomposed into their x- and y-components, expressed as Δx and Δy. The direction of each pathway was defined as the acute angle between the pathway and the x-axis, in formula (see Fig. 6):

$$\alpha = \text{arc tangent } \frac{|\Delta x|}{\Delta y}$$

By means of linear regression analysis, the extent and direction of the metal marker pathways denotes as Δx_{metal}, Δy_{metal}, and α_{metal}, were compared with the nearest corresponding endocardial landmark pathways, denoted as Δx_{endo}, Δy_{endo}, and α_{endo}.

Results

Endocardial Wall Motion in Pigs

Haemodynamic data before and after marker insertion did not differ significantly. After the experiment the myocardium was inspected visually at the position of marker insertion. No significant damage was observed.

In Fig. 7 an example of the normalized systolic pathways of the endocardial landmarks in two individual animals (7a and 8a) is shown, with the systolic pathway of the implanted metal markers of the same ventricles (7b and 8b). A comparison of the x- and y-components of coresponding pathways of endocar-

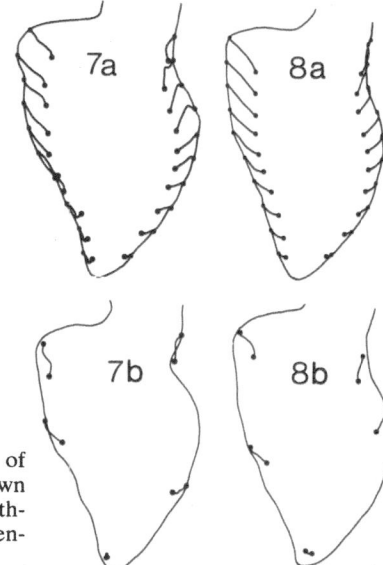

Fig. 7. Normalized left ventricular systolic pathways of the endocardial landmarks in two animals are shown (*7a* and *8a*), while *7b* and *8b* depict the systolic pathways of the implanted metal markers in the same ventricles

dial landmarks (Δx_{endo} and Δy_{endo}) and of metal markers (Δx_{metal} and Δy_{metal}) gives a correlation coefficient of $r = 0.74$ and $r = 0.86$, respectively, with linear regression equations expressed as:

$$\Delta x_{endo} = 0.16 \text{ cm} + 1.2 \mid \Delta x_{metal} \mid, \ \Delta y_{endo} = -0.13 \text{ cm} + \Delta y_{metal}, \ n = 41$$

The relation between the directions of the endocardial landmark pathways and of the metal marker pathways was similarly evaluated (see Fig. 8):

$$\alpha_{endo} = 0.86, \ \alpha_{metal} - 2.9°, \ r = 0.86, \ n = 33$$

In this comparison the apical segments were excluded, as the displacement of these segments is characterized by such short trajectories that accurate assessment of α is almost impossible.

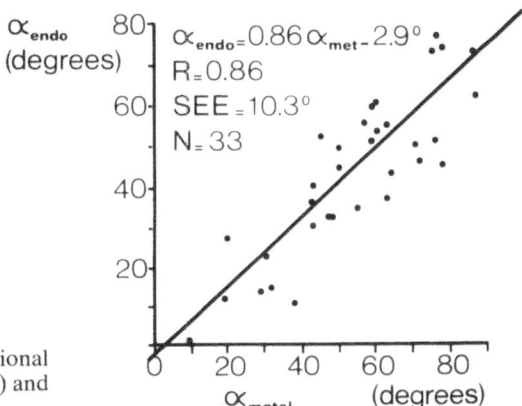

Fig. 8. Relation between the directional movement of endocardial markers (α_{endo}) and of metal markers (α_{metal})

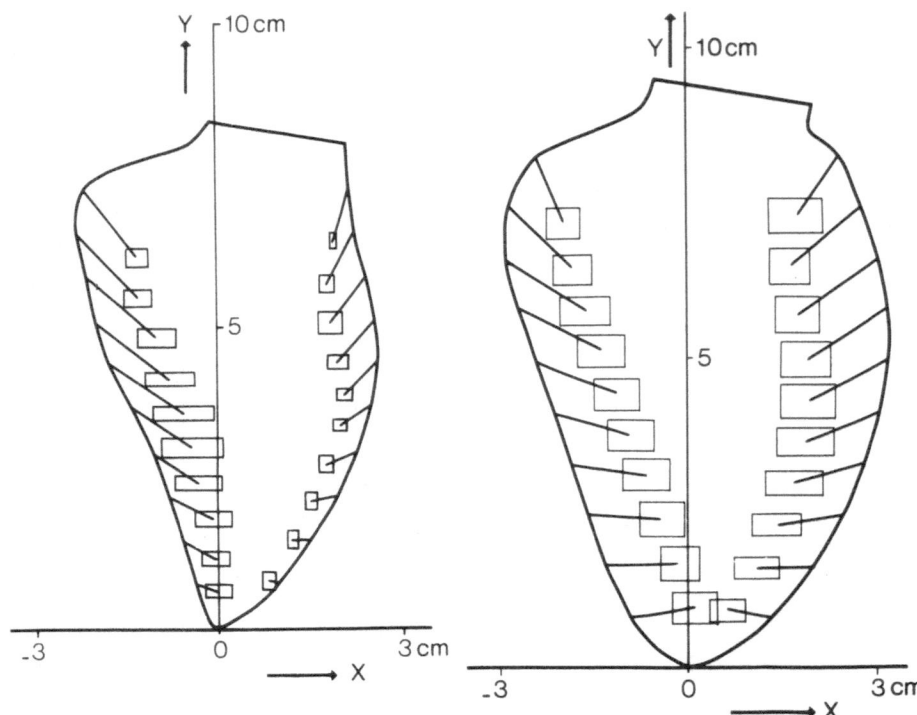

Fig. 9. Normalized shape of left ventricular end-diastolic contours in eight animals. Mean left ventricular long axis length is 7.3 ± 0.4 cm (mean ± SD). The mean systolic pathways of the endocardial landmarks are shown, while the rectangles represent the standard deviations

Fig. 10. Mean systolic left ventricular endocardial landmark pathways in normal human individuals. The rectangles represent the standard deviation

In Fig. 9 the normalized shape is shown of the end-diastolic left ventricular contours of the eight animals, together with the mean systolic pathways of the endocardial landmarks and their SD. Mean left ventricular long axis length was 7.3 ± 0.4 cm (mean ± SD).

Endocardial Wall Motion in Humans

The normalized starting point positions which define the normalized shape of the end-diastolic left ventricular contour together with the mean systolic pathways of the endocardial landmarks in the 23 normal human subjects are provided in Fig. 10. Mean left ventricular long axis length was 8.3 ± 1.3 cm (mean ± SD). The standard deviations are expressed in the figure by rectangles. The points of intersection of the pathways extending from the ten pairs of opposing starting points are depicted in Fig. 11 with the *x*- and *y*-coordinates of the

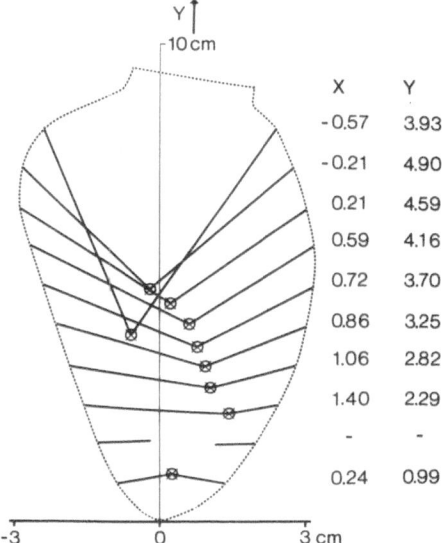

X	Y
-0.57	3.93
-0.21	4.90
0.21	4.59
0.59	4.16
0.72	3.70
0.86	3.25
1.06	2.82
1.40	2.29
-	-
0.24	0.99

Fig. 11. Points of intersection of the pathways extending from the 10 pairs of opposing starting points. The x- and y-coordinates of the intersection points are given

intersection points. In one case no point of intersection could be found within the ventricular cavity because of an almost parallel course of the facing trajectories.

To make the observed motion pattern applicable to the analysis of regional wall motion in other subjects, it was formulated as a generalized mathematical expression.

The midpoints of corresponding opposite end-diastolic starting points were used to obtain a simple but still accurate approximation of the successive x-coordinates of the true points of intersection. In formula:

$$X_{PI} = 0.5 \, (X_{SP_a} + X_{SP_i})$$

where X_{PI} is the x-coordinate of the point of intersection, X_{SP_a} ist the x-coordinate of the starting point at the anterior wall, and X_{SP_i} ist the x-coordinate of the starting point at the inferoposterior wall.

A good approximation of the y-coordinates of the points of intersection (Y_{PI}) is obtained from the y-coordinate of the corresponding anterior and inferoposterior starting points (Y_{SP}) and from left ventricular end-diastolic long axis length (LA), according to the formula:

$$Y_{PI} = LA \left[0.57 - 0.53 \left| 1 - 1.1 \, \frac{Y_{SP}}{LA} \right|^{1.4} \right]$$

where Y_{PI} is the y-coordinate of the point of intersection, Y_{SP} is the y-coordinate of the starting points, and LA is the end-diastolic left ventricular long axis length.

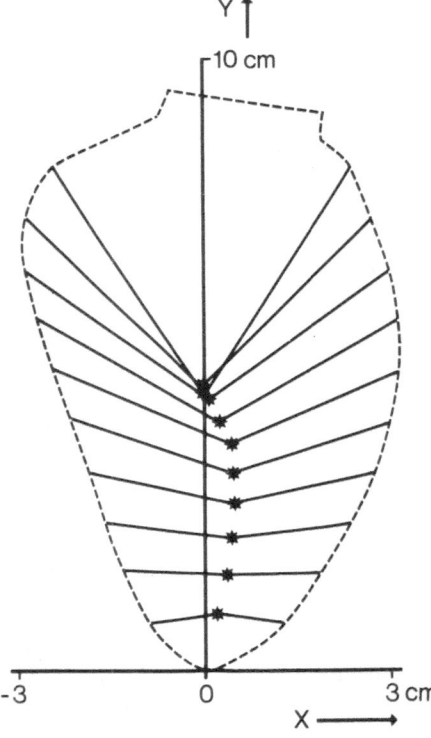

Fig. 12. Points of intersection of the trajectories and direction of regional wall motion as derived from the normalized end-diastolic contour using the mathematical expression described in the text

In Fig. 12 the points of intersection and the direction of the regional wall motion as derived from the normalized end-diastolic contour (Fig. 10) are shown using the mathematical expressions given above. Comparison of Fig. 11 with Fig. 12 clearly shows that this mathematical description provides a good approximation of the direction of the actually measured endocardial wall motion trajectories.

Discussion

Quantitative analysis of left ventricular endocardial wall motion from angiocardiograms has been hampered in humans by the lack of an accurate and generally accepted procedure to track specific sites at the endocardial border. Early experience with an automated endocardial outlining system [19] suggested the existence of endocardial landmarks which reappeared so regularly in consecutive frames of the cineangiogram that they could be followed over the entire cardiac cycle. The aim of this study is to test the hypothesis that the motion pattern of these landmarks reflects the motion pattern of actual anatomical structures at the endocardial border and that they can therefore be used as natural markers.

It is obvious that in humans no direct proof of this hypothesis could be reached as this would require endocardial marker implantation, the only accurate method to assess local endocardial wall motion. The animal experiment was therefore chosen to compare the motion pattern of these endocardial landmarks with that of metal markers. These were inserted via a percutaneous retrograde transvascular approach, in order to minimize the damage afflicted to the myocardium. Analysis of the haemodynamic variables and the ECG before and after marker insertion indeed showed no sign of significant cardiac damage resulting from the procedure. In one pig a minor change of the T-wave was observed. Visual inspection of the myocardium at autopsy in no case revealed significant damage at the position of the marker insertion.

Linear regression analysis of the endocardial landmark and metal marker pathways in pigs shows an acceptable correlation coefficient of the y-components ($r = 0.86$), but a much lower correlation coefficient oft the x-components ($r = 0.74$). This discrepancy can be explained by the apparent and exaggerated endocardial inward motion, which is observed on the contrast angiogram. This overestimation of systolic wall motion is caused by squeezing contrast media out of the intertrabecular spaces, something also observed by other authors [2, 7, 11, 20–22]. The discrepancy in percentage overall wall thickening between the contrast media methods [23–25] the bead and clip [7] and the ultrasonic crystal methods [26, 27] also points in this direction. Comparison of the motional direction of the endocardial landmarks and metal marker pathways shows a rather high correlation ($r = 0.86$) with a small standard error of the estimate of 10.3°. Taken together, these data imply that the landmark trajectories indeed represent the motion of actual anatomical landmarks and thus can serve as a non-invasive marker method.

In humans as well as in the animals, the y-components of the endocardial landmark trajectories show a gradually decreasing extent of motion as one reaches the apex. This agrees with the systolic descent of the base of the heart which has been observed by many authors in animal experiments [6, 28–30] as well as in humans [11, 12, 31]. The apical landmark motion in the y-direction is in fact very small, although in many cases visual inspection of the contrast angiogram would suggest a considerable apical upward motion towards the base. This seeming contradiction is caused by complete extrusion of contrast media from the apex in late systole. From the analysis of contrast angiograms, many authors came to the erroneous conclusion that the apex moves considerably towards the base during systole [32, 33], and consequently overestimated long axis shortening [31, 33]. In addition, contrast angiograms in the RAO projection in particular suggest a substantial rotation of the apex along the left ventricular long axis, a phenomenon which is partially due to extrusion of dye by the posterior papillary muscle. However, earlier studies with epicardial and endocardial markers had shown unmistakenly that the apex is remarkably stationary during systole [6, 11, 12, 28]. In keeping with this, the systolic motion of the apical metal markers, as displayed in Fig. 7, is minute, although the contrast angiogram in many instances would suggest a considerable apical upward motion and rotation, as is evident from inspection of Fig. 13.

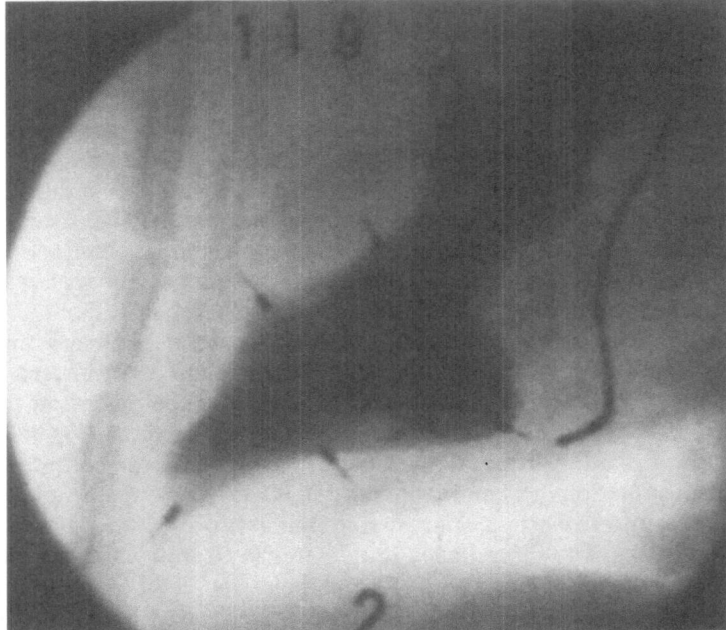

Fig. 13. End-systolic frame of left ventricular cine angiocardiogram after marker insertion. The corresponding end-diastolic frame is shown in Fig. 2. Squeezing of contrast from the apex may result in an apparent rotation and upward motion of the apex as observed on the contrast angiogram, while the end-diastolic and end-systolic metal marker positions are almost identical

Therefore, models for quantitative analysis of the angiogram, particularly those proposed for the assessment of endocardial wall motion, should take into account these observations. The generalized mathematical description of the anatomical landmark pathways serves will as one more step towards the achievement of a reliable approach for the quantification of endocardial wall motion in routine clinical work.

To conclude: the motion pattern of landmarks appearing at the endocardial border, as detected with an automated technique for the analysis of cine angiograms, reflects the motion pattern of actual anatomical structures. From this technique, a detailed description of normal endocardial wall motion has been derived, which provides the basis for the further development of methods to quantify regional left ventricular function in clinical practice.

Acknowledgements: The authors gratefully acknowledge the assistance of Mr. R. H. van Bremen and Mrs. A. M. Rutteman in performing the animal experiments, Mr. J. van Oosten of the University of Technology at Delft who with great craftmanship constructed the marker insertion device, an Mrs. C. de Bruijn in preparing the manuscript.

References

1. Chaitman BR, Bristow JD, Rahimtoola SH (1973) Left ventricular wall motion assessed by using fixed external reference systems. Circulation 48:1043
2. Herman MV, Heinle RA, Klein MD, Gorlin R (1967) Localized disorders in myocardial contraction. N Eng J Med 227:222
3. Leighton RF, Wilt SM, Lewis RP (1974) Detection of hypokinesis by a quantitative analysis of left ventricular cineangiograms. Circulation 50:121
4. Harris LD, Clayton PD, Marshall HW, Warnet HR (1974) A technique for the detection of asynergistic motion in the left ventricle. Comput Biomed Res 7:380.
5. Rickards A, Seabra-Gomes R, Thurstone P (1977) The assessment of regional abnormalities of the left ventricle by angiography. Eur J Cardiol 5:167
6. Rushmer RF, Crystal DK, Wagner C (1953) The functional anatomy of ventricular contraction. Circ Res 1:162–170
7. Mitchell JH, Wildenthal K, Mullins CB (1969) Geometrical studies of the left ventricle utilizing biplane cinefluorography. Fed Proc 28:1334–1343
8. Carlsson E, Milne ENC (1967) Permanent implantation of endocardial tantalum screws. A new technique for functional studies of the heart of the experimental animal. J Assoc Can Radiol 19:304–309
9. Ingels NB, Daughters GT, Stinson EB, Alderman EL (1975) Measurement of midwall myocardial dynamics in intact man by radiography of surgically implanted markers. Circulation 52:859
10. Harrison DC, Goldblatt A, Braunwald E, Glick G, Mason DT (1963) Studies on cardiac dimensions in intact, unanaesthetized man. I. Description of techniques and their validation. Circ Res 13:448
11. McDonald IG (1970) The shape and movements of the human left ventricle during systole. Am J Cardiol 26:221
12. McDonald IG (1972) Contraction of the hypertrophied left ventricle in man studied by cineradiography of epicardial markers. Am J Cardiol 30:587–594
13. Brower RW, ten Katen HJ, Meester GT (1978) Direct method for determining regional myocardial shortening after bypass surgery from radiopaque markers in man. Am J Cardiol 41:1222
14. Wildenthal K, Mitchell JH (1969) Dimensional analysis of the left ventricle in unanaesthetised dogs. J Appl Physiol 27:115
15. Slager CJ, Reiber JHC, Schuurbiers JCH, Meester GT (1978) Contouromat: hardwired left ventricular angioprocessing system. I. Design and application. Comput Biomed Res 11:491–502
16. Chapman CB, Baker O, Reynolds J, Bonte FJ (1958) Use of biplane cinefluorography for measurement of ventricular volume. Circulation 18:1105–1117
17. Slager CJ, Hooghoudt TEH, Reiber JHC, Schuurbiers JCH, Booman F, Meester GT (1979) Left ventricular contour segmentation from anatomical landmark trajectories and its application to wall motion analysis. Computers in Cardiology, Vol 6. IEEE Computer Society, Long Beach, pp 347–350
18. Brower RW (1980) Evaluation of patient recognition rules for the apex of the heart. Cathet Cardiovasc Diagn 6:145–157
19. Slager CJ, Reiber JHC, Schuurbiers JCH, Meester GT (1978) Automated detection of left ventricular contour. Concept and application. In: Heintzen PH, Buersch JH (eds) Roentgen-Video-Techniques. Thieme, Stuttgart, pp 158–167
20. Chapman CB, Baker O, Mitchell JH (1966) Experience with a cinefluorographic method for measuring ventricular volume. Am J Cardiol 18:25
21. Mitchell JH, Mullins CB (1967) Dimensional analysis of left ventricular function. In: Tanz RD, Kavaler F, Roberts J (eds) Factors influencing myocardial contractility. Academic, New York, p 177
22. Hugenholtz PG, Kaplan E, Hill E (1969) Determination of left ventricular wall thickness by angiocardiography. Am Heart J 78:513
23. Sandler H, Dodge HT (1963) Left ventricular tension and stress in man. Circ Res 13:91

24. Eber LM, Greenberg HM, Cooke JM, Gorlin R (1969) Dynamic changes in left ventricular free wall thickness in the human heart. Circulation 39:454
25. Dumensnil JG, Ritman EL, Frye RL, Gau GT, Rutherford BD, Davies GD (1974) Quantitative determination of regional left ventricular wall dynamics by roentgen videometry. Circulation 50:700
26. Sasayama S, Franklin D, Ross J Jr, Kemper WS, McKown D (1976) Dynamic changes in left ventricular wall thickness and their use in analysing cardiac function in the conscious dog. Am J Cardiol 38:870–879
27. Osakada G, Sasayama S, Kawai C, Hirakawa A, Kemper WS, Franklin D, Ross J Jr (1980) The analysis of left ventricular wall thickness and shear by an ultrasonic triangulation technique in the dog. Circ Res. 47:173
28. Hamilton WF, Rompf JH (1932) Movements of the base of the ventricle and the relative consistency of the cardiac volume. Am J Physiol 102:559–565
29. Tsakiris AG, van Bernuth G, Rastelli GC, Bourgolis MJ, Titus JL, Wood EH (1971) Size and motion of the mitral valve annulus in anaesthetized intact dogs. J Appl Physiol 30:611–618
30. Hinds JE, Hawthorne EH, Mullins CB, Mitchell JH (1969) Instantaneous changes in the left ventricular lengths occurring in dogs during the cardiac cycle. Fed Proc 28:1351–1357
31. Brower RW, Meester GT (1976) Computer based methods for quantifying regional left ventricular wall motion from cine ventriculograms. Computers in Cardiology Vol 3. IEEE Computer Society, Long Beach, pp 55–62
32. Leighton RF, Wilt SM, Lewis RP (1974) Detection of hypokinesis by a quantitative analysis of left ventricular cineangiograms. Circulation 50:121
33. Rickards A, Seabra-Gomes R, Thurston P (1977) The assessment of regional abnormalities of the left ventricle by angiography. Eur J Cardiol 5:167–182

Quantitation of Regional Left Ventricular Function Using the Endocardial Landmark Model – Clinical Results

T. E. H. Hooghoudt, C. J. Slager, J. H. C. Reiber, and P. W. Serruys

Thoraxcenter, Erasmus University, P. O. Box 1738, 3000 DR Rotterdam, The Netherlands

Introduction

Since coronary heart disease is often regional in character, the assessment of regional left ventricular function under resting conditions and during intervention studies may elicit both the functional significance of coronary artery stenosis and the extent of jeopardized areas of myocardium [1]. Such assessment may be of great importance in the selection of patients for bypass surgery. Although ejection fraction [2] and the isovolumic indices of contractility [3] are useful parameters of global cardiac function, in these measurements regional dysfunction may be masked by compensatory action of healthy wall segments.

Regional pump and contractile function may be derived from regional wall motion itself. To assess regional wall motion, a number of methods have been proposed [4–8], which almost all introduce a considerable error, both in extent and direction of determined wall motion [9]. The temporal aspects of left ventricular performance also bear important information [10, 11], although their analysis is often omitted because manual frame by frame analysis is so tedious.

For all these reasons, a system for automated quantitative analysis of regional left ventricular wall motion, pump and contractile function, and their temporal aspects, was developed. For the accurate assessment of regional endocardial wall motion a new wall motion model was devised which relies on the actual trajectories of endocardial anatomical structures [12].

In the present study the findings in 20 normal human hearts are described. Two further examples of the application of the method to clinical research are given.

Patient Population and Methods

The first study group consisted of 20 patients who, after a complete right and left heart catheterization including coronary arteriography, showed completely normal hemodynamic findings, normal coronary angiograms, and normal left ventricular wall motion as judged by a least two experienced observers. Most patients had been submitted to cardiac catheterization to exclude coronary artery disease or because of murmurs which required investigation. Left ventriculography was performed in the 30° RAO projection with 0.75 ml/kg Urografin 76 (Schering, Berlin) at a flow rate of 18 ml/s and was recorded with an Arriflex 35-mm camera (Arnold and Richter, Munich) at a rate of 50 frames/s. The cycle with the maximum contrast of the left ventricle – excluding extrasystolic and postextrasystolic beats – was chosen for analysis; usually this was the 3rd–5th beat after the start of contrast injection. This excluded a significant volume load from the injected contrast agent [13].

For the second part of the study, data were collected from five patients catheterized because of suspected coronary artery disease. All of them proved to have normal coronary arteries with an ejection fraction well within the normal range. After informed consent was obtained from each patient to participate in the remainder of the study, an additional left ventricular cineangiogram was obtained 30 s after a bolus injection of 0.075 to 0.15 mg nifedipine into the left main coronary artery. The injection was made only after the values for left ventricular end-diastolic pressure and the various isovolumic parameters of contractility were again identical with those recorded before the initial angiogram. In all cases the interval between the two angiograms was at least 20 min. Care was taken to maintain the patients' position constant in relation to the X-ray equipment during both angiograms. Diaphragm movement was excluded by shallow inspiration taking care to prevent Valsalva maneuver.

The third study group consisted of 28 patients, catheterized within the first 6 h after the onset of symptoms of acute myocardial infarction (AMI), who were treated with intracoronary infusion of a thrombolytic agent, and of whom two sequential left ventriculograms (during the acute event and during follow up, 2–3 weeks later) of sufficient quality to permit automated analysis could be obtained. The diagnosis of AMI was based on an anamnesis of typical chest pain, ECG changes, and serial CPK values. In all patients the ECG at admission showed changes compatible with acute myocardial ischemia. After informed consent was obtained, coronary arteriography was performed via the retrograde brachial [14] or femoral [15] approach. In 25 of 28 patients injection of contrast medium into the infarct related artery (IRA) showed a total occlusion. Recanalization of the IRAs was attempted with intracoronary infusion of streptokinase (Behring) or urokinase (Abbott Laboratories, North Chicago) 2000–4000 U/min for 10–90 min. In 17 out of 25 patients the IRA could be recanalized and was still patent during the control study. Eight patients had sustained an anterior myocardial infarction (IRA, left anterior descending coronary artery), seven an inferior infarction (IRA, right coronary artery), two a lateral wall infarction (IRA, left circumflex coronary artery). In three other patients the IRA was already patent at the time of the first coronary angiogram and remained so during follow up. In eight patients the IRA could not be recanalized or was reoccluded at the time of the control study. Quantitative hemodynamic data were assessed in the eight patients with "unsuccessful recanalization" and the 20 patients with "successful recanalization" of the IRA. In eight patients with an anterior infarction and seven with an inferior infarction with successful recanalization of the IRA, detailed analysis of regional left ventricular function was performed.

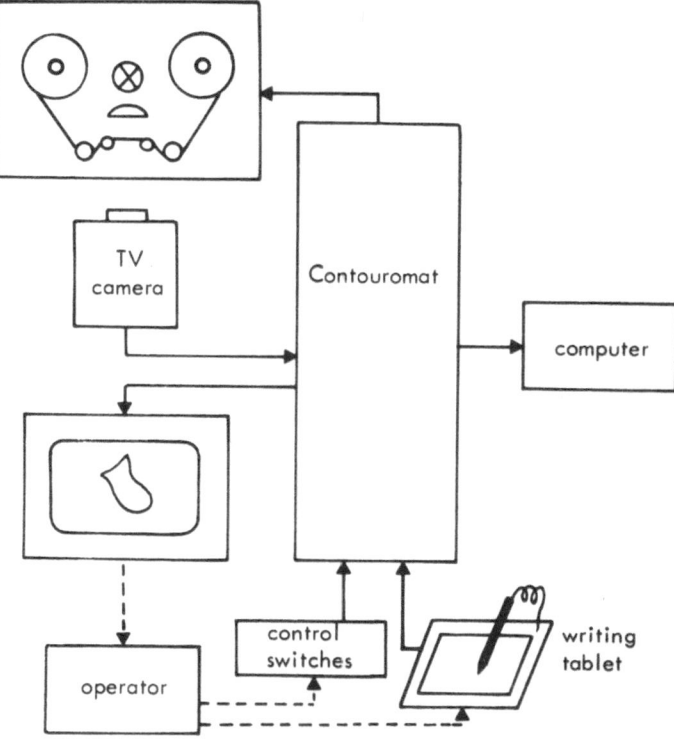

Fig. 1. Simplified block diagram of the automated endocardial outlining system

Analysis of the left ventriculograms was performed with a dedicated hard-wired system, the video-contour detector, Contouromat. A simplified block diagram of this automated outlining system is shown in Fig. 1. Films are projected with a Vanguard projector (Vanguard Instruments, Melville, N. Y.) and are converted into video format with a Philips video camera (Philips, Eindhoven). The cineangiogram is rotated such that the long axis of the left ventricle is about perpendicular to the direction of the video scanlines. With this optimized orientation there will never be more than two contour points on a videoline, one for the left and one for the right border. Contour detection is based upon a refined thresholding technique which uses an analog comparator to compare the video signal with the reference level. As soon as the video signal crosses the reference level, the comparator changes state, indicating the presence of a border point.

The reference level is determined by three factors:
1. The local brightness of structures surrounding the detected border, assessed on a line to line basis.
2. The "expectation window," a narrow window which adapts dynamically to the ventricular shape. The center of this window is defined as having the

same x-coordinate as the last detected border point in the previous videoline. The comparator is enabled during the expectation window period only. During this period, the calculated reference level is assigned a probability function such that the center of the expectation window has the highest probability to be the next border point.

3. The endocardial border in the last detected frame. Because the border position changes little from frame to frame, the margin in the current frame can be approximated with the margin of the previous frame. During contour detection the stored border positions of the previous contour are used to assign a probability function to the reference level.

The great advantage of this complex method of contour detection is that the detection process is rather insensitive to shading, nonhomogeneous mixing of contrast agent in the left ventricle, and overlapping of roentgen-opaque structures such as diaphragm, ribs, and catheters, because the reference level is adjusted accordingly. The left ventricular contour is detected at a rate of 50 TV fields/s. Including operator interaction, mean processing time is 7–10 s per frame or 3–15 min per cardiac cycle [16].

All data from the Contouromat are coded in a special purpose interface and stored with a PDP-11/34 minicomputer onto a RK-05 disk (Digital Equipment,

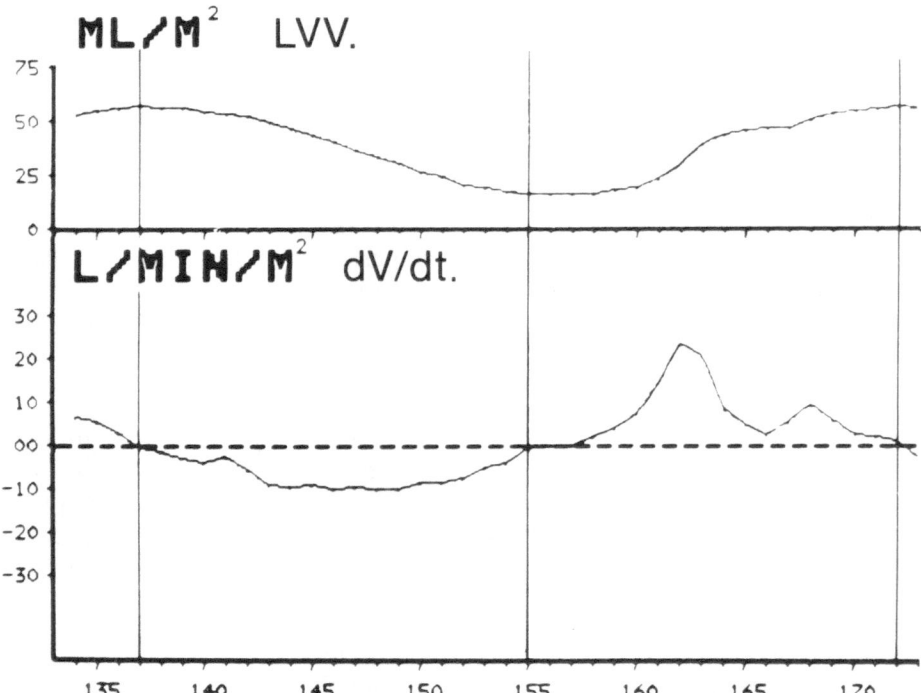

Fig. 2. Graphic display of the time course of left ventricular volume (LVV), corrected for body surface area, and its time derivative. *Vertical lines* indicate the end-diastolic and end-systolic frames

Maynard, Mass.). The first step in processing these data is the calculation of left ventricular volume from all analyzed cineframes according to Simpson's rule and the graphical display of instantaneous volume and its time derivative (Fig. 2). The end-diastolic and end-systolic frames, defined as the frames with the maximal and minimal volume respectively, are so marked by the operator via the writing tablet. From the left ventricular volume data over the systolic period, ejection fraction, stroke volume, and total cardiac output are computed. The end-diastolic and end-systolic contours are displayed on the computer video monitor with the computed values for ejection fraction, stroke volume, and cardiac output. Next the computer generates a system of coordinates along which regional left ventricular wall motion is determined (Fig. 3). This method to analyze left ventricular wall motion is based on the endocardial landmark trajectories as previously established in a group of normal individuals. Over a full cardiac cycle, starting in end-diastole, segmental wall displacement is determined in 20 segments, ten in the anterior and ten in the inferoposterior wall. Regional wall velocity is calculated as the first derivative of the instantaneous displacement function after a three-point smoothing function has been applied to the data (Fig. 4). From these data mean systolic velocity is calculated for each segment. For all 20 segments the regional contribution to global ejection fraction (CREF) is derived from systolic wall displacement data and left ventricular long axis shortening.

ED :137
ES :155

EDV:	57.6	ML/M^2
ESV:	16.4	ML/M^2
SV:	41.1	ML/M^2
EF:	71.4	%
HR:	88	B/MIN
TCI:	3.6	L/MIN/M^2
BSA:	1.6	M^2
WTH:		CM

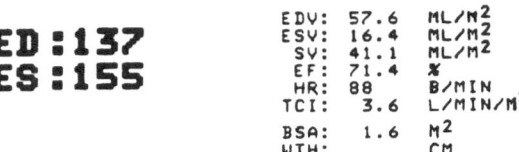

Fig. 3. Example of the computer output showing the end-diastolic and end-systolic contours of the 30° RAO angiogram in their relative proportions and place. The corresponding volume data, ejection fraction, and other parameters are shown in the *upper right* corner. Left ventricular segmental wall motion is determined along a system of coordinates derived from the endocardial landmark trajectories in normal subjects and is studied in 20 separate segments, ten in the anterior and ten in the inferoposterior wall

11.   1.
12.   2.
13.   3.
14.   4.
15.   5.
16.   6.
17.   7.
18.   8.
19.   9.
20.   10.

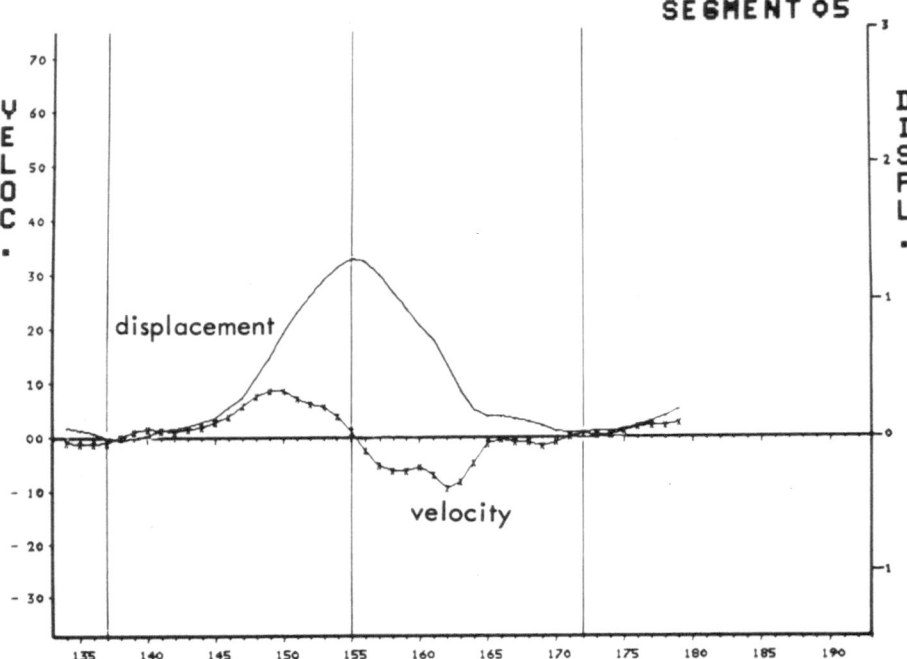

Fig. 4. For every segment a plot is generated showing left ventricular wall displacement and velocity as a function of time

To achieve this, the end-diastolic lumen – from the level of the mitral valve edge to the apex – is divided into ten slices of equal height, each corresponding to two opposite segments of the model (Fig. 5). Each slice is divided into halves by the left ventricular axis of symmetry. The volume of each half slice is computed in end-diastole (ED) and end-systole (ES) according to the formula:

$$\frac{1}{2} \times \pi R^2 \times \frac{1}{10} L = \frac{1}{20} \pi R^2 L,$$

where R is the radius of a particular slice and L the left ventricular long axis length, extending from base to apex. During systole the volume of a particular half slice decreases, mainly as a consequence of the decrease of radius which is determined by the x-component (x) of the displacement vector (d) (Fig. 6), and only slightly by left ventricular long axis shortening. In normal individuals a 14% long axis shortening, as previously assessed [12], is applied to the calculations. The CREF is defined as the change of volume during ejection of a particular segment normalized for global left ventricular end-diastolic volume:

$$\frac{\text{ED half slice volume (ml) – ES half slice volume (ml)}}{\text{Global left ventricular end-diastolic volume (ml)}} \times 100 = \text{CREF (\%)}$$

The sum of CREF data of all 20 segments (SUMCREF) will be approximately equal to global ejection fraction.

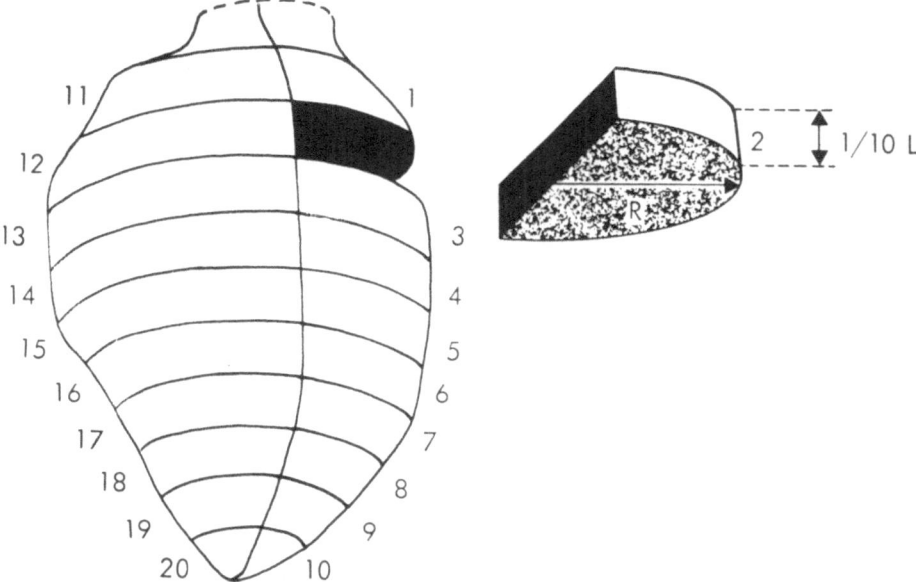

Fig. 5. The regional contribution to global ejection fraction (CREF) is determined in 20 half slices of equal height, each corresponding to a segment of the wall motion model shown in Fig. 3

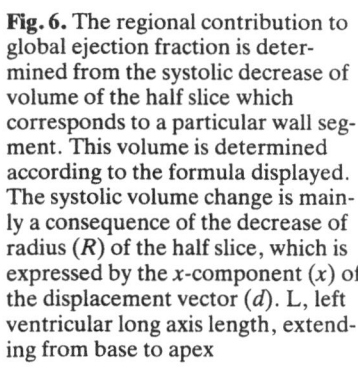

Fig. 6. The regional contribution to global ejection fraction is determined from the systolic decrease of volume of the half slice which corresponds to a particular wall segment. This volume is determined according to the formula displayed. The systolic volume change is mainly a consequence of the decrease of radius (R) of the half slice, which is expressed by the x-component (x) of the displacement vector (d). L, left ventricular long axis length, extending from base to apex

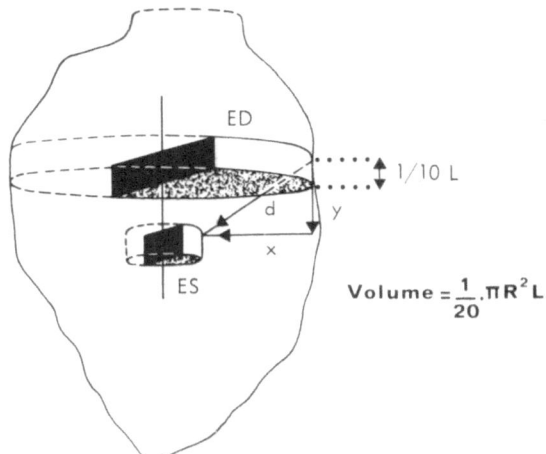

$$\text{Volume} = \frac{1}{20} . \pi R^2 L$$

From the systolic volume change, the regional ejection fraction (REF) is determined according to the formula:

$$\frac{\text{ED half slice volume (ml)} - \text{ES half slice volume (ml)}}{\text{ED half slice volume (ml)}} \times 100 = \text{REF (\%)}$$

For the last part of the study, 20 left ventriculograms coded 1–20 were processed with the contour detector by two independently working observers X and Y.

After an interval of 1 week to 3 months, the same films, provided with a new randomly alloted number, were processed for the second time by the same observers. The intra- and interobserver variability in the assessment of global left ventricular volume, ejection fraction and SUMCREF values, were evaluated by computation of the correlation coefficient and the standard error of the estimate (SEE). The relation between ejection fraction and SUMCREF was also evaluated twice by each observer.

Results

In the 20 normal individuals, calibrated displacement (cm) and velocity (cm/s) values were determined in all 20 segments. The 10% and 90% limits of segmental wall displacement in cm as well as the median are shown in Fig. 7. When segments 1 and 11, which are in some cases less reliable due to interference from aortic and mitral valve motion, are excluded, correlation coefficients of −0.99 and −0.98 are found between median values of local displacement of specific segments in the anterior and inferoposterior wall, respectively, and their distance to the base (Fig. 8). Normal values of mean systolic wall velocity (MSV) are displayed in Fig. 9 and in Table 1. Here again a linear decrease is observed in the median values viewed from base to apex (MSV vs distance to base, $r =$ −0.98 and −0.97 in the anterior and inferoposterior wall, respectively). The normal range of values for the regional contribution to global ejection fraction (CREF) is shown in Fig. 10 and Table 2, while in Fig. 11 the normal values of regional ejection fraction are given. The time between end-systole (ES) and the moment of maximal inward wall displacement in 20 segments of the 30° RAO left ventriculogram is shown in Fig. 12.

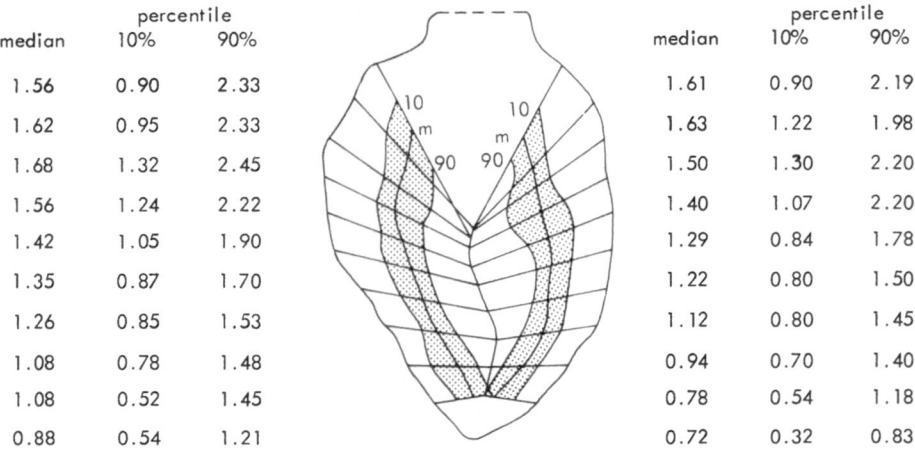

median	percentile 10%	90%		median	percentile 10%	90%
1.56	0.90	2.33		1.61	0.90	2.19
1.62	0.95	2.33		1.63	1.22	1.98
1.68	1.32	2.45		1.50	1.30	2.20
1.56	1.24	2.22		1.40	1.07	2.20
1.42	1.05	1.90		1.29	0.84	1.78
1.35	0.87	1.70		1.22	0.80	1.50
1.26	0.85	1.53		1.12	0.80	1.45
1.08	0.78	1.48		0.94	0.70	1.40
1.08	0.52	1.45		0.78	0.54	1.18
0.88	0.54	1.21		0.72	0.32	0.83

�⌴⌴⌴⌴⌴⌴⌴⌴ = 1 cm

Fig. 7. Median, 10th, and 90th percentile values of left ventricular wall displacement (cm) in normal subjects. The ventriculograms were made in the 30° RAO position

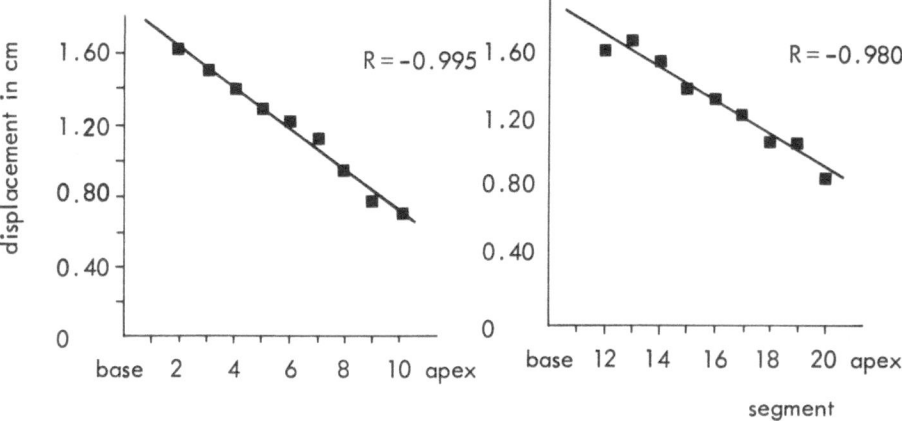

Fig. 8. In this group of normal subjects an approximately linear relationship has been found between the median value of displacement of a particular segment and its distance to the base

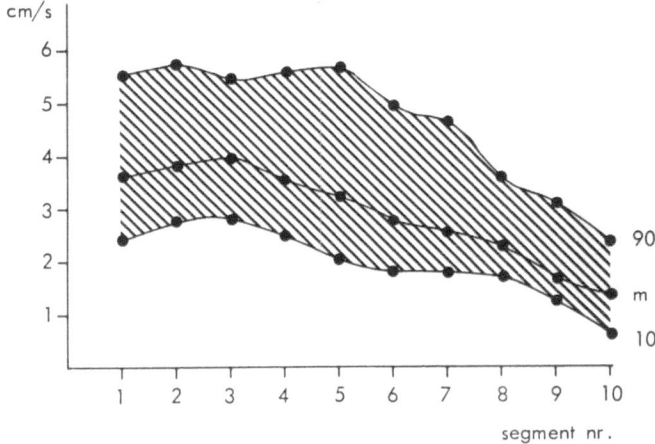

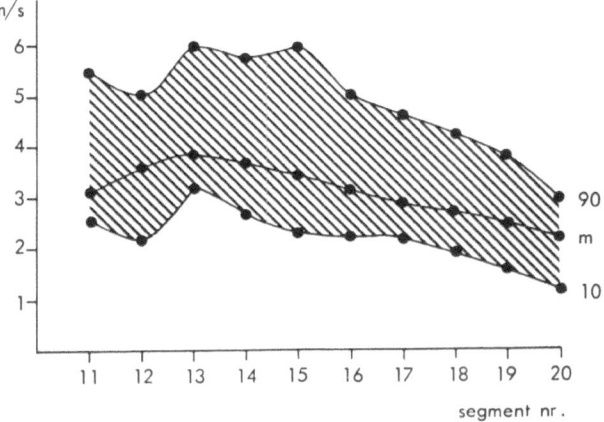

Fig. 9. Mean systolic velocity for all 20 segments in 20 normal subjects. The median, 10th, and 90th percentile are shown. The *upper panel* gives the data for the anterior segments, the *lower panel* for the inferoposterior segments

Table 1. Mean systolic wall velocity values in 20 left ventricular wall segments of 20 normal individuals

Segment	10th Percentile (cm/s)	Median (cm/s)	90th Percentile (cm/s)
1	2.40	3.65	5.55
2	2.75	3.83	5.75
3	2.80	4.00	5.50
4	2.50	3.60	5.60
5	2.05	3.30	5.70
6	1.85	2.80	5.00
7	1.85	2.60	4.70
8	1.74	2.30	3.60
9	1.25	1.65	3.16
10	0.60	1.40	2.40
11	2.55	3.15	5.50
12	2.10	3.65	5.00
13	3.20	3.85	6.00
14	2.65	3.70	5.78
15	2.25	3.45	6.00
16	2.25	3.13	5.00
17	2.25	2.88	4.62
18	1.90	2.75	4.25
19	1.55	2.50	3.86
20	1.20	2.20	3.00

Table 2. Values of regional contribution to global ejection fraction (CREF) in 20 normal individuals

Segment	10th Percentile (%)	Median (%)	90th Percentile (%)
1	1.7	3.1	4.8
2	3.2	4.2	5.5
3	4.0	4.9	5.9
4	3.9	5.0	6.3
5	3.2	4.7	5.7
6	3.0	4.1	4.9
7	2.9	3.5	4.5
8	2.0	2.7	3.5
9	1.2	1.8	2.9
10	0.5	0.9	1.5
11	2.0	2.7	4.2
12	2.8	4.4	5.3
13	4.4	5.4	6.5
14	4.5	5.2	6.3
15	4.0	4.9	6.1
16	3.0	4.5	5.3
17	2.9	3.9	4.4
18	2.0	2.7	3.8
19	1.4	1.9	3.2
20	0.7	1.0	1.7

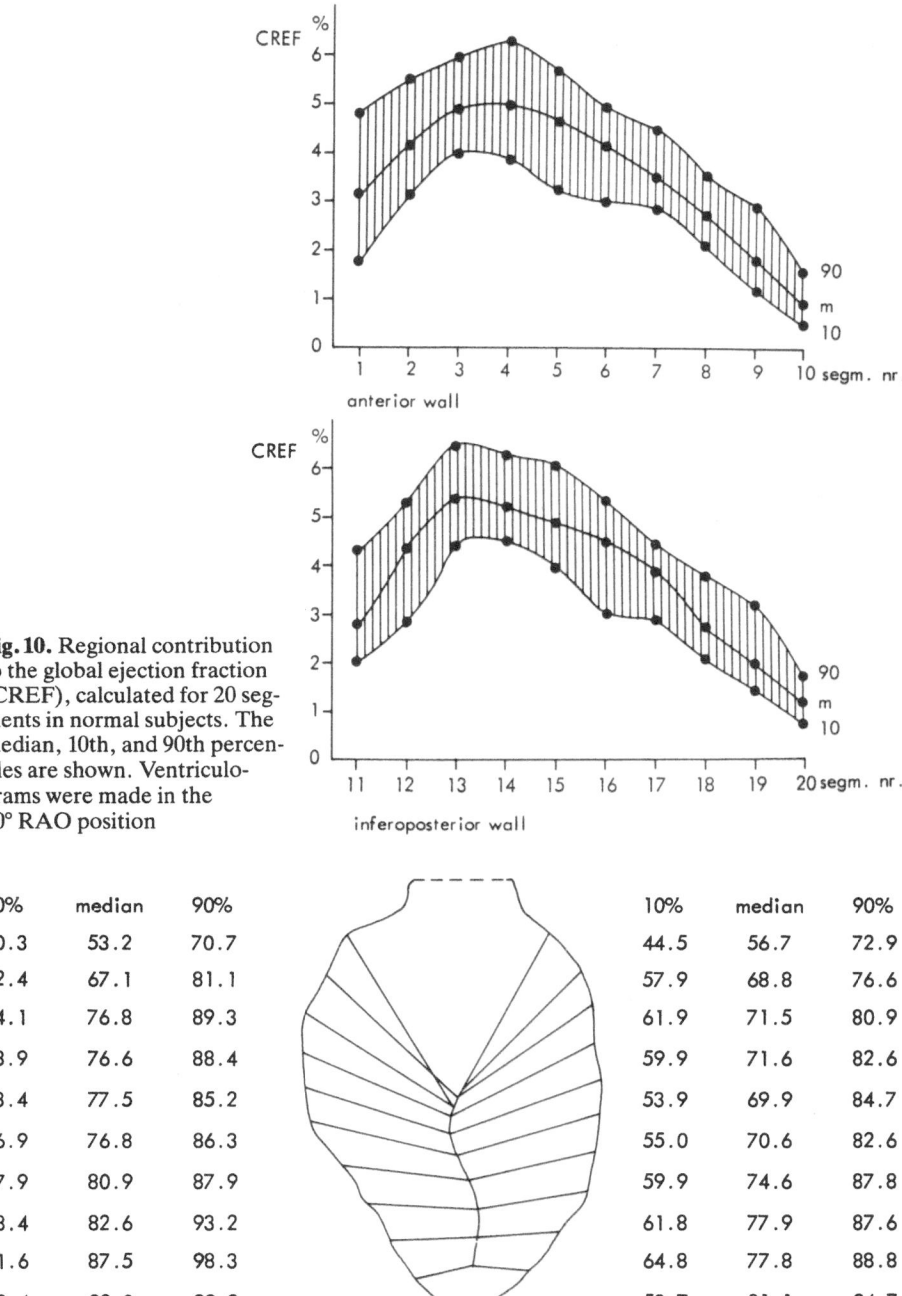

Fig. 10. Regional contribution to the global ejection fraction (CREF), calculated for 20 segments in normal subjects. The median, 10th, and 90th percentiles are shown. Ventriculograms were made in the 30° RAO position

10%	median	90%		10%	median	90%
40.3	53.2	70.7		44.5	56.7	72.9
42.4	67.1	81.1		57.9	68.8	76.6
64.1	76.8	89.3		61.9	71.5	80.9
63.9	76.6	88.4		59.9	71.6	82.6
63.4	77.5	85.2		53.9	69.9	84.7
56.9	76.8	86.3		55.0	70.6	82.6
67.9	80.9	87.9		59.9	74.6	87.8
68.4	82.6	93.2		61.8	77.9	87.6
61.6	87.5	98.3		64.8	77.8	88.8
79.4	92.0	99.9		53.7	81.1	94.7

Fig. 11. Percentage of blood ejected (regional ejection fraction) as calculated in 20 left ventricular segments in normal subjects. The ventriculograms are of the 30° RAO projection. Notice that the apical segments in systole practically occlude their part of the ventricular lumen, though their contribution to global ejection fraction is small (Fig. 10)

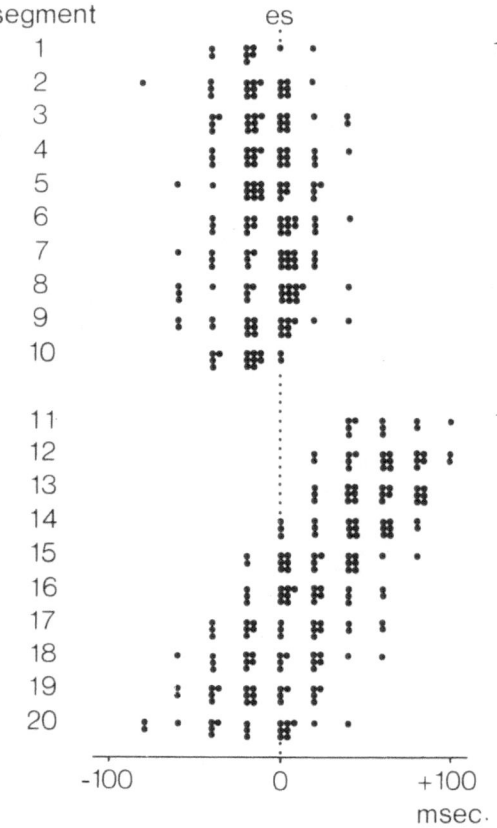

Fig. 12. Time between end-systole (es) and the moment of maximal inward displacement in 20 segments of the 30° RAO left ventriculogram of 20 normal subjects. A consistent delay of relaxation is observed in the posterobasal segments. In 33 of 400 segments the moment of maximal displacement could not be determined accurately. The data of these segments are not displayed, but their occurrence is indicated by a number in the respective segment

Table 3. Regional contractile and pump function and time-relationship in five patients before (C) and after (N) intracoronary administration of nifedipine

	Delay of onset of displacement (ms)		Temporal relation between AVC and max. wall displacement (ms)		$\overline{V}_{ed\text{-}es}$ (cm/s)		CREF (%)	
	C	N	C	N	C	N	C	N
An-terior wall seg-ments	29 ± 27	144 ± 95 $P<10^{-10}$	-11 ± 31	60 ± 56 $P<10^{-10}$	3.5 ± 1.2	1.9 ± 1.2 $P<10^{-10}$	3.33 ± 1.46	2.46 ± 1.29 $P<10^{-8}$
Inferior wall seg-ments	28 ± 27	72 ± 70 $P<10^{-4}$	10 ± 44	22 ± 76 NS	3.5 ± 1.1	2.3 ± 1.0 $P<10^{-8}$	3.32 ± 1.34	2.85 ± 1.26 $P<10^{-4}$

C, control values; N, values 30 s after nifedipine; $\overline{V}$, mean velocity; ed, end diastolic (based on pressure measurement); es, end systolic (based on pressure measurement); CREF, regional contribution to global ejection fraction; P, Students t-test (paired data); Values are expressed as means $\pm$ SD

The profound effect of intracoronary nifedipine on left ventricular wall motion and its time sequence is shown in Fig. 13. The delay in onset of displacement with respect to the end-diastole (Table 3) is illustrated in Fig. 14 for each of the 20 segments. Prior to administration of nifedipine, the onset of displacement of the anterior and inferior wall are observed 29 and 28 ms respectively, after end-diastole. After injection of nifedipine into the main stem of the left

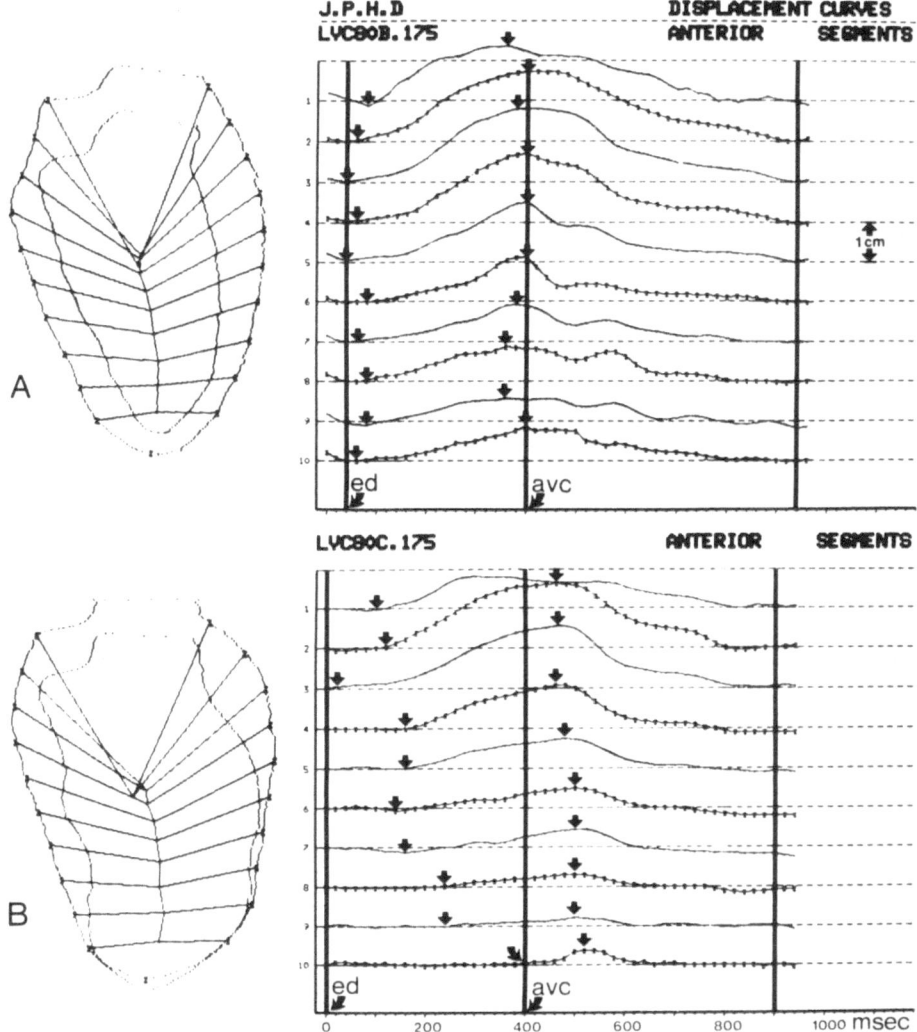

Fig. 13. Effect of nifedipine into the left main coronary artery on left ventricular anterior wall motion and its time sequence. *Arrows* indicate onset and the moment of maximal wall displacement. Nifedipine induces a delay in onset of displacement, a decrease in the extent of segmental wall motion, and a delay of the maximal wall displacement. *A* control left ventriculogram. *B* postnifedipine left ventriculogram. ed, end-diastole; avc, aortic valve closure

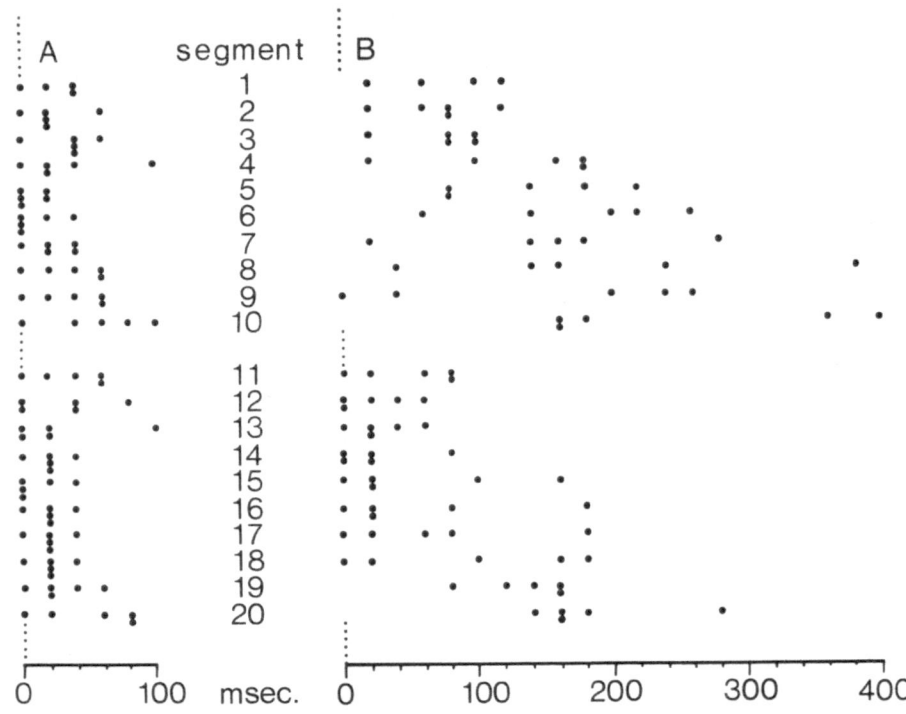

Fig. 14a,b. Delay (ms) in onset of displacement for the 20 individual wall segments with respect to end-diastole (time zero) *a* before and *b* after intracoronary nifedipine. In two (segment 1) out of 200 segments the moment of onset of displacement could not be determined accurately. These data are omitted in the figure

coronary artery, the onset of displacement of the anterior wall is delayed by 115 ms ($P<0.001$), while the inferior wall is delayed by only 44 ms ($P<0.001$). For each segment the timing relationship between the aortic valve closure and the occurrence of the maximal wall displacement is demonstrated in Fig. 15. Before nifedipine, the maximal displacement of the anterior wall occurs 11 ms before the aortic valve closure (AVC). In contrast with the anterior wall segments, the inferoposterior wall segments do not reach their maximal wall displacement synchronously. The maximal displacement of the five posterobasal segments (nos. 11–15) occurs between 20 and 100 ms after the aortic valve closure, so that the maximal wall displacement of the entire inferior wall falls, on average, 10 ms after the aortic valve closure. After nifedipine, the moment of maximal wall displacement for the anterior wall shifts from end-systole (11 ms before AVC) to early diastole (60 ms after AVC). The anterolateral and the apical segment of the anterior wall and the apical segment of the inferior wall appear to be the most affected. On the contrary, the posterobasal wall segments reach their maximum in end-systole, instead of early diastole.

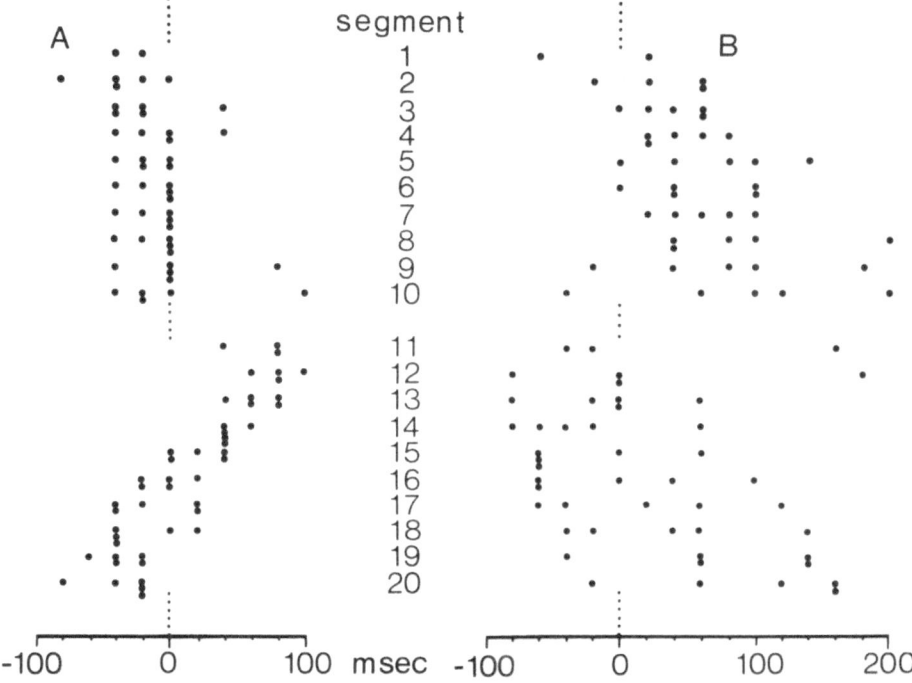

Fig. 15a, b. Time relationship between aortic valve closure (time zero) and the occurrence of maximal wall displacement *a* before and *b* after intracoronary nifedipine. In 13 out of 200 segments the moment of maximal wall displacement could not be determined accurately. These data are omitted in the figure

Mean wall velocity after nifedipine shows a decrease which is again more pronounced in the anterior wall segments (Table 3) than in the inferior wall segments. Figure 16 shows a typical example of such a regional depression of contractility. The individual regional pump function data for all 20 segments before and after the intracoronary administration of nifedipine are given in Fig. 17. Although these data demonstrate a myocardial depression affecting the whole ventricle, the anterolateral and apical segments are the most severely affected. Two patients with a left dominant coronary artery exhibit an impressive reduction of the pump function of their posterobasal wall segments as well. Under the influence of nifedipine, the mean CREF values decrease from 3.30% to 2.46% ($P<0.001$) for the anterior wall and from 3.32% to 2.85% ($P<0.001$) for the inferior wall (Table 3).

In Tables 4 and 5 the hemodynamic data of the patients with acute myocardial infarction (AMI) during the first heart catheterization (acute) and during the follow-up study (chronic) are shown. In Table 4 the data of eight patients with unsuccessful recanalization are shown. Most prominent are the decrease in stroke volume (SV), cardiac index (CI), and ejection fraction (EF). In Table 5 the results of 14 patients with successful opening and persistent patency of the

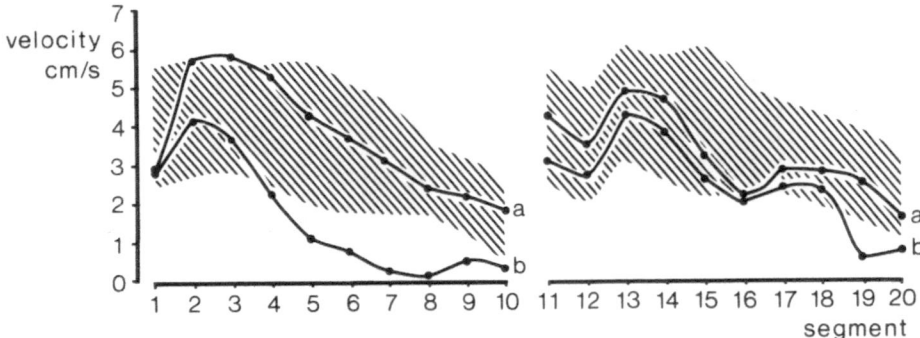

Fig. 16a,b. Example of changes in mean wall velocity in 20 wall segments *a* before and *b* after nifedipine. *Shaded areas* indicate the normal range. After injection of nifedipine into the left main coronary artery, a reduction of wall velocity is observed in the anterior (1–8) and apical (9, 10 and 19, 20) segments

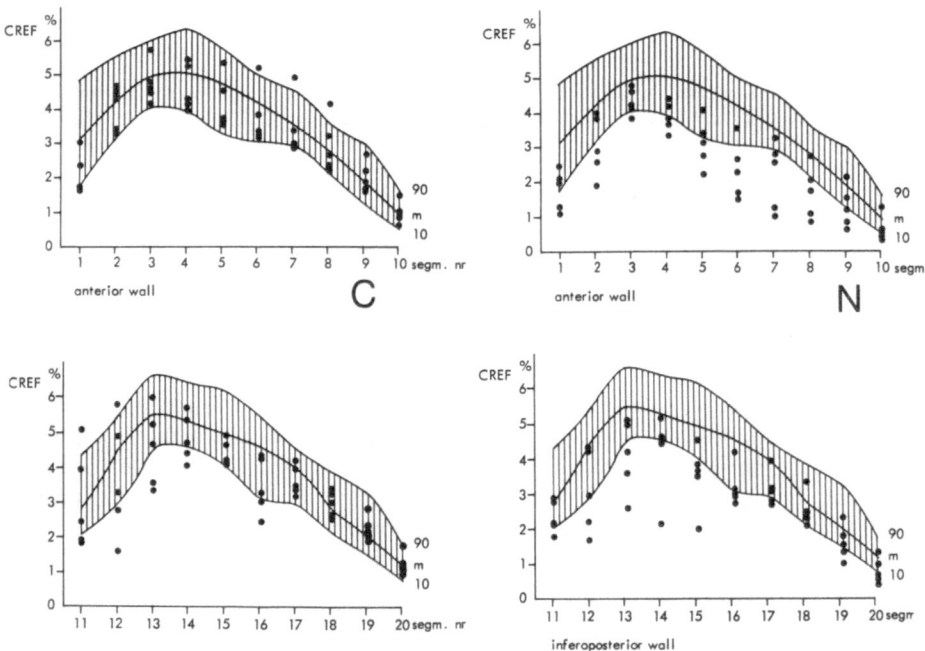

Fig. 17. Effect of nifedipine injection into the left main coronary artery on regional contribution to global ejection fraction (CREF). *Left panels*, individual CREF values (five patients) in the anterior and inferoposterior wall segments before nifedipine injection. *Shaded areas* represent the normal range of CREF values. *Right panels*, after nifedipine an overall depression of regional pump function is observed which is more pronounced in the anterior (1–8) and apical (9, 10 and 19, 20) segments

Table 4. Hemodynamic data of eight patients with "unsuccessful recanalization" of the occluded coronary artery

	Acute	Chronic	P-value
Heart rate (bpm)	79 ± 18	82 ± 17	NS
Mean AoP (mmHg)	84 ± 20	90 ± 13	NS
LVEDP (mmHg)	16 ± 7	21 ± 11	NS
CI (l/m²)	3.7 ± 1.3	3.05 ± 1.4	<0.09
LVEDV (ml/m²)	96 ± 20	100 ± 30	NS
LVESV (ml/m²)	49 ± 14	66 ± 32	NS
SV (ml/m²)	47 ± 15	35 ± 12	<0.02
Ejection fraction (%)	49 ± 11	37 ± 14	<0.001
Akinetic segments (%)	16 ± 16	20 ± 19	NS

AoP, aortic pressure; LVEDP, end diastolic pressure; CI, cardiac index; LVEDV, end diastolic volume; LVESV, end systolic volume; SV, stroke volume; P-value, Students t-test (paired data); NS, not significant; Values expressed as means ± SD

Table 5. Hemodynamic data of 20 patients with "successful recanalization" of the occluded coronary artery

	Acute	Chronic	P-value
Heart rate (bpm)	79 ± 13	72 ± 14	<0.03
Mean AoP (mmHg)	91 ± 14	96 ± 13	NS
LVEDP (mmHg)	22 ± 8	20 ± 10	NS
CI (l/m²)	3.1 ± 0.7	3.2 ± 0.6	NS
LVEDV (ml/m²)	80 ± 27	82 ± 13	NS
LVESV (ml/m²)	40 ± 21	36 ± 11	NS
SV (ml/m²)	40 ± 10	45 ± 9	<0.04
Ejection fraction (%)	52 ± 10	56 ± 10	<0.02
Akinetic segments (%)	18 ± 16	13 ± 13	NS

AoP, aortic pressure; LVEDP, end diastolic pressure; CI, cardiac index; LVEDV, end diastolic volume; LVESV, end systolic volume; SV, stroke volume; P-value, Students t-test (paired data); NS, not significant; Values expressed as means ± SD

IRA are shown. Global ejection fraction increases significantly ($P<0.02$) from 52% to 56%. The individual CREF data of a patient with anterior infarction, during the acute event and during the follow-up study, are shown in Fig. 18. A few hours after the onset of infarction, regional pump function is severely depressed in the anterior and apical wall segments (segments 3–10 and 19, 20), but is only slightly affected in the inferoposterior wall (segments 11–18). Three weeks after successful recanalization regional pump function is improved in both the anterior and the inferoposterior wall segments. In Fig. 19 the CREF values (mean ± SD) in five wall regions of eight patients with anterior infarction, during the acute event (first bar) and after an interval of 2–3 weeks (second bar) are shown. The interrupted lines represent the 10th percentile (lower)

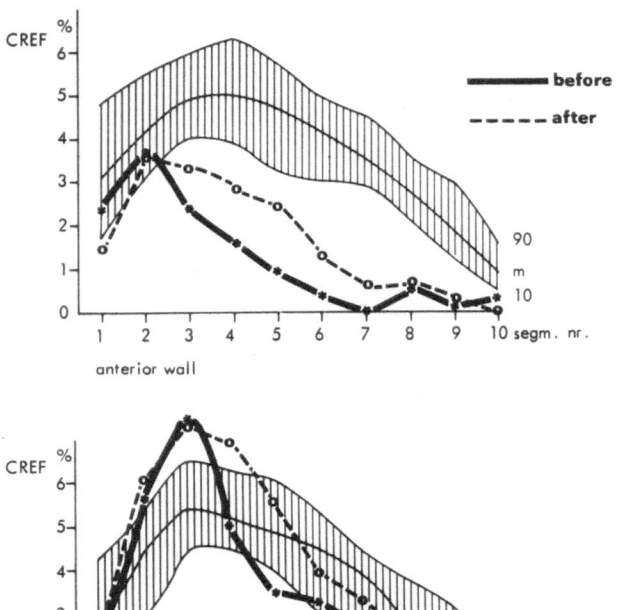

Fig. 18. Regional contribution to global ejection fraction (CREF) in 20 segments of the 30° RAO left ventriculogram, before (*continuous line*) and 3 weeks after recanalization of an occluded left anterior descending coronary artery in a patient with acute anterior myocardial infarction. CREF values are severely depressed in the anterior and apical wall segments (3–10, 19 and 20) and approximately normal in the inferior and posterobasal segments (11–18). After coronary recanalization, regional pump function improves, not only in the anterior, but also in the inferior wall. *Shaded areas* represent CREF values in normal individuals (*10*, 10th percentile; *90*, 90th percentile; *m*, median)

border of regional pump function in normal individuals. In particular, the anterolateral and apical wall regions' subnormal CREF values are observed, as would be expected in anterior infarction. Analysis using the paired t-test shows a significant improvement of regional pump function in the anterolateral and apical segments, which is accompanied by a significant increase of CREF values in the inferior ($P<0.001$) and posterobasal ($P<0.05$) wall regions. In Fig. 20 the changes in regional pump function after recanalization of the right coronary artery are shown. At the time of acute inferior infarction a severe depression of pump function is observed in the inferoposterior wall, while CREF values in the anterior wall remain within normal limits. After successful recanalization of the IRA a significant ($P<0.01$) increase of CREF is observed in the inferior wall segments.

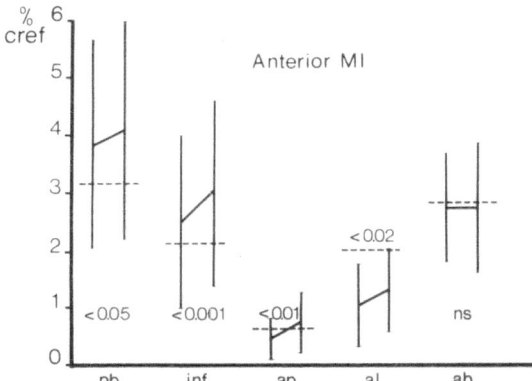

Fig. 19. Mean CREF values ± SD (*bars*) of eight patients with acute anterior wall infarction before (*first bar*) and 2–3 weeks after (*second bar*) recanalization of the left anterior descending coronary artery with streptokinase. Interrupted lines represent the 10th percentile border of CREF in normal individuals in the posterobasal (*pb*), inferior (*inf*), apical (*ap*), anterolateral (*al*), and anterobasal (*ab*) wall segments. Before recanalization regional pump function is severely depressed in the anterior and apical wall segments. After recanalization, a significant improvement of pump function in the anterolateral and apical segments is paralleled by a very significant increase of pump function in the inferoposterior wall

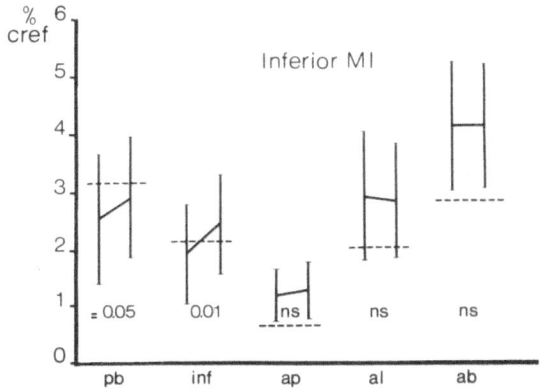

Fig. 20. Mean CREF values ± SD (*bars*) of seven patients with acute inferior wall infarction, before (*first bar*) and 2–3 weeks after (*second bar*) thrombolytic recanalization of the right coronary artery. Before recanalization regional pump function is severely depressed in the inferior and posterobasal wall and normal in the anteroapical wall segments. After recanalization a significant improvement of regional pump function is observed in the inferior wall

With this method of analysis the intraobserver variability in the quantitative assessment of left ventricular volume and ejection fraction is small: the standard error of the estimate (SEE) is 1.2–1.5 ml/m^2 and 1.6%–1.8%, respectively (Table 6). Interobserver variability is only slightly greater (SEE 1.5–2.3 ml/m^2 and 1.9%–2.3%, respectively). Computation of SUMCREF is subject to an SEE

Table 6. Intra- and interobserver variability in the assessment of left ventricular end-diastolic volume, ejection fraction, and SUMCREF in 20 patients

Comparison between observations	LVEDVI (73.1 ± 27.6 ml/m²)		Ejection fraction ($58.3 \pm 17.2\%$)		SUMCREF ($58.3 \pm 15.6\%$)	
	Correlation coefficient	SEE (ml/m²)	Correlation coefficient	SEE (%)	Correlation coefficient	SEE (%)
Xa – Xb	0.99	1.5	0.99	1.8	0.99	2.5
Ya – Yb	0.99	1.2	0.99	1.6	0.99	1.8
Xa – Ya	0.99	1.6	0.99	2.2	0.99	2.2
Xa – Yb	0.99	1.5	0.99	1.9	0.98	2.9
Xb – Ya	0.99	2.2	0.99	2.3	0.98	3.1
Xb – Yb	0.99	2.3	0.99	2.3	0.97	3.6

LVEDVI, left ventricular end-diastolic volume corrected for body surface area; SUMCREF, summated CREF values; SEE, standard error of the estimate; X, observation of observer X; Y, observation of observer Y; a, first observation; b, second observation

Table 7. Correlation between ejection fraction assessed from global left ventricular volume change and the SUMCREF

Observations of EF and SUMCREF	Correlation coefficient	SEE (%)
Xa – Xa	0.99	1.9
Xb – Xb	0.97	3.9
Ya – Ya	0.99	2.5
Yb – Yb	0.99	2.6

EF, ejection fraction

of 1.8%–2.5% for the intraobserver variability and 2.2%–3.6% for the interobserver variability. The correlation between ejection fraction computed from global left ventricular volume change and SUMCREF is liable to an SEE of 1.9%–3.9% (Table 7).

Discussion

In the present study a new method to determine regional wall motion is introduced and applied to the assessment of regional left ventricular pump and contractile function. The search for this new wall motion model was initiated by the inadequacy of the currently available methods [4–8]. The very existence of these different methods to analyze left ventricular wall motion indicates that no exact and generally accepted procedure is available to track fixed points along the endocardial wall.

Nearly all methods show a considerable error of determined wall motion in comparison with midwall markers [9], and are liable to introduce artifacts, as most approaches include procedures to "correct" for translation and rotation.

Daughters et al. [17] showed, however, that sustained respiration and a fixed geometric position of the patient with regard to the X-ray equipment reduces translation to a minimum, and that long axis rotation may be neglected. These problems were circumvented with the aid of an automated contour detector. This high resolution outlining system detects small irregularities at the endocardial border and thus preserves information which is lost with manual analysis of a ventriculogram. The hypothesis that these irregularities represent specific anatomical structures has been tested in cadaver hearts [12] and in pigs (see Slager et al., this volume). The mean systolic pathways of these "anatomical landmarks" were measured in normal individuals. This forms the basis for the definition of the wall motion model applied in this study (Fig. 3). As segmental wall motion is determined according to these mean pathways, the direction and extent of measured wall motion will be very accurate in normal subjects, although it is obvious that even this method will not track the actual motion of all endocardial points. In fact, the method will introduce some error when applied to abnormally contracting hearts. However, in general, a subnormal regional contraction will cause a decrease of both the x- and the y-component of the displacement vector d (Fig. 21), which results in a decrease in the extent, but not a major change in direction of wall motion. Thus, the normal pattern of wall motion may be the closest general approximation applicable to the abnormal ventricle. The right anterior oblique projection was selected for analysis of the ventriculogram. This implies that the septal and posterolateral wall are not visualized. Coronary heart disease however is seldom confined to these wall segments [18]. Analysis of the left anterior oblique angiogram is less rewarding because of technical limitations, such as the foreshortening effect of the septal and posterolateral wall and the imperfect delineation of the ventricular silhouette at the level of the mitral valve. Although most authors normalize regional wall motion for the end-diastolic diameter, we opted for absolute displacement values, which then remain applicable for further calculations. With this method, displacement is shown to have a narrow range (Fig. 7), while

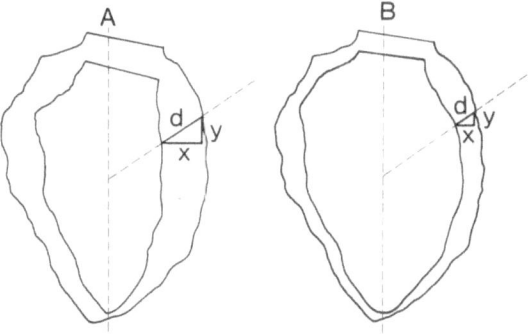

Fig. 21. The end-diastolic and end-systolic endocardial contours of a normally contracting and a hypokinetic left ventricle are shown. Although the extent of displacement (d) is decreased in the latter case, the direction of wall motion is not essentially changed since both the x- and the y-component of the displacement vector d are diminished

a close relationship is observed between the data of neighboring segments, as is reflected by a smooth decrease of displacement data from base to apex (Fig. 8). A comparative study of other wall motion models shows on the contrary a very irregular distribution of the extent of wall motion over the left ventricular silhouette [19]. We consider this a strong argument in favor of this method, as it is hardly conceivable that wall motion in normal subjects would show major differences between adjoining segments. In this study, segmental wall velocity, the time derivative of segmental displacement, is introduced as an index of regional left ventricular performance reflecting the inotropic state. The myocardial inotropic state is commonly assessed from the isovolumic indices of contractility. However, these indices disregard the regional character of left ventricular (dys)function, while their capacity to discriminate between normal and abnormal function is inferior to that of the ejection phase indices [20]. Since their theoretical basis is violated when contraction is asynchronous or when the mitral valve is insufficient, the isovolumic parameters are further disadvantaged. To what extent these conditions also affect the present method must be further investigated.

Gault et al. [21] showed that the myocardial contractility may be assessed during the ejection phase. At peak stress, the circumferential fiber-shortening velocity (V_{cf}) – computed as $2\,dR/dt$ – equals the contractile element velocity (V_{CE}) and thus can be regarded as an index of the contractile state. Mean V_{cf} [22] was shown to reflect the inotropic state with almost the same accuracy, although it lacks the fundamental base of instantaneous velocity at peak stress. As V_{cf} assessed in the RAO view is the mean of velocities of the anterior and inferoposterior wall, depressed contractile function in one wall segment may still be obscured by normal function of the other.

Determination of segmental wall velocity – computed as dR/dt – solves this problem. The mean circumferential velocity data described by Gault et al. [21] show, after correction for the computational method (i.e., division by 2π), excellent agreement with the mean systolic velocity (MSV) data in the current study. The average radial wall velocity in their group of individuals without left ventricular disease was $23.3/6.28 = 3.7$ cm/s, while we find median MSV values of 3.3–4.0 cm/s in the midventricular wall segments.

In patients with coronary heart disease, a subnormal ejection fraction, or a decrease of ejection fraction during interventions such as rapid atrial pacing [23], is often caused by a regional disturbance of pump function. Although regional ejection fraction [24] may be used as a determinant of regional performance, the contribution of a given wall segment to global ejection cannot be assessed with this method, as the "end-diastolic volume" contained in each segment may differ considerably. Normalization of regional volume displacement for end-diastolic volume yields a new parameter of regional pump function (CREF), which expresses quantitatively to what extent a particular segment contributes to global ejection fraction. CREF values in normal subjects (Fig. 10, Table 2) show that the midventricular segments are of prime importance for the ejection of blood: segments 4, 5, 14, and 15 contribute 15.6%–24.4% to global ejection fraction, whereas the apical segments 9, 10, 19, and 20 contribute only 3.8%–9.3%. Though the apical segments contribute only little to global ejection fraction, blood is ejected from this area more completely than from the midventricular segments, as is expressed by the regional ejection fraction (Fig. 11). The basal segments 1, 2, 11, and 12, which, because of their relation to the noncontractile structures of aortic and mitral valve, are restricted in their inward excursions, have the lowest values of regional ejection fraction, but still contribute importantly (9.7%–19.8%) to global ejection fraction. A number of studies show that analysis of the time course of left ventricular performance may reveal left ventricular dysfunction even when quantitative analysis of the end-diastolic and end-systolic contours shows no abnormality [25, 26]. The ejection fraction in the first third of systole appears to be a particularly sensitive determinant of left ventricular function [27]. To study the asynchrony of contraction, which is a typical consequence of coronary heart disease [10], frame-by-frame analysis of the left ventriculogram is indispensable. Our system tracks the regional endocardial motion throughout the entire cardiac cycle at 20-ms intervals and may provide data on global ejection fraction and CREF at any moment during the cardiac cycle.

Although left ventricular contraction in normal man is essentially synchronous, some variability in the time sequence of regional wall motion may be observed.

In Fig. 14 the time measured between end-systole (determined from volume measurements) and the moment of maximal inward wall displacement for the 20 segments in the 20 patients of the study group is shown: inward wall motion proceeds in the posterobasal area beyond end-systole, defined as the frame with minimal volume.

After intracoronary administration of nifedipine, a decrease in the extent of segmental wall motion, a delay in the onset of wall displacement, and a delay of maximal wall displacement is observed..Mean systolic wall velocity (Table 3) is significantly reduced in both the anterior and inferior wall. Furthermore, regional pump function (CREF) of the anterior and inferior wall segments decreases by 27% and 14%, respectively. It is concluded that intracoronary nifedipine not only delays and prolongs the segmental contraction, but also slows and depresses it.

As shown in Tables 4 and 5, unsuccessful recanalization of an occluded coronary artery appears to be associated with depressed global left ventricular function, while successful recanalization and persistent patency of the IRA improves ejection fraction. This finding is in agreement with the results of similar studies by Rentrop et al. [28], Ganz et al. [29], and Mathey et al. [30]. However, such improvement may be due not only to enhancement of regional function in the reperfused "infarct zone" but also by compensatory action of other wall segments. The results of this study suggest that, although significant improvement of regional function in the infarct zone is observed, at least part of the increase of ejection fraction is caused by compensation of other wall regions.

However, these results must be interpreted with care, first, because the number of patients studied is small, and second, because angiograms made during the first hours of myocardial infarction provide only one "snapshot" of what must be a rapidly changing situation. Also, analysis of ejection fraction with conventional methods has proved to be subject to substantial variation

[31], which makes any interpretation of small changes of ejection fraction in sequential angiograms a dubious affair. Computer-assisted analysis of the angiograms reduces the variability significantly. In fact, with the system used in this study, intra- and interobserver variability of repeated assessment of ejection fraction was only 1.6%–2.3%. Even so, variations of ejection fraction in sequential left ventriculograms may still be due to changes in pre- and afterload and in heart rate [32].

While in this study no significant changes in left ventricular end diastolic pressure (EDP), volume (EDV), or mean aortic pressure (mean AoP) were observed, heart rate decreased slightly in the successfully recanalized group. It would have been interesting to perform a similar analysis of the angiograms of patients with unsuccessful recanalization. However, the heterogeneity of this small group with respect to localization of infarction and IRAs would have made interpretation very difficult.

To conclude, in this paper we have introduced and discussed a new method to quantify regional left ventricular function and given two examples of its application in clinical research.

References

1. Popio KA, Gorlin R, Bechtel D, Levine JA (1977) Postextrasystolic potentiation as a predictor of potential myocardial viability: preoperative analyses compared with studies after coronary bypass surgery. Am J Cardiol 39:944–953
2. Nelson GR, Cohn PF, Gorlin R (1975) Prognosis in medically-treated coronary artery disease. Influence of ejection fraction compared to other parameters. Circulation 52:408–412
3. Hugenholtz PG, Ellison RC, Urschel CW, Mirsky I, Sonnenblick EH (1970) Myocardial force-velocity relationships in clinical heart disease. Circulation 41:191–202
4. Herman MV, Heinle RA, Klein MD, Gorlin R (1967) Localized disorders in myocardial contraction. N Engl J Med 227:222–232
5. Leighton RF, Wilt SM, Lewis RP (1974) Detection of hypokinesis by quantitative analysis of left ventricular cineangiograms. Circulation 50:121–127
6. Harris LD, Clayton PD, Marshall HW, Warner HR (1974) A technique for the detection of asynergistic motion of the left ventricle. Comput Biomed Res 7:380–394
7. Rickards A, Seabra-Gomes R, Thurston P (1977) The assessment of regional abnormalities of the left ventricle by angiography. Eur J Cardiol 5:167–182
8. Chaitman BR, Bristow JD, Rahimtoola SH (1973) Left ventricular wall motion assessed by using fixed external reference systems. Circulation 48:1043–1054
9. Ingels NB Jr, Daughters GT, Stinson EB, Alderman EL (1980) Evaluation of methods for quantitating left ventricular segmental wall motion in man using myocardial markers as standard. Circulation 61:966–972
10. Holman BL, Wyne J, Idoine J, Neill J (1980) Disruption in the temporal sequence of regional ventricular contraction. I. Characteristics and incidence in coronary artery disease. Circulation 61:1075–1082
11. Slutsky R, Karliner JS, Battler A, Peterson K, Ross J Jr (1980) Comparison of early systolic and holosystolic ejection phase indexes by contrast ventriculography in patients with coronary artery disease. Circulation 61:1083–1090
12. Slager CJ, Hooghoudt TEH, Reiber JHC, Schuurbiers JCH, Booman F, Meester GT (1979) Left ventricular contour segmentation from anatomical landmark trajectories and its application to wall motion analysis. Computers in cardiology, IEEE Computer Society, Long Beach, pp 347–350

13. Vine DL, Hegg TD, Dodge HT, Stewart DK, Frimer M (1977) Immediate effect of contrast medium injection on left ventricular volumes and ejection fraction. Circulation 56:379–384
14. Sones FM (1962) Cine coronary angiography. Mod Concepts Cardiovasc Dis 31:735
15. Judkins MP (1967) Selective coronary arteriography. Part I. A percutaneous transfemoral technique. Radiology 89:815
16. Reiber JHC, Slager CJ, Schuurbiers JCH, Meester GT (1978) Contouromat – a hard-wired left ventricular angio processing system. II. Performance evaluation. Comput Biomed Res 11:503–523
17. Daughters GT, Ingels NB Jr, Jang GC, Alderman EL, Stinson EB (1977) Left ventricular long axis rotation assessed by cinefluoroscopy of implanted myocardial markers. Fed Proc 36:447
18. Sullivan W, Vlodaver Z, Tuna N, Long L, Edwards JE (1978) Correlation of electrocardiographic and pathologic findings in healed myocardial infarction. Am J Cardiol 42:724
19. Brower RW, Meester GT (1976) Computer based methods for quantifying regional left ventricular wall motion from cine ventriculograms. Computers in cardiology, IEEE Computer Society, Long Beach, pp 52–62
20. Peterson KL, Skloven D, Ludbrook P, Uther JB, Ross J Jr (1974) Comparison of isovolumic and ejection phase indices of myocardial performance in man. Circulation 49:1088
21. Gault JH, Ross J Jr, Braunwald E (1968) Contractile state of the left ventricle in man. Instantaneous tension-velocity-length relations in patients with and without disease of the left ventricular myocardium. Circ Res 22:451–463
22. Karliner JS, Gault JH, Eckberg D, Mullins CB, Ross J Jr (1971) Mean velocity of fiber shortening. A simplified measure of left ventricular myocardial contractility. Circulation 44:323–333
23. Dwyer EM Jr (1970) Left ventricular pressure-volume alterations and regional disorders of contraction during myocardial ischemia induced by atrial pacing. Circulation 42:1111–1122
24. Maddox DE, Wynne J, Uren R, Parker JA, Idoine J, Siegel LC, Neill JM, Cohn PF, Holman BL (1979) Regional ejection fraction: a quantitative radionuclide index of regional left ventricular performance. Circulation 59:1001–1009
25. Leighton RF, Pollack ME, Welch TG (1975) Abnormal left ventricular wall motion at mid-ejection in patients with coronary heart disease. Circulation 52:238–244
26. Johnson LL, Ellis K, Schmidt D, Weiss MB, Cannon PJ (1975) Volume ejected in early systole. A sensitive index of left ventricular performance in coronary artery disease. Circulation 52:378–389
27. Battler A, Slutsky R, Karliner J, Froelicher V, Ashburn W, Ross J Jr (1980) Left ventricular ejection fraction and first third ejection fraction after acute myocardial infarction: value for predicting mortality and morbidity. Am J Cardiol 45:197–202
28. Rentrop P, Blanke H, Karsch KR, Kaiser H, Kostering H, Leitz K (1981) Selective intracoronary thrombolysis in acute myocardial infarction and unstable angina pectoris. Circulation 63:307
29. Ganz W, Buchbinder N, Marcus H, Mondkar A, Maddahi J, Charuzi Y, O'Connor L, Shell W, Fishbein MC, Kass R, Miyamoto A, Swan HJC (1981) Intracoronary thrombolysis in evolving myocardial infarction. Am Heart J 101:4
30. Mathey DG, Kuck K-H, Tilsner V, Krebber H-J, Bleifeld W (1981) Nonsurgical coronary artery recanalization in transmural myocardial infarction. Circulation 63:489
31. Cohn PF, Levine JA, Bergeron GA, Gorlin R (1974) Reproducibility of angiographic left ventricular ejection fraction in patients with coronary artery disease. Am Heart J 88:713
32. Yang SS, Bentivoglio LG, Maranhao V, Goldberg H (eds) (1978) From cardiac catheterization data to hemodynamic parameters. Davis, Philadelphia, p 264

Analysis of Left Ventricular Function Using Midwall Myocardial Markers

I. Amende, R. Simon, K. Heim, R. Hetzer, and P. R. Lichtlen

Medical University Hannover, Karl-Wiechert-Allee 9, D-3000 Hannover 61, FRG

Introduction

Contrast ventriculography is used routinely to quantify left ventricular global and regional function. However, this method is not suitable for frequently repeated or continuous measurements of dimensions and volumes, due to the known hemodynamic effects of the contrast material. Radiopaque markers implanted during the time of surgery provide an alternative method of quantitating changes in left ventricular volume and regional dimensions in man [1, 5, 6]. It has been demonstrated in animal studies that epicardial markers do not necessarily reflect ventricular dynamics [7]. In contrast, several studies indicate that markers implanted into the midwall of the ventricle offer a sensitive method for accurate and repeatable determinations of ventricular global and segmental myocardial dynamics [2, 3, 4].

In Hannover, since 1975, two types of midwall myocardial markers have been implanted in patients: either a pair of markers during bypass surgery within the grafted region, or a set of seven markers outlining the left ventricle.

Methods

In 40 patients who had received a saphenous vein bypass graft to the anterior descending coronary artery (LAD), a pair of markers (small metallic spheres, 1.2 mm in diameter) were implanted in the midwall of the myocardium within the grafted region. The markers were placed at a depth of 5 mm, about 2 cm apart in the transverse direction (Fig. 1).

In 35 patients the markers were filmed postoperatively in a 10°–20° left anterior oblique projection at 150 frames/s. Changes in marker distance were determined frame by frame over several heart cycles, using a computer-assisted video system. From maximal and minimal marker distances the shortening fraction was calculated (Fig. 2).

In another group of 30 patients, seven markers – tiny helices (0.8 × 1.5 mm) of pure tantalum wire – had been implanted into the midwall of the myocardium at a depth of 5 mm during cardiac surgery: one at the left ventricular apex and three each along the anterolateral and inferior margins of the left ventricle, in a

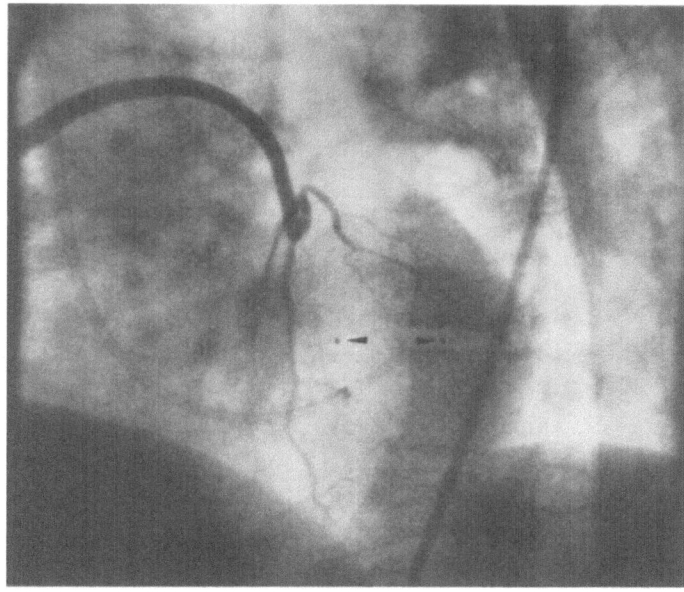

Fig. 1. Midwall myocardial marker pair in the grafted region (20° left anterior oblique projection)

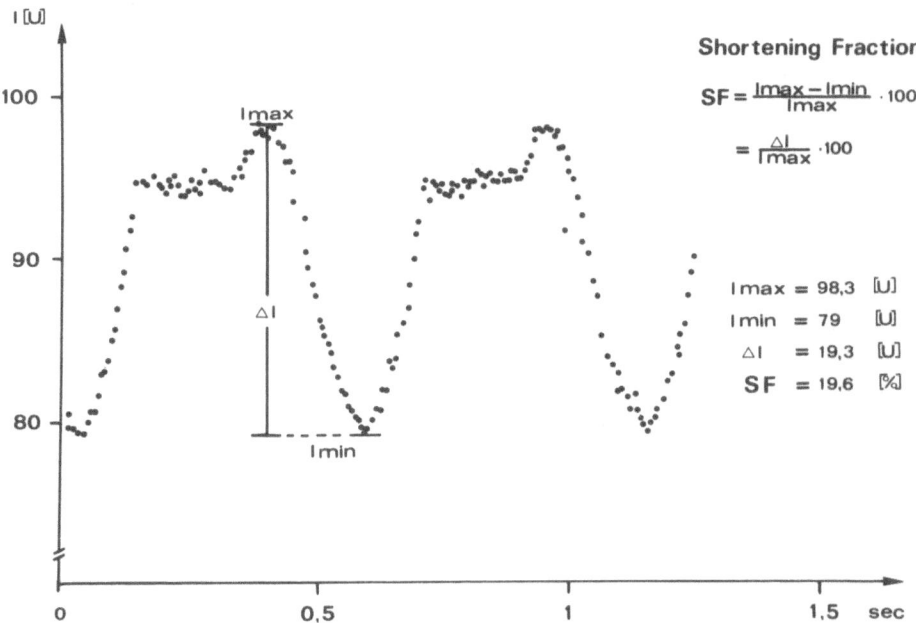

Fig. 2. Marker pair distance plotted frame by frame during two cardiac cycles. Shortening fraction was calculated from maximal (1 max) and minimal (1 min) segmental length. Marker distance in arbitrary units (U)

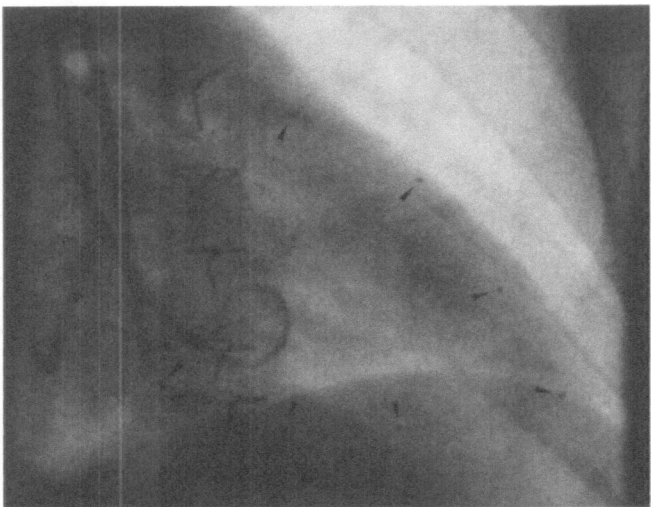

Fig. 3. Left ventricle outlined by seven midwall myocardial markers (30° right anterior oblique projection)

pattern outlining the ventricular chamber as seen in this 30° RAO projection (Fig. 3).

In six patients the myocardial markers were filmed at 150 frames/s before and 1 min, 3 min, 5 min, and 10 min following 0.1 mg intracoronary nifedipine infusion. Regional systolic function was evaluated in terms of percentage systolic shortening and mean shortening velocity of the transverse diameter between the middle pair of myocardial markers [3].

Results

Analysis of segmental wall motion was made using radiopaque markers.

Thirty-five patients were followed up for 18 months (Fig. 4). The shortening fraction was 16.4% two weeks postoperatively, 17.5% after 3 months, and did not change in the following months. As an estimate of regional function, the preoperative shortening fraction was obtained from coronary bifurcations located within the grafted region [2]. In seven of the followed-up patients, analysis of marker motion revealed a considerable reduction in regional myocardial shortening. Subsequent coronary angiography showed a closed LAD graft in these patients.

In four patients, stressing of the myocardium by handgrip demonstrated an early relaxation of the anterior wall not present at rest. Figures 5 and 6 show such an example. At rest, there was a normal pattern of segmental lengthening and shortening. The pressure-length loop looks normal (Fig. 5). Stressing the heart by isometric exercise, however, produced segmental early relaxation. The

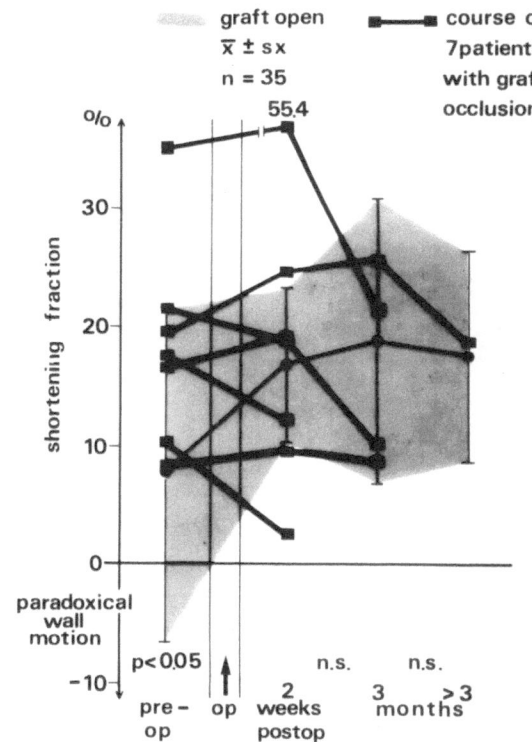

Fig. 4. Shortening fraction over the 18 months follow-up period. In seven patients (*squares*) with reduced marker motion coronary angiography revealed a closed LAD graft

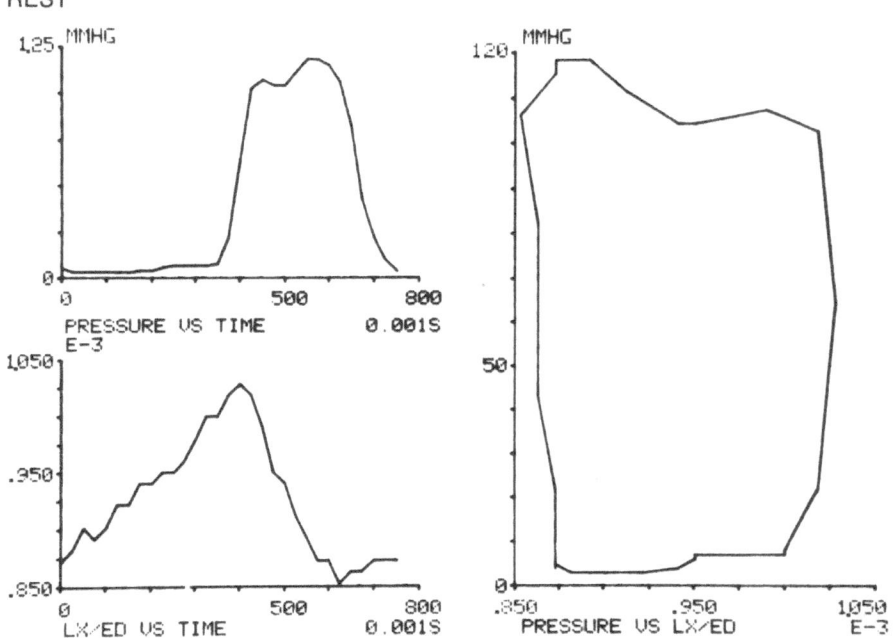

Fig. 5. Frame-by-frame plot of left ventricular high-fidelity pressure and segmental length vs time and pressure-segmental length relation at rest. *LX/ED*, segmental length normalized for end-diastolic length

HANDGRIP

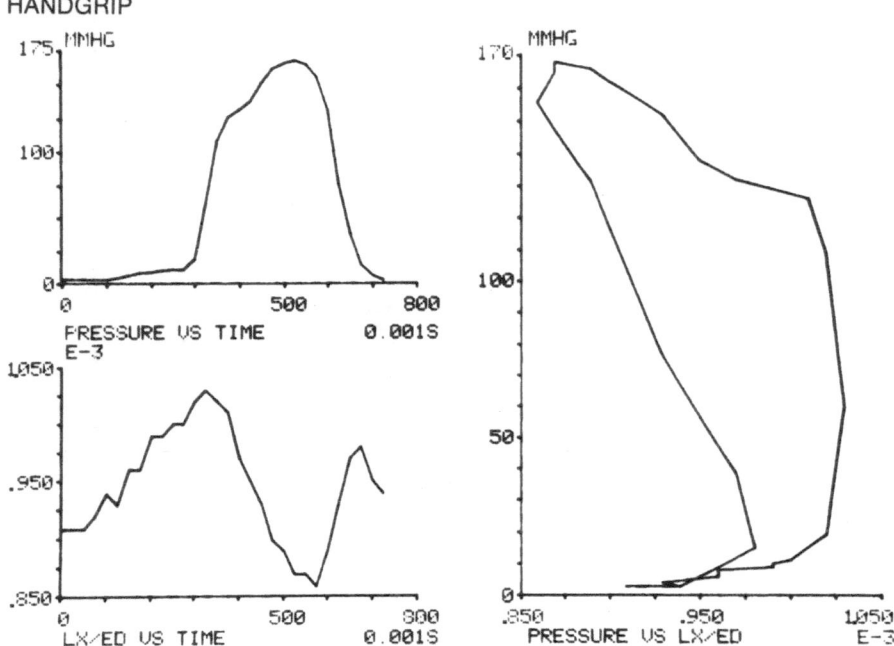

Fig. 6. Segmental early relaxation produced by isometric exercise. Same patient as in Fig. 5

pressure-length loop showed an asymmetrical wall movement during the isovolumic relaxation period (Fig. 6). This patient's coronary angiogram revealed a patent LAD graft, but there were significant obstructions in the grafted vessel.

Analysis of Regional and Global Function Using Radiopaque Markers

Figure 7 shows the effects of intracoronary nifedipine infusion on percentage systolic shortening and mean shortening velocity. Following intracoronary nifedipine, both parameters were significantly reduced at 1 min but had returned to baseline by 3 min, indicating a transient depressant effect of the drug on the myocardium.

During this period of drug-induced reduction in regional systolic performance, the effects of intracoronary nifedipine on diastolic function were analyzed. Midwall circumference obtained from the markers was plotted frame by frame against pressure throughout diastole (Fig. 8). One minute following nifedipine infusion there was a significant upward shift of the diastolic pressure-circumference curve and a change in slope indicating an increase in diastolic stiffness.

Using contrast ventriculography, chamber volume assessed by myocardial markers was calibrated and volume and derived parameters obtained in absolute terms.

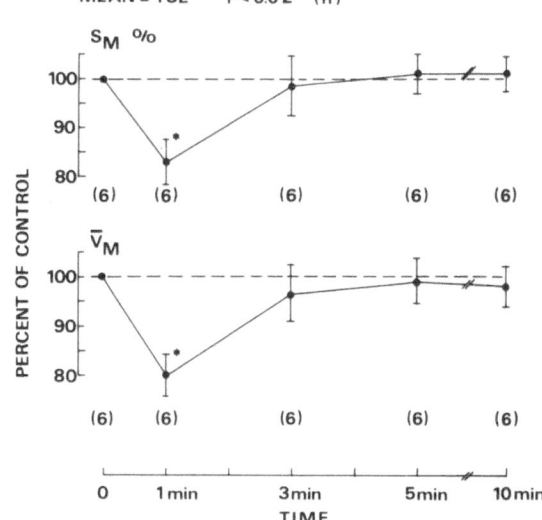

Fig. 7. Effects of 0.1 mg intracoronary nifedipine on percentage systolic shortening ($S_M\%$) and mean shortening velocity ($\overline{V}_M$)

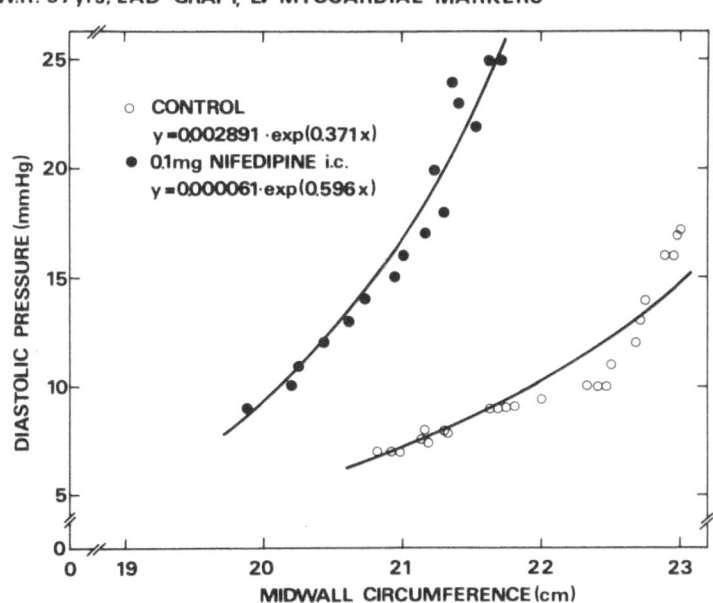

Fig. 8. Effects of intracoronary (*i.c.*) nifedipine on diastolic pressure-circumference relationship. Midwall circumference was derived from myocardial markers

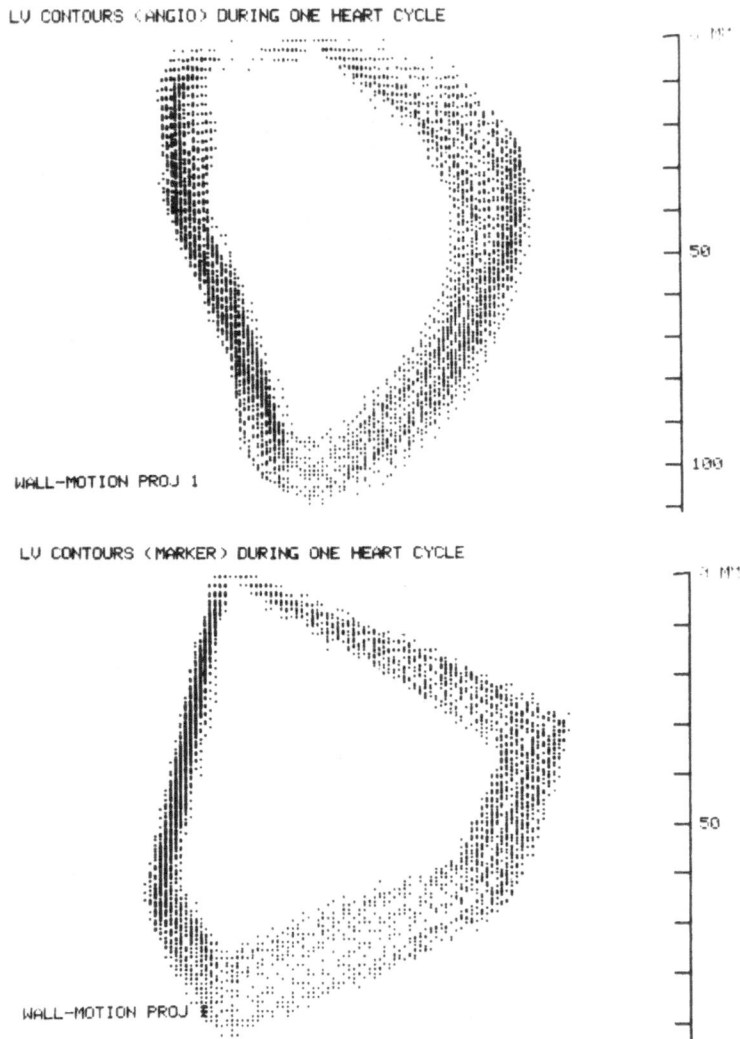

LU CONTOURS (ANGIO) DURING ONE HEART CYCLE

WALL-MOTION PROJ 1

LU CONTOURS (MARKER) DURING ONE HEART CYCLE

WALL-MOTION PROJ

Fig. 9. Left ventricular contours obtained using angiography (*upper panel*) and midwall myocardial markers (*lower panel*) during one cardiac cycle

Figure 9 shows the superimposed contours of an opacified left ventricle during one cardiac cycle and the corresponding contours formed by the seven myocardial markers from the same beat. The regression equation obtained from the relationship between the angiographically determined volumes and the volumes computed from the midwall myocardial markers over one cardiac cycle was used for volume correction. Simpson's rule was applied for volume calculations.

Figure 10 illustrates that the angiographically determined left ventricular volume curve and the volume curve calculated using the regression equation

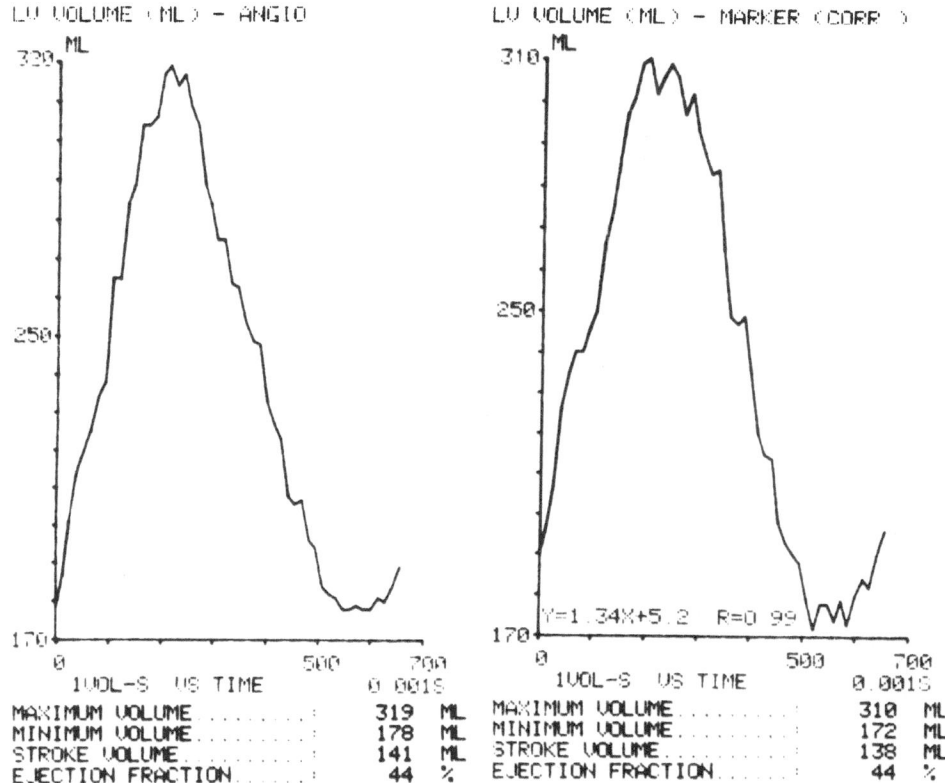

Fig.10. Left ventricular volume curve determined by angiography (*left*) and the corrected volume curve computed from midwall myocardial markers (*right*)

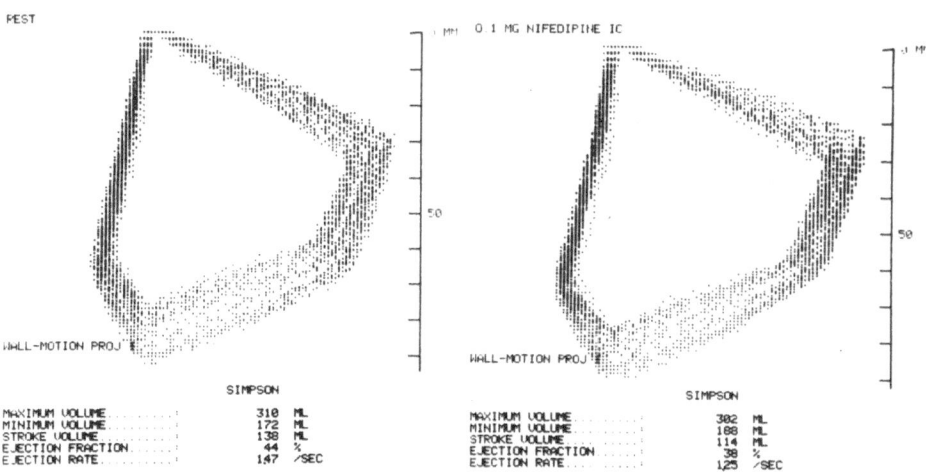

Fig.11. Left ventricular contours derived from midwall myocardial markers and indices of global ventricular function at rest (*left*) and after intracoronary (*ic*) nifedipine (*right*)

($y = 1.34 \ x + 5.2; \ r = 0.99$) and marker measurements from this patient are similar. The ejection fractions are identical.

Figure 11 demonstrates the effects of intracoronary nifedipine on volumes and indices of left ventricular global function computed from midwall myocardial markers in the same patient. Contours before and 1 min after intracoronary nifedipine infusion are shown. Following nifedipine there was an increase in end-systolic volume and a decrease in ejection fraction and normalized systolic ejection rate, indicating the depressant action of the drug on left ventricular global function.

It is concluded that midwall myocardial markers provide a sensitive method of determining left ventricular global and regional myocardial dynamics during follow-up studies and drug-induced interventions. Once calibrated by means of a postoperative ventriculogram, volumes and derived parameters can be obtained in absolute terms and no further heart catheterization or application of contrast material is required.

References

1. Brower RW, ten Katen HJ, Meesters GT (1978) Direct method for determining regional myocardial shortening after bypass surgery from radiopaque markers in man. Am J Cardiol 41:1222
2. Hetzer R, Heim K, Borst HG, Amende I, Sigwart U (1976) Cineradiographical studies of local ventricular motility before and after aorto-coronary bypass. Thoraxchir 24:296
3. Ingels NB, Daughters GT, Stinson EB, Alderman EL (1975) Measurement of midwall myocardial dynamics in intact man by radiography of surgically implanted markers. Circulation 52:859
4. Ingels NB, Daughters GT, Stinson EB, Alderman EL (1980) Evaluation of methods for quantitating left ventricular segmental wall motion in man using myocardial markers as a standard. Circulation 61:966
5. Serruys PW, Brower RW, ten Katen HJ, Bom AH, Hugenholtz PG (1981) Regional wall motion from radiopaque markers after intravenous and intracoronary injections of nifedipine. Circulation 63:584
6. Vine DL, Dodge HT, Frimer M, Stewart DK, Caldwell J (1976) Quantitative measurement of left ventricular volumes in man from radiopaque epicardial markers. Circulation 54:391
7. Wildenthal K, Mitchel JH (1969) Dimensional analysis of the left ventricle in unanesthetized dogs. J Appl Physiol 27:115

Pulmonary Angiography: Recent Advances in Technique, Indications, and Methods of Interpretation

J. S. Alpert[1] and J. E. Dalen[2]

[1] Division of Cardiovascular Medicine, University of Massachusetts Medical School, Worcester, Massachusetts, USA
[2] Department of Medicine, University of Massachusetts Medical School, Worcester, Massachusetts, USA

Introduction

Pulmonary angiography has become a routine procedure in most hospitals as part of the evaluation of patients for pulmonary embolism [1–3]. Although radiologic examination of the pulmonary vascular tree has been performed since the middle of the 1930s, pulmonary angiography has only been a routine diagnostic procedure for the last 15 years. Pulmonary embolism is an elusive diagnostic entity in which clinical acumen may result in a correct diagnosis in as few as 50% of cases. The advent of routinely available pulmonary angiography has considerably improved the accuracy of diagnosis for this disease. In recent years, pulmonary angiography has been performed as part of the diagnostic evaluation of patients with a variety of other pulmonary and cardiovascular conditions. Moreover, a number of new techniques have improved and expanded the information obtained from the pulmonary angiogram.

Pulmonary angiography is a low-risk procedure which can be performed in a reasonably short period of time. Right heart catheterization is performed simultaneously with pulmonary angiography in order to obtain important physiologic information concerning the response of the heart and pulmonary vasculature to the embolic insult or other pathologic condition.

The earliest pulmonary angiograms were performed following injection of contrast medium into the inferior vena cava. Since the early 1960s, however, selective pulmonary angiography, with injection of contrast medium directly into the pulmonary vascular tree, is performed exclusively [1–6]. Earlier angiographic studies were filmed with large size cut film in the anteroposterior projection. During the last 10 years other film modalities (105 mm "spot" films, 35-mm cineangiography) and projections (oblique, lateral, and angulated views) have been used to supplement the standard anteroposterior view [7–11]. This review will examine the changes that have evolved in the technique, diagnostic criteria, complication rate, and frequency of use of pulmonary angiography in the last 18 years, during which time period we have utilized this procedure routinely in the diagnostic evaluation of patients with suspected pulmonary embolism.

Indications

Because of the vagaries of the clinical diagnosis of pulmonary embolism, particularly in patients with preexisting heart and/or lung disease, it is often appropriate to perform pulmonary angiography to confirm or deny the clinical diagnosis of pulmonary embolism [1–3]. However, in recent years, the advent of increasingly accurate nuclear medical diagnostic procedures such as ventilation/perfusion lung scanning, taken together with increased knowledge of the clinical presentation and natural history of pulmonary embolism, has reduced the need to perform pulmonary angiography in these patients [12–13]. Often, the diagnosis can be confirmed or denied on the basis of clinical information combined with analysis of arterial blood gases, chest X-ray, electrocardiogram, and most importantly, ventilation/perfusion lung scanning [6, 12, 13]. In addition, tests of venous patency have also been shown to increase the accuracy of the noninvasive work-up of patients suspected of having pulmonary embolism. If there is still any question in the mind of the clinician concerning the diagnosis of pulmonary embolism at the conclusion of the noninvasive evaluation, then pulmonary angiography should be performed, since the risk of this procedure (even in critically ill patients) is far less than the risk of therapy (anticoagulation, fibrinolysis, embolectomy, venous interruption) for pulmonary embolism. Moreover, a sizeable percentage of such patients have angiograms which are negative for pulmonary embolism; the angiogram has spared such individuals the risks of therapy.

Because of the remarkable increase in quality and accuracy of pulmonary ventilation/perfusion scintigraphy and noninvasive tests of venous thrombosis, the number of pulmonary angiograms performed has declined markedly during the last 5–7 years (Table 1). During the period 1964–1973, when pulmonary angiography was considered essential in the diagnostic work-up of patients with suspected pulmonary embolism, we performed 544 angiograms. During the most recent period (1976–1981), only 69 angiograms were carried out. This represents an 80% decrease in the number of angiograms per year: 54.5 angiograms/year during 1964–1972; 11.5 angiograms/year during 1976–1981.

During the period 1964–1973, pulmonary angiography was performed almost exclusively in patients with suspected pulmonary embolism. During the period 1976–1981, suspicion of pulmonary embolism was still the commonest indication for pulmonary angiography. However, patients with a variety of other pulmonary and cardiovascular diseases were evaluated by pulmonary angiography [14, 15]. Individuals with suspected primary pulmonary hypertension were studied to be sure that chronic, unresolved pulmonary embolism was not the cause of their severe pulmonary hypertension. Patients with congenital heart disease and marked pulmonary hypertension had angiographic evaluation of the severity of anatomical changes in the pulmonary vascular bed. Individuals with pulmonary arteriovenous malformations, bullous emphysema, and pulmonary neoplasms were evaluated by pulmonary angiography before surgical resection of the lesion. The current indications for pulmonary angiography are:

1. Suspected pulmonary embolism
2. ?Primary pulmonary hypertension; unresolved, chronic pulmonary embolism (subselective injections) ruled out
3. Evaluation of anatomical changes in pulmonary vasculature in patients with congenital heart disease and marked pulmonary hypertension
4. Presurgical evaluation of anatomy in patients with arteriovenous malformation, bullous emphysema, and malignant neoplasms of the lung

Techniques

Catheterization techniques employed for pulmonary angiography have developed during the last 20 years. During the period 1964–1973, almost all studies were performed in the anteroposterior supine position with injection of contrast medium (usually 60 cc) into the main pulmonary artery [1–3]. All of these angiograms were recorded on large (14 × 14 in.), cut film with the aid of an automatic film changer. In contrast, most studies obtained during the period 1976–1981 were selective views frequently recorded in rotated (RAO, LAO, lateral) or angulated positions [8]. The location of the catheter and the view obtained was guided by the location of defects on the pulmonary scintigram and by frequent small test injections of contrast medium recorded on videotape for review. Most studies were recorded on 35-mm cineangiographic film rather than on large, cut film. Occasional studies were performed using 105-mm "spot" films taken at short (0.5-s) intervals. It is our feeling that cineangiographic studies often enable us to identify intraluminal filling defects more readily than can be done with large, cut-film angiograms [7, 9]. Similar observations have recently been reported for angiographic studies of patients with dissection of the aorta, in whom the intimal flap is more easily identified with cineangiography than with cut-film studies. Younger patients with high cardiac output, however, may be best studied with mainstream contrast medium injection and large, cut film. Finally, selective angiographic studies can be performed with a smaller amount of contrast medium (generally about 30 cc) than is necessary for mainstream pulmonary arterial injections. Thus, two views can be obtained with the same amount of contrast medium as would have been required for one mainstream injection.

Our current protocol for pulmonary angiography consists of a venous cutdown on the right arm with right heart catheterization performed by means of a 7F or 8F Eppendorf (USCI, Billerica, Massachusetts) catheter. Occasional studies are performed from the right groin with injection of contrast medium into the right femoral vein through the sheath before introduction of the catheter to be sure that the vein is not filled with thrombus. Right heart pressures and oxygen saturations for measurement of cardiac output are recorded before angiography. Intraarterial pressure is obtained only if the patient is felt to be hemodynamically compromised by pulmonary embolism or preexisting heart disease. The angiographic catheter is then positioned in that pulmonary lobar artery which is felt to be supplying a region of lung parenchyma that demonstrates abnormal perfusion on the pulmonary scintigram. Test injections of contrast medium are performed and recorded on videotape for immediate review. Three-quarters of our angiographic studies are then recorded on 35-mm cineangiographic film; 10%–15% are recorded on large, cut film; and approximately 10% of studies are recorded using both film modalities. All films are developed and reviewed before the catheter is removed. Repeat studies or further films in other views are obtained as deemed necessary.

Complications

Complications were reported in 4% of patients undergoing pulmonary angiography during the period 1964–1973 and in 3% of patients during the period 1976–1981 (Table 1). Minor complications included pyrogen reactions, self-limited arrhythmias, transient bronchospasm, and mild angioneurotic edema [1–3]. These minor complications were not observed during 1976–1981: disposable catheters eliminated pyrogenic reactions, improved contrast medium formulations, and eliminated bronchospasm and allergic reactions; further increase in technical expertise and experience with pulmonary angiography avoided the precipitation of arrhythmias. Cardiac perforation was the only serious complication observed during 1976–1981. Both of these perforations occurred during catheter manipulation in the right ventricle following introduction of the catheter into the right femoral vein. It is more difficult to place a catheter in the pulmonary artery using the groin approach than with an arm approach; this may have contributed to the two cardiac perforations observed during 1976–1981, since the arm approach was used exclusively during 1964–1973. Pyrogen reactions accounted for one-third of all complications during 1964–1973 [1–3]. As noted earlier, pyrogen reactions no longer occur when disposable catheters are employed. Two patients died as a result of complications of pulmonary angiography during 1964–1973. No deaths occurred from pulmonary angiography during 1976–1981.

Diagnostic Criteria for Pulmonary Embolism

Only three findings are felt to be definitive for the diagnosis of pulmonary embolism using angiography: filling defects, tracking, and cut-offs (Table 2) [16, 17]. Intravascular filling defects are the most specific sign of pulmonary embolism on the angiogram. In some individuals, incompletely obstructing thrombus may not be detected on the angiogram because it is obscured in a particular view by contrast medium that flows around the clot. Other rotated or angulated views usually demonstrate the thrombus, often with contrast medium on both sides, so-called tracking. Pulmonary arterial cut-offs are observed if embolism completely obstructs a pulmonary artery. A more common finding, however, is an embolus straddling a bifurcation of a pulmonary artery with partial obstruction of the two branches. Occasionally, an artery is totally occluded at its origin and the resultant angiographic cut-off may be recognized only if it is noted that a

Table 1. Pulmonary angiography (1964–1981)

	1964–1973	1976–1981
Number of studies performed	544 (54.4/year)	69 (11.5/year)
Percentage of studies interpreted as normal	45%	68%
Percentage of studies interpreted as equivocal	14%	0%
Minor complication rate	31% (16 patients)	0%
Serious complication rate	1% (8 patients)	3% (2 patients)
Fatality rate	0.4% (2 patients)	0%

Table 2. Results of pulmonary angiography

Findings	Readings 1964–1973 (%)	Readings 1976–1981 (%)
Definite embolism	41	32
Equivocal for emboli	14	0
Negative for embolism	45	68

specific artery is absent or a specific zone of pulmonary parenchyma is hypovascular. During the period 1964–1973, two findings on the pulmonary angiogram were said to be suggestive of pulmonary embolism: areas of oligemia and asymmetry of flow. With the advent of rotated and angulated views, we now feel that filling defects or cut-offs can be demonstrated in virtually all patients with pulmonary embolism. Consequently, areas of oligemia and asymmetry of flow on the pulmonary angiogram are no longer interpreted as suggestive of pulmonary embolism. The findings of oligemia or asymmetry of flow on the pulmonary angiogram led to an equivocal diagnosis of pulmonary embolism in 14% of pulmonary angiograms performed during 1964–1973. With the increased use of special views during angiography during 1976–1981, equivocal readings were eliminated.

Correlation of Pulmonary Angiography with Pathological Findings and Hemodynamic Measurements

Validation of the pulmonary angiographic diagnosis of pulmonary embolism requires comparison of the radiographic diagnosis with operative or pathological material. This validity has been demonstrated both experimentally and clinically [1–6]. Angiography has been repeatedly shown to demonstrate accurately the presence of thrombus in the pulmonary vascular bed. False positive and false negative diagnosis of pulmonary embolism by pulmonary angiography is exceedingly rare. Comparison of the extent of embolic occlusion is estimated from the pulmonary angiogram, while hemodynamic measurements made at that time have demonstrated several aspects of the pathophysiology of pulmonary embolism. First, mean pulmonary arterial pressure correlates with the extent of pulmonary angiographic obstruction as estimated from the angiogram [18–20]. Thus, increasingly severe pulmonary hypertension is associated with progressively more severe obstruction of the pulmonary vascular bed by thrombus. Secondly, pulmonary arterial systolic pressures in excess of 50 mmHg are often associated with the development of right ventricular failure (right atrial pressure in excess of 7 mmHg; cardiac index less than 2.5 l/min/m^2) [19, 20]. Finally, estimates of pulmonary blood volume reveal that this variable decreases progressively with increasingly severe pulmonary embolism judged angiographically (J. S. Alpert, unpublished observations).

Conclusions

Pulmonary angiography is a useful and safe diagnostic procedure that can be employed in the evaluation of patients with suspected pulmonary embolism as well as a variety of other cardiovascular and pulmonary disorders. Recent advances have increased the accuracy of pulmonary angiography while decreasing the risk associated with this procedure. The last 20 years have witnessed widespread dissemination of this procedure.

References

1. Alpert JS, Dalen JE (1974) Pulmonary angiography in the diagnosis of pulmonary embolism. Int Med Digest 9:17
2. Dalen JE (1970) Pulmonary angiography in pulmonary embolism. Bull Physio-Path Resp 6:45
3. Dalen JE, Brooks HL, Johnson LW, Meister SG, Szucs MM Jr, Dexter L (1971) Pulmonary angiography in acute pulmonary embolism: indications, techniques, and results in 367 patients. Am Heart J 81:175
4. Dalen JE, Mathur VS, Evans H, Haynes FW, Pur-Shahriari AA, Stein PD, Dexter L (1966) Pulmonary angiography in experimental pulmonary embolism. Am Heart J 72:509
5. Mathur VS, Dalen JE, Evans H, Haynes FW, Pur-Shahriari AA, Stein PD, Dexter L (1967) Pulmonary angiography one to seven days after experimental pulmonary embolism. Invest Radiol 2:304
6. Stein PD, Willis PW, Dalen JE (1979) Importance of clinical assessment in selecting patients for pulmonary arteriography. Am J Cardiol 43:669
7. Meister SG, Brooks HL, Szucs MM, Banas JS Jr, Dexter L, Dalen JE (1972) Pulmonary cineangiography in acute pulmonary embolism. Am Heart J 84:33
8. Kattan KR (1970) Angled view in pulmonary angiography. A new roentgen approach. Radiology 94:79
9. Raphael MJ, Steiner RE (1966) Selective cine-fluoroscopic studies of pulmonary circulatory disorders. Br Heart J 28:523
10. Orta DA Jr, Eisen S, Yergin BM, Olsen GN (1979) Segmental pulmonary angiography in the critically ill patient using a flow-directed catheter. Chest 76:269
11. Dougherty JE, LaSala AF, Fieldman A (1980) Bedside pulmonary angiography utilizing existing Swan-Ganz catheter. Chest 77:43

12. Bell WR, Simon TL (1976) A comparative analysis of pulmonary perfusion scans with pulmonary angiograms. From a national cooperative study. Am Heart J 92:700
13. Moses DC, Silver TM, Bookstein JJ (1974) The complimentary roles of chest radiography, lung scanning, and selective pulmonary angiography in the diagnosis of pulmonary embolism. Circulation 49:179
14. Tsuiki K, Miyazaws K, Ishikawa K, Matsunaga A, Haneda T, Katori R, Nakamura T (1971) Correlation of magnifying pulmonary wedge angiogram and pulmonary hemodynamics. Am Rev Resp Dis 104:899
15. Greenough WG (1972) Role of pulmonary angiography in carcinoma of the lung. Chest 62:206
16. Lowman RM, Reardon J, Hipona FA, Stern H, Toole AL (1967) The role of pulmonary angiography in pulmonary embolism. Angiology 18:291
17. Stein PD, O'Connor JF, Dalen JE, Pur-Shahriari AA, Hoppin FG Jr, Hammond DT, Haynes FW, Fleischner FG, Dexter L (1967) The angiographic diagnosis of acute pulmonary embolism: evaluation of criteria. Am Heart J 73:730
18. Alpert JS, Godtfredsen J, Ockene IS, Anas J, Dalen JE (1978) Pulmonary hypertension secondary to minor pulmonary embolism. Chest 73:795
19. Sasahara AA (1967) Pulmonary vascular responses to thromboembolism. Mod Concepts Cardiovasc Dis 36:55
20. McIntyre KM, Sasahara AA (1974) Hemodynamic and ventricular response to pulmonary embolism. Prog Cardiovasc Dis 17:175

Computer-Generated Index of the Severity of Coronary Disease

R. Balcon, M. Cattell, and K. Wong

The London Chest Hospital, Bonner Road, London E2 9 JX, UK

The coronary artery tree is classically divided into three vessel systems and patients are categorised according to lesions involving 50% or more reduction of lumen diameter in the branches of these systems – thus, heart patients are described as having one-, two- or three-vessel disease. There are, however, a number of major branches in the coronary circulation and it is, for instance, often possible to perform coronary bypass surgery on a number of terminal vessels in each of the coronary systems. Each of these individual vessels is important and has to be evaluated if the extent of disease is to be accurately described. Furthermore, the effects of multiple stenoses are probably more than additive, so attention to only the severest stenosis does not give an adequate representation of the reduction of myocardial blood flow, one of the critical factors in determining the symptoms of ischaemic heart disease. A second critical factor is the amount of myocardium prejudiced by stenosis, which must determine the outcome of sudden events such as infarction resulting from changes related to that stenosis. These factors are to a variable extent ameliorated by collateral blood flow. It is very important, therefore, to take all of them into account when assessing the coronary circulation.

Scoring Systems

Friesinger and his colleagues (1970) introduced a scoring system whereby each of the main coronary trunks was scored from 0 to 5, with 0 representing no disease, 5 total occlusion, and 2–4 increasing degrees of severity. These intervening scores represented a combination of the diffuseness and severity of the disease. The maximum total score possible was 15. They showed that in a follow up of up to 7 years, survival was related to the coronary score. This type of scoring system has been used by many authors for the purposes of one particular study to help categorise the patients according to the severity of their coronary disease. No other examples of the use of a scoring system for long-term evaluations could be found, apart from the classical studies using the one-, two- and three-vessel disease classifications (Bruschke et al. 1973). More complex systems for recording coronary angiographic data have been published by Austen et al. (1975) and Brandt et al. (1977), but as yet, these data have not been analysed in terms of correlations with prognosis.

A scoring system has been designed which takes into account the site and severity of all lesions in the coronary circulation (Balcon 1980). In addition, it adds weight to lesions that occur in series in any vessel or vessel system and scores vessels that are normal. Each lesion is graded from 1 to 4, 4 being total occlusion. Grade 1 is stenosis of less than 50%, grade 2 is 51%–75%, and grade 3 is 76%–99%. The coronary circulation is coded for 13 branches, the left main stem and three main trunks, right, anterior descending, and circumflex. Nine possible terminal branches are described, three inferior left ventricular branches from the right coronary artery, three circumflex branches, the diagonal, and the anterior descending before and after its major septal branch. Not all branches are identified in all patients. The index is mathematically computed by weighting each arterial lesion according to its severity with weights increasing by 25% for each stenosis grade. Lesions in parallel are then added and lesions in series multiplied. The right and left coronary artery systems start with a numerical score of 1 which is then reduced by the lesions as described. The average of the two final figures for right and left systems is expressed as a percentage. High percentage scores represent minor disease and low scores severe disease. The angiographic data from which these scores are derived are recorded on computer mark-sense cards, together with clinical and follow-up data. Information is available on more than 4000 patients followed for up to 11 years.

It is well recognised that in individual cases there may be a poor correlation between the angiographically judged severity of disease and clinical variables. There is, however, an overall correlation in large groups of patients that may be helpful and provide general management guidelines.

Angina end point and marked ST-segment depression during exercise testing, for instance, have been shown to indicate severe disease (Ellestad et al. 1979). This correlation holds for the coronary index. It is known for example, that angina or ST depression of at least 2 mm terminate the test in 62% of patients with an index of below 25, compared with 27% for patients with indices between 51 and 99. Interestingly enough, these end points also terminated the test in 14% of patients with normal coronary arteries. There is also a general correlation between the index and maximum exercise levels. The patients whose maximum level was 450 kpm/min or less have a significantly ($P < 0.05$) lower index than the remainder. This general correlation holds good for the state of the left ventricle as judged by resting end-diastolic pressure or the number of abnormally contracting segments seen angiographically.

These correlations serve only as a form of validation of the index. The more important considerations relate to prognosis, since management of patients with ischaemic heart disease, especially with regard to surgical treatment, depends to a great extent on an accurate prognosis and how it is affected by surgery. Survival data depend on full mortality reporting. The mortality figures in this study are derived from indexing all patients with the Registrars General of Great Britain, to whom all deaths must be reported, so that they are 100% for all deaths that occur there. Noncardiac deaths are excluded if it is possible to make a decision from the death certificate.

The value of the index as a predictor was tested in a pilot study of 205 patients all receiving medical therapy and all followed for at least 3 years or until death.

Survival curves emphasise the importance of the site of lesions. The worst prognosis is for patients with left main stem lesions (1st generation), then for patients with main trunk lesions (2nd generation), and finally for distal disease only (3rd generation). Lesions of 50% or more were required to enter these categories. Patients with minor lesions, wherever sited, had a better prognosis

The curves for our 205 patients were redrawn according to quartiles of the coronary index. The separation is as expected, with the greatest difference between first and second quartiles. The former had a prognosis similar to that for left main stem stenosis, but was a larger group of patients. It seemed, therefore, that the index was helpful at least in defining more patients at high risk who might therefore be considered for prophylactic surgery.

The following 5-year survival data concerns 1512 patients treated medically. There were 178 deaths in this time (11.8%). Survival curves can be calculated in two different ways. On the one hand, patients are divided according to the presence of stenoses of at least 50% in one, two, or all three of the main trunks. On the other hand curves can also be shown for patients with lesions in distal branches only and those with left main stem stenosis. The curves are significantly ($P < 0.01$) different from each other (Wilcoxon rank sum test). Curves of survival rates for the patients grouped according to their coronary index can be divided into quartiles for convenience. Both sets of curves show similar trends. The left ventricle has been scored from the right oblique ventriculogram. The anterior, apical and inferior walls are considered to contract normally or to be hypokinetic, akinetic or dyskinetic. The average number of abnormally contracting segments in each subgroup of patients is important. The number increases significantly with increasing severity of disease except for the left main stem group, which is not worse than the three-vessel disease group. This also applies for subgroups of coronary index. The effect of the left ventricular abnormality seems, at least to a certain extent, to be contained in coronary angiographic data, although an additional independent effect cannot be excluded. These two types of curves contain different information. The distribution of patients relates to the number of vessels diseased within the coronary index quartiles. Patients with three-vessel disease, for instance, appear in the first three quartiles. An attempt has therefore been made to combine the information available from the different types of data. An analysis for patients with proximal (main trunk) three-vessel disease shows that of these patients, 98% had indices below 50%. The left panel compares survival curves of the first and second coronary index quartiles within the three-vessel disease group. The patients with the higher indices have a significantly better survival rate than the whole group and those with the lower indices a survival rate which is significantly worse. This division by coronary index level also produces a significant difference in left ventricular score, again suggesting that the effect on mortality due to the left ventricle is not entirely separate. It might be argued that the low coronary index group included more severe proximal lesions which wholly accounted for the lower score, and that the presence of other lesions played no part in the increased mortality. The same separation exists, but at even lower survival levels. Left ventricular abnormality follows as before. The best survival for a three-vessel disease subgroup is 71% and the worst 26%, a difference of

45% for patients who are usually classified in one group. Similar information can be gained for single- and double-vessel disease, respectively. A similar separation exists for single-vessel disease, with one group with a high index and a better prognosis and one with a low index with a worse survival than the whole group with double-vessel disease. The best subgroup had a 93% 5-year survival and the worst 61%, a difference of 32%. The left ventricle again follows. The patients with double-vessel disease are rather surprising in that they appear to be more homogeneous than the others. It was however, possible to select a small subgroup with a significantly better prognosis by examining further subdivisions of the coronary index.

These data confirm that all of the following are important factors to take into account when assessing survival from angiographic data:

1. Proximal site of the lesion
2. Severity of stenosis – an arbitrary division at 50% is not adequate
3. Presence of multiple lesions in distal coronary branches
4. Degree of left ventricular damage – ?independent variable

It may seem that the above is nothing more than a statement of the obvious; however, there is considerable controversy concerning angiographically judged prognosis. Single lesions in the left anterior descending coronary artery, for instance, are considered benign by some, and to be "widow makers" by others. Equally, the controversy that exists concerning the prophylactic effect of coronary bypass surgery may be merely a function of inadequate classification of patients. It is not thought to be necessary to use a relatively complicated computer-generated index, as discussed here to evaluate angiograms, but these data emphasise the need to take into account all of the known adverse angiographic factors, particularly when comparing groups of patients.

References

Austen WG, Edwards JE, Frye RL, Gensini GG, Gott VL, Griffith LSC, McGoon DC, Murphy ML, Roe BB (1975) A reporting system on patients evaluated for coronary artery disease. Report of the ad hoc committee for grading coronary artery disease, council on cardiovascular surgery. Circulation 51:4

Balcon R (1980) Prognostic significance of coronary arteriography. Acta Med Port [Suppl] 1:9

Brandt PWT, Partridge JB, Wattie JW (1977) Coronary arteriography; method of presentation of the arteriogram report and a scoring system. Clin Radiol 28:361

Bruschke AVG, Proudfit WL, Sones FM (1973) Progress study of 590 consecutive nonsurgical cases of coronary disease followed 5–9 years. Arteriographic correlations. Circulation 47:1147

Ellestad MH, Cooke BM, Greenberg PS (1979) Stress testing: clinical application and predictive capacity. Prog Cardiovasc Dis 21:431

Friesinger GC, Page EE, Ross RS (1970) Prognostic significance of coronary arteriography. Trans Assoc Am Physicians 83:78

Comparison of Stenosis as Obtained Using Coronary Angiography and Postmortem Coronary Measurements

H. FREUDENBERG and P. R. LICHTLEN

Medizinische Hochschule, Hannover, Karl-Wiechert-Allee 9, D-3000 Hannover 61, FRG

There is no question that at present coronary angiography is the only method which allows detailed presentation of the coronary anatomy.

To examine its sensitivity with regard to detection of sclerotic alterations in the wall of the large coronary arteries, we compared the degree of stenosis as estimated from the coronary angiogram with measurements in the histologic cross sections of the arteries. Similar investigations on this point have as yet been published only in limited number [1–8]. We tried to find answers to the following questions:

1. How often and to what degree is coronary sclerosis unrecognized, underestimated, or correctly estimated from the angiogram?
2. What can be quantified from the angiogram?

Materials

In 87 cases with valve replacement, bypass operation, coronary heart disease, cardiomyopathy, and nonoperable valve disease, collected between 1975 and 1981, the coronary angiograms could be compared with the complete histological cross sections of the large coronary arteries at 5-mm intervals obtained after pressure injection of the arteries to prevent postmortem collapse of the vessel wall as a precondition for planimetric measurements in histology. Additionally, postmortem coronary angiograms (CA) from different projections were performed in order to recognize new angiographic alterations – possibly developed during the interval between intravital and postmortal angiography, an interval that ranged from 10 days to 2 years (5 months on average) – and to complete missing intravital projections. The results were as follows: group I, normal CA, normal histology (H) (18%; $n = 16$); group II, normal CA, at H stenoses up to 60% (33%; $n = 29$); group III, stenoses in CA underestimated (28%; $n = 25$); group IV, stenoses in CA estimated as in H (19%; $n = 17$).

The term "up to 60%" should not be misunderstood. There were some cases up to 60%, but it was about 30% on average.

The same results may be written in another way. Compared with H the sclerotic alterations were 38% judged correctly in the CA (I + IV, $n = 33$); 28% underestimated (III), and 33% not detected (II) in the CA.

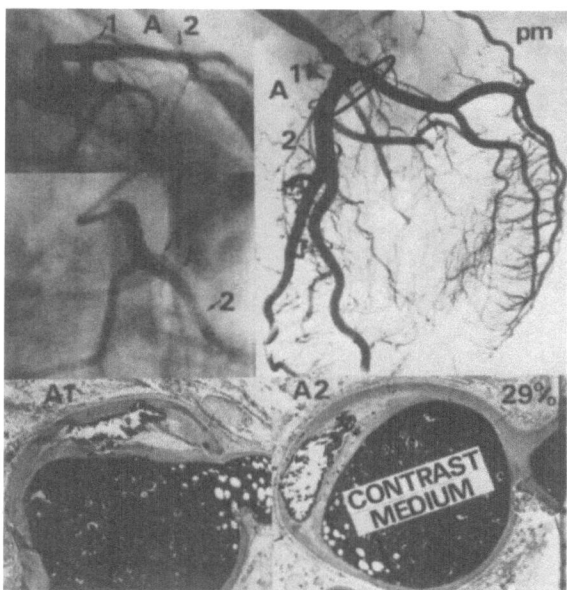

Fig. 1. Angiographically normal LAD in the intravital (*left*) and postmortal (*right*) coronary angiograms

Histologic degree of stenosis up to 60% by areas is compatible with a "normal coronary angiogram" (I + II).

It is necessary for better understanding of these results to demonstrate one example of each group. It also seems necessary to remind the reader that the coronary angiogram delineates the vessel lumen primarily and that all descriptions of wall alterations are made indirectly.

Figure 1 presents an angiographically normal LAD in the intravital (left) and postmortal (right) coronary angiograms. The histologic cross sections from points 1 and 2 show some degree of sclerosis up to 29% by areas, already with calcification, that could not be detected in the angiograms (group II).

Figure 2 demonstrates a right coronary artery from group III. Some degree of sclerosis can be detected from the angiograms, especially at 4 and 5, but it was underestimated when compared with the histology which shows a more diffuse sclerosis of up to 50% by areas. It is not quite clear whether sclerosis led to narrowing of the lumen, to dilatation of the whole cross section, or to both. Besides, some degree of sclerosis will be missed when the artery is cut in the longitudinal way, as is normally done. The cross section after pressure injection demonstrates the degree of sclerosis quite clearly.

Finally, Fig. 3 shows a case that may be representative for group IV: an angiographically isolated stenosis of the LAD that can be detected quite well. Nevertheless, different cardiologists gave different answers to the questions: What is the degree of this stenosis, and Is it an eccentric or a concentric one? The histologic cross sections show an eccentric stenosis up to 75% in number 2, with a narrowing of 40% already in the earliest proximal part of the LAD and even with some degree of sclerosis in the left main artery, that could not be detected from the angiogram.

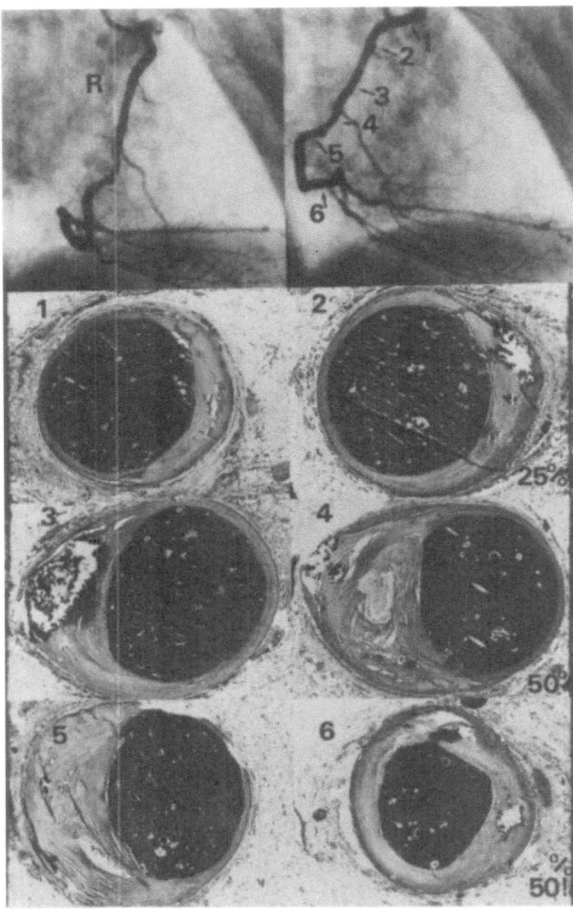

Fig. 2. A right coronary artery from group III

In our material we have clearly seen the development of sclerosis – beginning more focally, distributing around the cross section, and at the same time proximally and distally. Especially in high degree stenoses of the proximal LAD – with more than 70% – the sclerotic process was never isolated but extended to more than three histologic segments, which means to more than 15 mm. Normally not only the proximal LAD but also the left main artery was involved to some degree. That means that even in angiographically isolated stenoses, the sclerotic process is already more diffuse than can be detected from the angiogram.

When estimating or quantifying the degree of stenosis, the diameter or cross-sectional area of stenosis should be compared with that of a nearby prestenotic region which seems to be without sclerotic alterations. This precondition is seldom fulfilled in the high-degree proximal stenoses of our material.

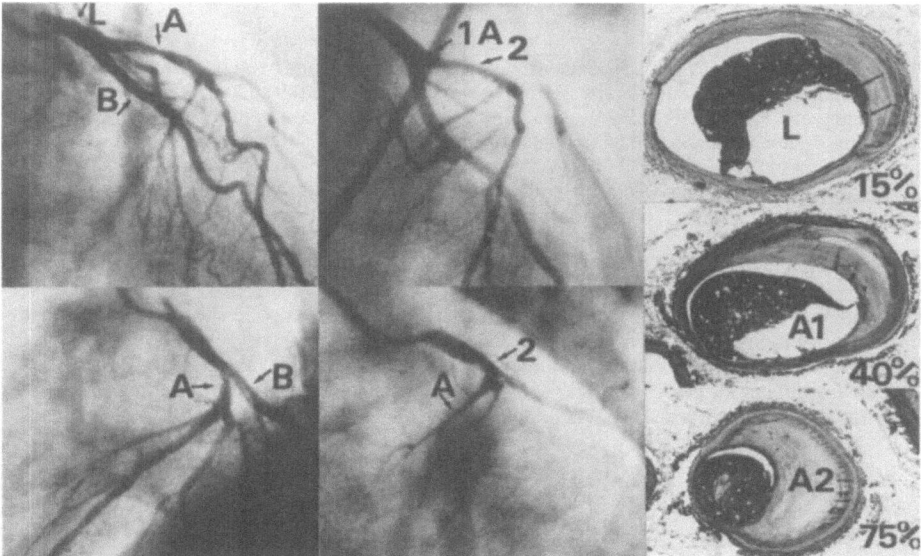

Fig. 3. A case representative of group IV, including an angiographically isolated stenosis of the LAD

Conclusions

With regard to this comparison between intravital angiography and postmortem histology, the following conclusions about the limitations of coronary angiography can be drawn:
1. Diffuse thickening of the intima is often recognized only in a late stage, especially when the lumen is of a round and regular shape.
2. Short narrowings in the region of the ostia and of branching of the arteries, as well as in the proximal LAD, are often underestimated due to the fact that natural reduction of diameter in these locations is overlapped by coronary disease.
3. Significant obstructions (more than 75%) of major coronary branches, typical for bypass surgery, are usually well recognized. However, coronary disease in the poststenotic segment is often underestimated.
4. A "normal coronary angiogram" does not exclude histologically abnormal arteries.
5. One should always take into account that coronary angiography delineates only the vessel lumen and that all descriptions of wall alterations are made indirectly – especially when estimating or quantifying the degree of stenosis.

References

1. Arnett EN et al. (1979) Coronary artery narrowing in coronary heart disease: comparison of cineangiographic and necropsy findings. Ann Intern Med 91 (3):350
2. Barmeyer J et al. (1971) Morphologie und postmortales Angiogramm bei Koronarsklerose. Eine vergleichende Studie. Z Kreislaufforsch 60 (8):679–683
3. Eustermann JH et al. (1962) Artherosclerotic disease of the coronary arteries: a pathologic-radiologic correlative study. Circulation 26:1288
4. Grey CR et al. (1962) Correlation of arteriographic and pathologic findings in the coronary arteries in man. Circulation 26:494–499
5. Hutchins GM et al. (1977) Correlation of coronary arteriograms and left ventriculograms with postmortem studies. Circulation 56 (1):32–37
6. Vlodaver Z et al. (1973) Correlation of the antemortem coronary arteriogram and the postmortem specimen. Circulation 47:162
7. Stolte M (1975) Morphologische Analyse der Koronarchirurgie. Witzstrock, Baden-Baden
8. Schwartz JN et al. (1975) Comparison of angiographic and postmortem findings in patients with coronary artery disease. Am J Cardiol 36:174–178

Flashing Tomosynthesis – A New Tomographic Technique for Quantitative Coronary Angiography

H. Woelke,[1] P. Hanrath,[1] M. Schlüter,[1] W. Bleifeld,[1] E. Klotz,[3] H. Weiss,[3] D. Waller,[2] and J. von Weltzien[2]

[1] Department of Cardiology, University Hospital, Hamburg, FRG
[2] Department of Pathology, University Hospital, Hamburg, FRG
[3] Philips GmbH Forschungslaboratorium, Hamburg, FRG

Introduction

Cine coronary angiography is a standard technique widely used in clinical cardiology. Yet there have recently been several reports on alternative recording methods [1, 2] improving on some of the limitations of coronary angiography. In this paper we report on the evaluation of coronary artery stenoses with flashing tomosynthesis as a new tomographic technique, first applied to neuroradiological problems [8, 9].

Principles of Flashing Tomosynthesis

The procedure consists of a recording and a reconstruction step.

In the recording step (Fig. 1), the three-dimensional object is recorded on a large-size film (60×60 cm) by means of 24 stationary X-ray tubes (Fig. 2). During exposure all X-ray tubes are fired simultaneously. Exposure time is about 50 ms.

The X-ray image thus produced is decoded in a subsequent image processing step (Fig. 3). The coded image is placed in front of a lightbox and imaged 24 times by an array of lenses mounted according to the distribution of the X-ray tubes. Because of this multiprojection, a real three-dimensional image of the object is reconstructed. If a screen is now inserted in any arbitrary position within the reconstruction volume, the corresponding tomographic layer is isolated from the object. This offers the possibility of continuously "going through the object."

Layer depth is about 1 mm. Due to the optical superposition of 24 single recordings, image contrast is considerably enhanced, and the reconstructed layer images are less "noisy" than single cine frames.

By proper choice of layer orientation an undistorted focused display of stenotic areas with no superposition of vessels is obtained. A special device (Fig. 4) then projects the reconstructed layers onto a TV monitor which can consequently be photographed.

More recent developments enable a true three-dimensional image reconstruction, apart from the two-dimensional display of tomographic layers (Fig. 5).

This can be achieved by oscillating the ground glass screen in the image region of interest at 25 Hz with an amplitude of 50 mm.

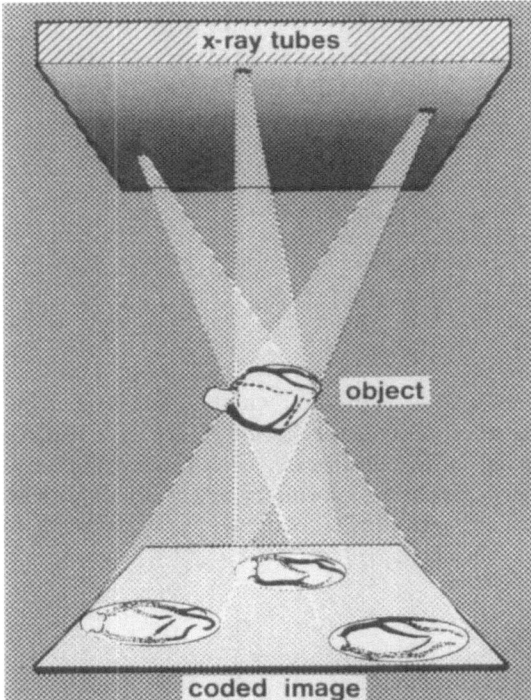

Fig. 1. Flashing tomosynthesis: principle of the recording step. An array of X-ray tubes projects the object onto different locations on the recording film. During exposure all X-ray tubes are fired simultaneously

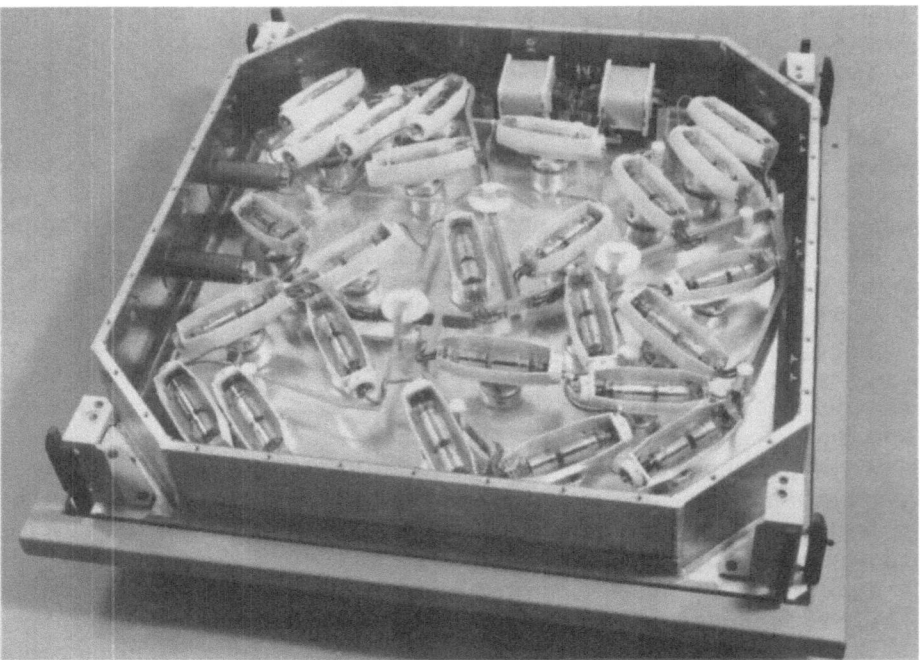

Fig. 2. Multiple X-ray source consisting of 24 small X-ray tubes

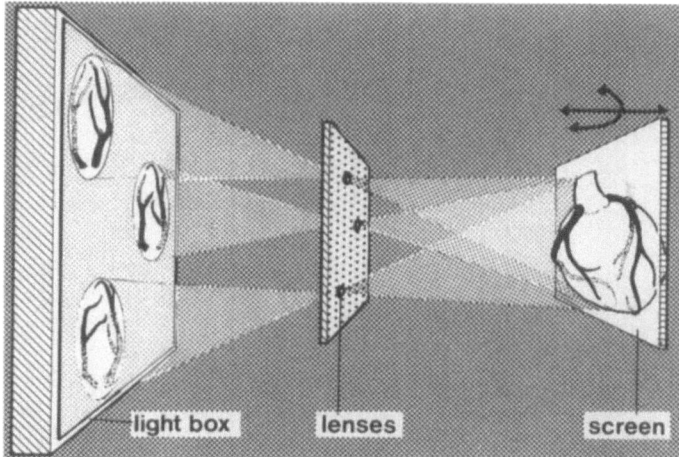

Fig. 3. Principle of optical decoding: a special array of lenses produces a truly three-dimensional image. By inserting a screen which can be shifted and tilted, complex object structures are isolated

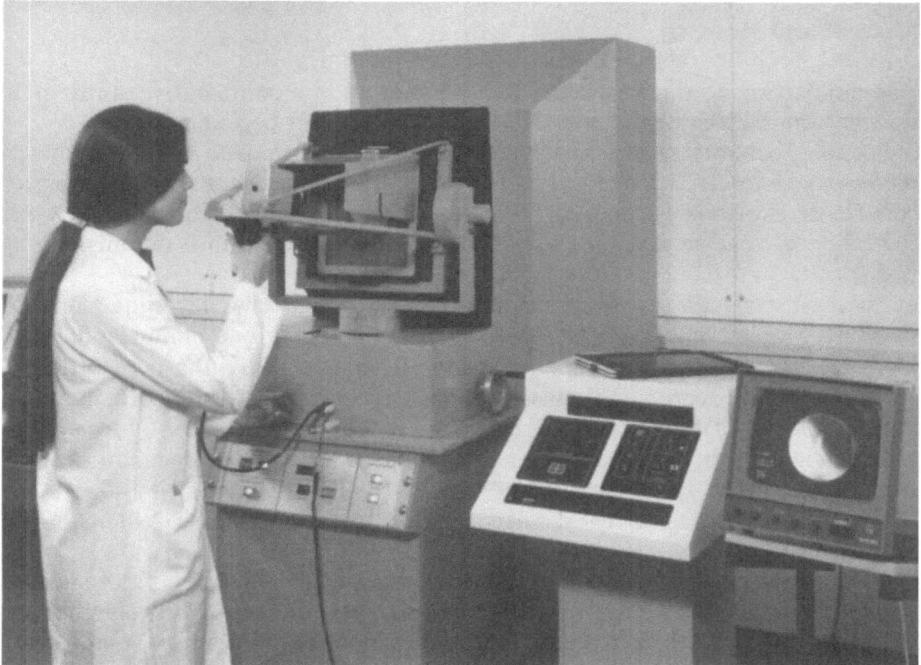

Fig. 4. The decoding hardware. The large apparatus on the *left-hand side* contains the optical postprocessing unit. The orientation of the ground-glass screen can be externally manipulated. Reconstructed image layers are electronically transfered to a TV monitor (*right-hand side*) and photographed using a special camera unit (*center*)

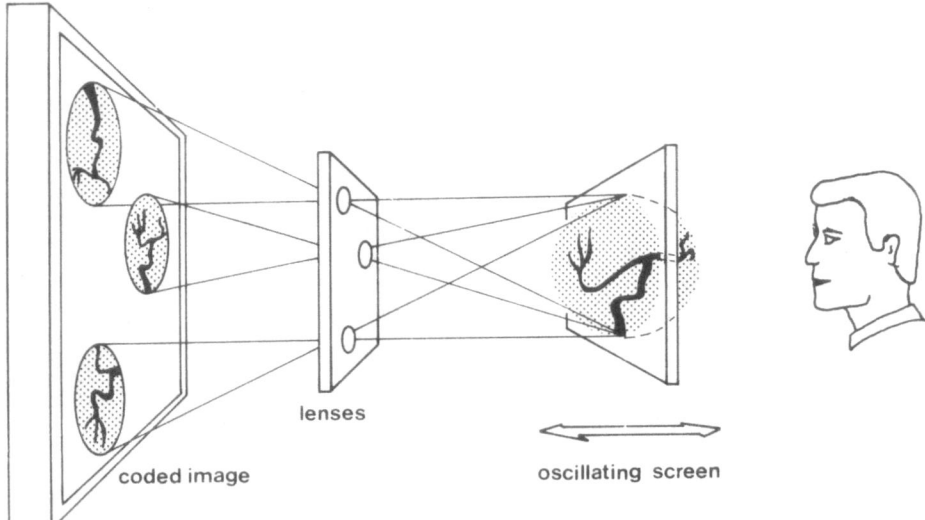

coded image

lenses

oscillating screen

Fig. 5. Principle of true three-dimensional image reconstruction. In the image region of interest, the ground glass screen is oscillating at 25 Hz with an amplitude of 50 mm

Material and Methods

The application of this new technique was tested in a comparative study of 10 postmortem human hearts with 20 stenoses of the left coronary artery.

For the postmortem examination the hearts were removed in toto. Contrast medium was injected into the left coronary artery by means of a special procedure, as previously reported [3–6]. In order to simulate the normal X-ray recording as realistically as possible the heart was placed in a dummy thorax (3-M).

Thereafter recordings were made with the 35-mm cine technique in four standard projections (RAO 30°, LAO 40°, caudocranial, and craniocaudal projection). The same set-up was used for the flashing tomosynthesis recording.

To obtain the degree of stenosis, the cine recordings and the corresponding tomographic images were analysed in a tenfold magnification. From these enlarged images the vessel diameters in the narrowest and the prestenotic region were obtained by two independent observers. The actual calculation of the degree of stenosis was carried out according to the formula for a circular stenotic area.

Of the four cine projections, the one showing the highest degree of stenosis was taken for further analysis. Morphometric measurements of the corresponding parts of the vessels were made on serial sections at intervals of 2 mm using a special video system [7].

Results

The comparative study of 20 left coronary artery stenoses in a total of 10 postmortem hearts resulted in a correlation coefficient of $r = 0.92$ between the stenotic degree obtained using flashing tomosynthesis and that obtained using morphometric measurement. On the other hand, stenotic degree determined by conventional cine technique correlated to a lesser extent with morphometry ($r = 0.82$; Fig. 6).

In Figs. 7 and 8, corresponding tomographic and cine recordings of the same postmortem heart are shown as an example. Figure 7a reveals 75% stenotic changes at the origin of the first diagonal branch of the left anterior descendens in the tomographic layer image. The degree of stenosis is not as clearly appreciated in the corresponding cine image of Fig. 7b (69%). The degree of stenosis of the left anterior descending artery shown on Fig. 8 was determined as 60% from the tomographic layer image (Fig. 8a) and as 52% from the cine image (Fig. 8b).

Based on these experiments, we recently used this technique in a first clinical trial on five patients with angiographically proven coronary artery disease. Figure 9a represents an ECG-triggered flashing tomogram of a patient with a coronary artery bypass on the first marginal branch of the left circumflex artery. Details in the stenotic area are much more clearly visualized than in the corresponding cine image of Fig. 9b.

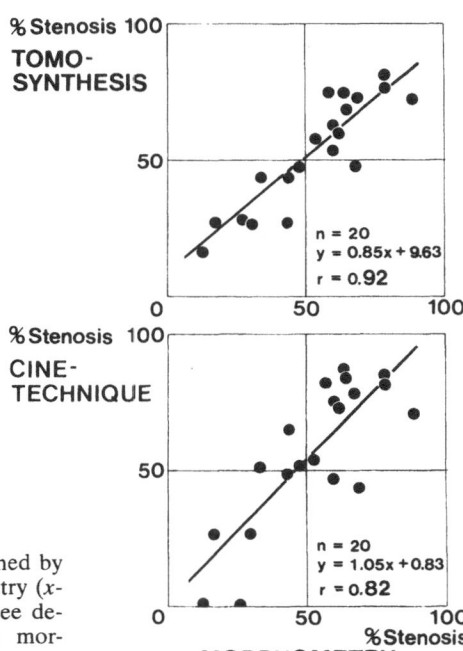

Fig. 6. *Upper panel*: stenotic degree determined by flashing tomosynthesis (*y*-axis) vs morphometry (*x*-axis); ($r = 0.92$). *Lower panel*: stenotic degree determined by cineangiography (*y*-axis) vs morphometry (*x*-axis); ($r = 0.82$)

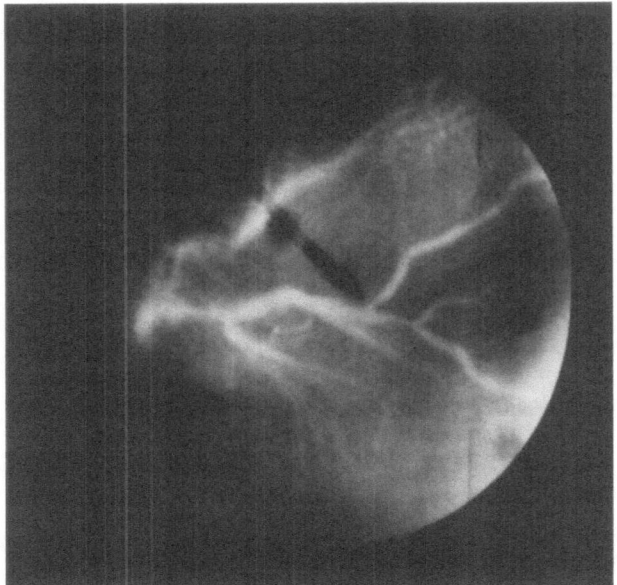

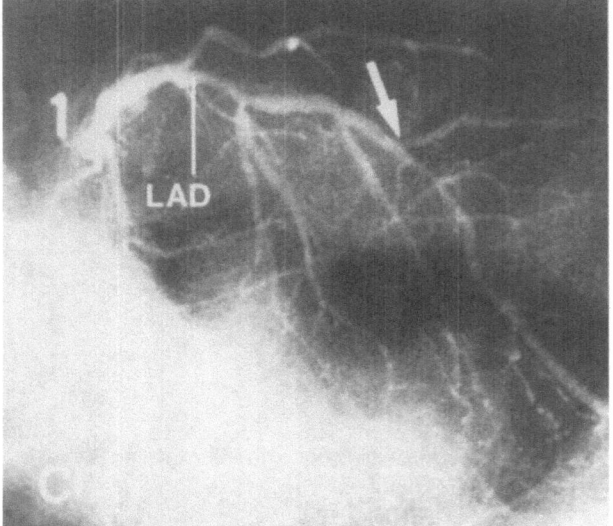

Fig. 7a, b. Comparative recordings of the first diagonal branch of the left anterior descendens (LAD) in a postmortem human heart. Stenotic degree obtained from the flashing tomogram (*a*) is 75%, whereas the craniocaudal cineangiogram (*b*) reveals only a 69% stenosis

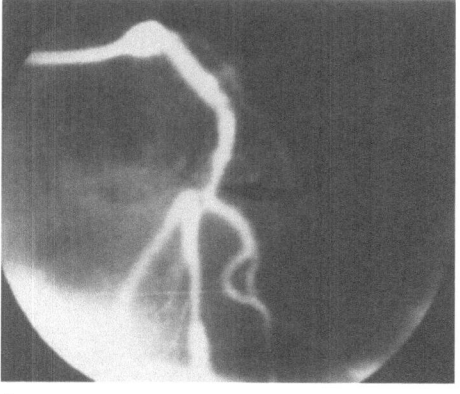

a

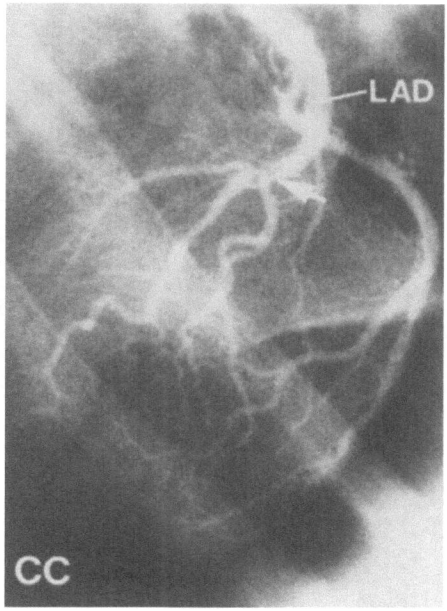

b

Fig. 8a, b. Comparative recordings of the left anterior descending coronary artery (LAD) in a postmortem human heart. Stenotic degree obtained from the flashing tomogram (*a*) is 60%. The same stenosis evaluated by cineangiography (*b*) revealed a degree of only 52%

Discussion

The main purpose of this paper was to report on the value of flashing tomosynthesis in the quantification of coronary artery stenoses in comparison with the standard techniques of cineangiography and morphometry. Taking morphometry as the reference, the present study revealed that flashing tomosynthesis allows a more accurate determination of stenotic degree than does cineangiography.

Several reasons for this can be given. Flashing tomosynthesis makes possible a distortion-free display of stenotic areas, disturbing superposition of different vessels is avoided, and image background noise is considerably reduced.

A major advantage of flashing tomosynthesis over cineangiography is the fact that the total three-dimensional information can be obtained in a single exposure. This is particularly important for in vivo examinations, since the amount of contrast agent is considerably reduced, as is the X-ray dose. Moreover, the time required for an investigation of the human coronary system is markedly shortened, thus reducing the risk for the patient.

At present there are still some limitations of this new technique. Dynamic blood flow behavior cannot be evaluated, although this is not important for the quantification of stenoses. Furthermore, the field of view is restricted to a circular area 9 cm in diameter.

Future developments will therefore comprise image processing techniques such as subtraction and automatic contour finding of vessels, as well as sequential ECG-triggered recording.

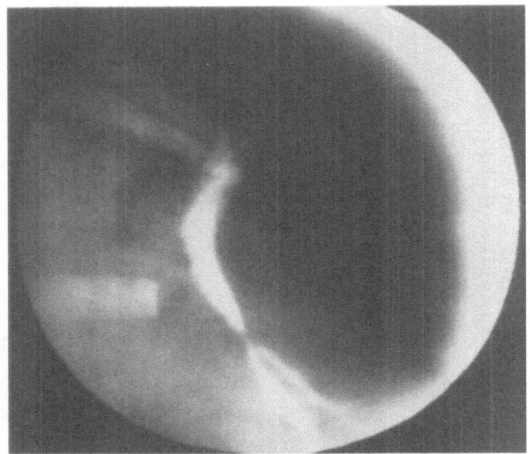

a

b

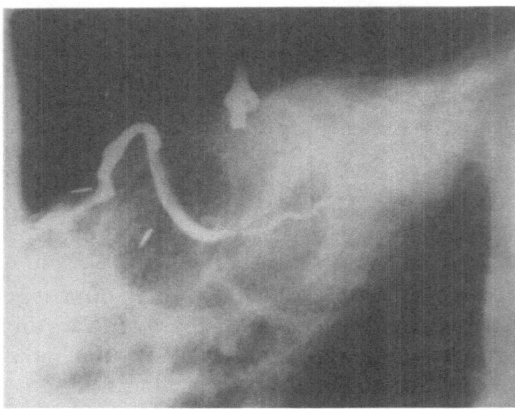

Fig. 9a, b. Comparative recordings of a 67-year-old patient with a coronary artery bypass on the first marginal branch of the left circumflex artery. *a* Flashing tomosynthesis recording. *b* Cine recording

References

1. Robb RA, Ritmann EL (1979) High speed synchronous volume computed tomography of the heart. Radiology 133:655–661
2. Haendle J, Sklebitz H (1981) Das elektrische Schichtbild. Röntgenpraxis 34:253–257
3. Schlesinger MJ (1938) An injection plus dissection study of coronary artery occlusion and anastomoses. Am Heart J 15:528
4. Gray CR, Hoffmann HA, Hammond WS et al. (1962) Correlation of arteriographic and pathologic findings in the coronary arteries in man. Circulation 26:494–499
5. Eusterman JH, Achor RWP, Kincaid OW et al. (1962) Atherosclerotic disease of the coronary arteries. A pathologic-radiologic correlative study. Circulation 26:1288–1295
6. Vlodaver Z, Frech R, van Tassel RA et al. (1973) Correlation of the antemortem coronary arteriogram and the postmortem specimen. Circulation 47:162–169
7. Kamm KF (1979) Angiographische Auswertungen mit einem Prozeßrechnersystem für das Herzkatheterlabor. Biomed Tech 24 [Suppl]:72–73
8. Nadjmi M, Weiss H, Klotz E, Linde R (1979) Kurzzeittomosynthese, erste klinische Erfahrungen. Röntgenstrahlen 42
9. Nadjmi M, Weiss H, Klotz E, Linde R (1980) Flashing tomosynthesis – a new tomographic method. Neuroradiology 19:113–117

Requirements for Coronary Probing and Intervention

U. Sigwart, A. Essinger, and M. Grbic

Centre Hospitalier Universitaire Vandois, 1011 Lausanne, Switzerland

The transluminal introduction of catheters into coronary arteries has become an important approach to the study and treatment of coronary artery disease.

Coronary catherization has the following uses:

1. Therapeutic
   - Transluminal angioplasty
   - Selective thrombolysis (reperfusion/venous retroperfusion?)
2. Diagnostic
   - Superselective angiography
   - Hemodynamic evaluation

Intracoronary catheters are used for superselective arteriography, hemodynamic measurements [1], administering vasoactive drugs, dissolving clots [2, 3] recanalizing obstructions [4, 5], and diminishing the degree of coronary artery stenoses [6]. Coronary venous retroperfusion via the coronary sinus to overcome acute ischemia has not yet gone beyond the experimental stage [7].

All these goals need manipulation of transluminally introduced catheters; these manipulations have to be directed and controlled through X-ray imaging techniques.

Since the dimensions of the coronary arterial tree are rather small compared with various other catheterizations, image resolution plays an important role in this particular diagnostic and therapeutic application. The three-dimensional nature of a coronary artery distribution also causes particular problems to the interpretation of X-ray images.

The objects to be visualized during intracoronary probing and intervention are:

1. Coronary artery
   - Curves
   - Bifurcations
   - Stenoses (0.8–1.5 mm in diameter)
2. Catheter
   - 0.8–1.1 mm in diameter
   - Metal markers (0.6 mm^2)
   - Metal guiding tip

In this paper we discuss some aspects of the problems encountered in applying these catheter techniques in human individuals.

Methods

At the present time, most intracoronary catheters are introduced into the coronary ostia using a coaxial system with large guiding catheters. These guiding catheters have an outer dimension of 8F or 9F and allow a 4F–4.5F catheter to be advanced through the lumen without getting trapped in peripheral bifurcating arteries. The guiding catheters are normally preshaped if employed from an entry in the groin and advanced via the femoral artery, or else constructed with minimal specific preshape when employed using the brachial technique. Intracoronary probes are normally fabricated from teflon, polyolefin, or other synthetic materials with an addition of radiopaque compounds. They feature one, two, or three lumina depending on the application. Evidently such a catheter cannot easily be manipulated, due to the lack of torque control and poor memory. In order to better identify the tip of the catheter with its 0.7- to 1.1-mm diameter, as well as pertinent points (for example, the limits of a balloon for dilatation), ring-shaped metal markers are currently employed. These metal markers have a projected surface of some $0.6 \, mm^2$. To verify the position of the distal catheter tip, the intracoronary catheter permits slow contrast injections through the lumen of up to 0.4 mm in diameter. This lumen normally also serves for pressure monitoring.

Geometric Resolution

Available X-ray equipment employing high-resolution image intensifiers makes it possible to resolve up to five lines/mm on a cineradiographic film. This would allow identification of small coronary artery branches like secondary septal branches, atrial branches, and terminal branches of the three large coronary arteries. The visualization on the television screen used to control catheter manipulations, however, is significantly worse. Standard equipment uses 625 TV lines on 38-cm monitors placed at a distance of between 1 and 2 m from the observer. This, of course, largely reduced the relatively satisfying resolution, to the extent that currently employed coronary catheters (with 0.8–1.1 mm diameter) are hardly visible.

Figure 1 shows an example of a coronary perfusion catheter (0.8 mm outer diameter) for direct thrombolysis introduced through a coaxial guiding system into the left anterior descending coronary artery. This picture was taken on 70-mm spotfilm using a $1.0 \, mm^2$ focus and a 17.0 cm high resolution cesium iodiate image intensifier. The patient weighed 74 kg and the film was exposed using 96 kV. Despite the rather optimal equipment and photographic imaging technique, the catheter is hardly visible during fluoroscopy. For control of catheter manipulations only the TV screen image with its rather poor resolution is

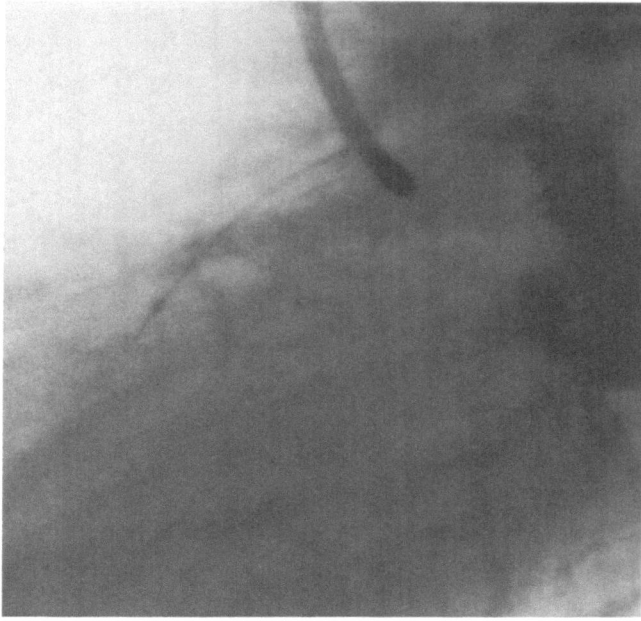

Fig. 1. Magnified 70-mm spot image of a coronary perfusion catheter introduced into the left anterior coronary artery (LAD)

available, and it is evident that these fine structures can barely be recognized on a standard TV screen.

It is necessary to identify the probe introduced into the lumen of the coronary arteries. However, the structure of coronary artery stenoses as well as recognition of intimal alterations is also of the utmost importance. Unfortunately there is no means of appreciating the shape of coronary artery stenoses from regular coronary angiograms. Superselective injections of contrast medium help somewhat to improve visualization of such stenoses (Fig. 2a, b), but even from multiple projections it is not yet possible to three-dimensionally reconstruct the geometry of stenoses. In tight lesions the chance of successfully passing a stenosis remains hazardous.

After successful dilatation of coronary artery stenosis, it is quite usual to find intimal tears and intramural hemorrhage [8]. The degree of these lacerations of the vessel wall is most important in predicting recovery after transluminal angioplasty.

Figure 3 shows one such intimal disruption after successful dilatation of a subtotal stenosis of the left anterior descending coronary artery; the hemodynamic result of this procedure was excellent, leaving only a minimal pressure gradient. The degree of dissection, however, could not be sufficiently judged from the TV image even after multiple repeated observations with the help of video tape storage. Since the cine film could not be developed the same night,

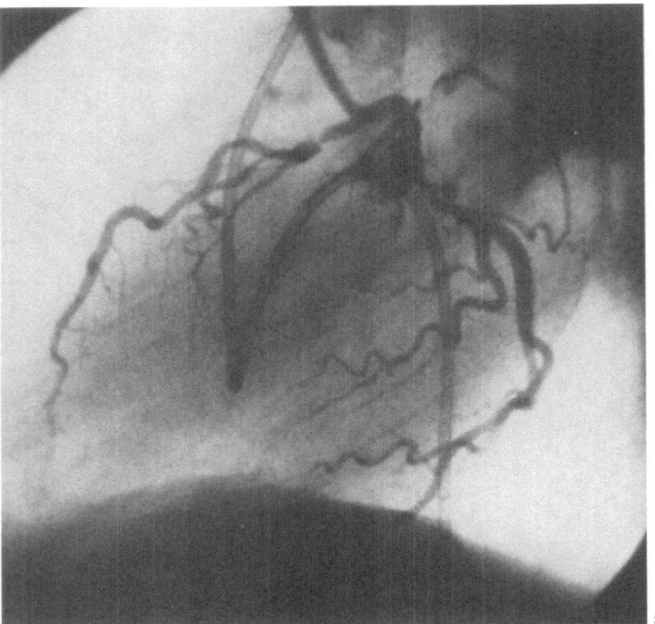

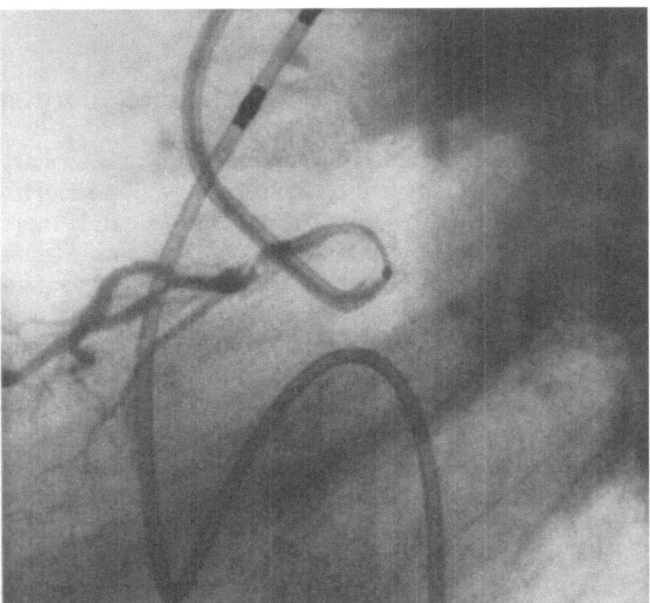

Fig. 2a,b. Subtotal LAD stenosis proximal to the first septal branch. **a** Regular coronary angiogram in lateral projection. **b** The same stenosis with superselective injection through an intracoronary 4.5F catheter. The latter method better shows of the amorphous geometry of the lesion

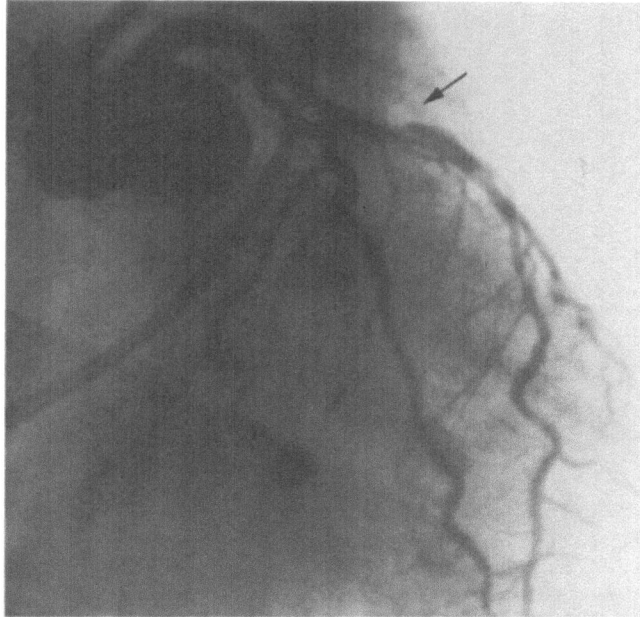

Fig. 3. Intimal dissection of LAD after successful dilatation of a 90% stenosis. Televized fluoroscopy did not allow the correct diagnosis

no particular precautions were taken in order to prevent further damage. The patient developed an acute myocardial infarction with complete obstruction of the coronary artery 8 h after the dilatation, at night. Higher resolution TV display and magnification of the area of interest would have helped to overcome this problem.

Sometimes the dilatation catheter is trapped within small side branches of major coronary arteries that are hardly or not at all visible on standard display equipment. In these cases, it cannot be decided with certainty whether the catheter is engaged in subintimal plaques or normal side branches; in the latter case, one would continue trying to advance the catheter more distally, in the first case the greatest caution would be advisable.

Figure 4 shows one such a case, in which the flexible metal tip of a balloon catheter always entered a small septal perforator branch within a stenosis of the anterior descending left coronary artery. The fact that this lesion was finally successfully dilated has to be attributed to pure chance; no rational decision was taken in selecting a differently curved tip of the balloon catheter, since the metal guiding tip of the catheter was not sufficiently visible on the TV screen during fluoroscopy.

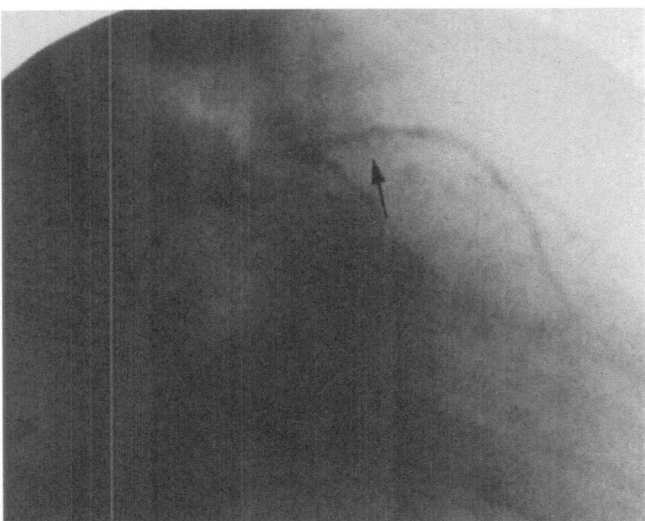

Fig. 4. The flexible metal tip of a 4.5F balloon catheter enters a small septal branch of the LAD. This phenomenon could not be seen during fluoroscopy

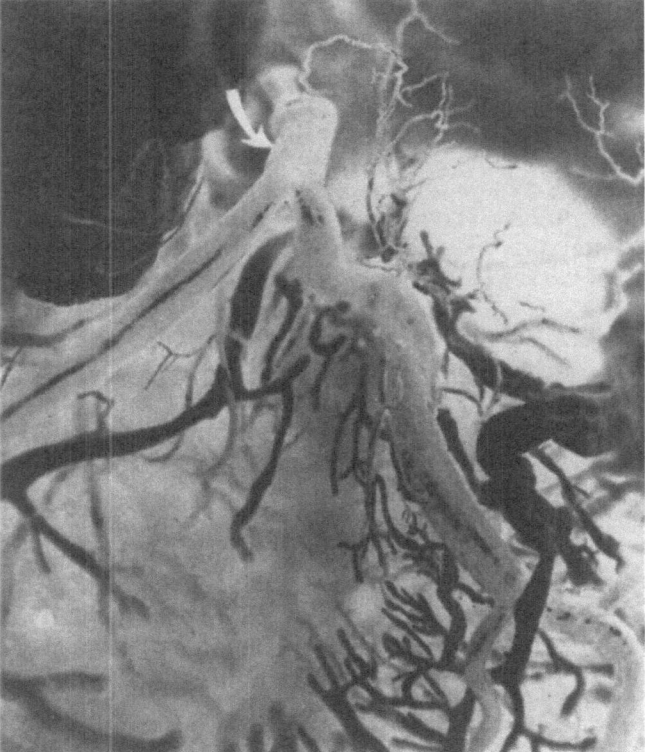

Fig. 5. Cast of the left coronary artery demonstrating the complex three-dimensional structure (from [10])

Problems Resulting from Two-Dimensional Display

Human coronary arteries are complicated three-dimensional structures (Fig. 5). The available imaging technique, however, provides only two-dimensional images at two simultaneous projections at its best. Therefore, it is often difficult to judge the angle of bifurcating arteries and to separate overlying vessels.

The first difficulty is normally encountered in catheterizing the left anterior descending branch of the left circumflex artery. From routine coronary angiograms, the spatial orientation of the main stem and the bifurcating main coronary arteries can only insufficiently be analyzed.

Figure 6 gives an example of a situation which at first glance looks relatively easy with respect to the off-set of the left anterior descending coronary artery with a 90% proximal stenosis. It was, however, extremely difficult to direct the catheter away from the circumflex branch and into the coronary artery; 45 min of manipulation and additional maneuvers including three different guiding catheters and two types of balloon catheters were needed to intubate the anterior descending branch and successfully dilate the stenosis. This difficulty could have been overcome with better resolution and higher magnification as well as adequate analysis of the orientation in space of the left main stem and the proximal left anterior descending coronary artery.

Such three-dimensional reconstruction might possibly be achieved with the aid of computer techniques which permit redrawing the course of the different coronary arteries from differently angulated regular coronary angiograms. A

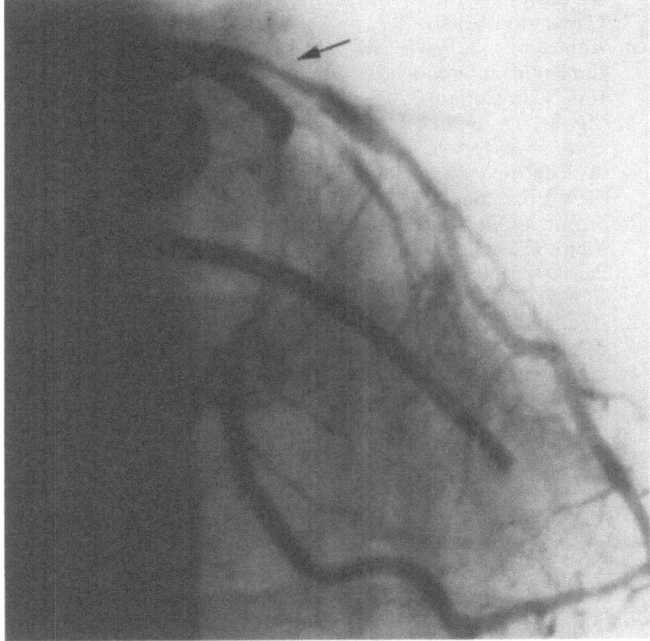

Fig. 6. Pitfall in LAD origin. Catheterization of LAD turned out to be extremely difficult despite its encouraging appearance

computer-generated three-dimensional graph [9] would permit selection of appropriately preshaped introducing catheters as well as proper choice of balloon catheters. The same technique could be applicable for all other coronary interventional procedures such as superselective angiography, selective thrombolysis or recanalization, and hemodynamic evaluation.

In conclusion, the currently available fluoroscopic radiographic equipment appears inadequate for intracoronary probing and intervention. High resolution television display may overcome some of the problems encountered; the disadvantage, however, includes problems with image storage and incompatibility with other currently used TV systems. Future improvement should be directed towards higher resolution, optical magnification for example, with zoom lenses), and spatial reconstruction of the coronary vascular tree.

References

1. Sigwart U, Essinger A, Sadeghi H, Rivier JL (1981) Objektivierung vermeintlicher Koronarstenosen durch transluminale Druckgradientenbestimmung. Z Kardiol 70:639
2. Ganz W, Buchbinder N, Markus H, Mondkar A, O'Connor L, Maddahi J, Berman D, Charuzi J, Beeber C, Peter T, Shah CK, Shell W, Swan HIC (1981) Intracoronary thrombolysis in involving myocardial infarction. In: Lichtlen PR, Engel HJ, Schrey A, Swan HJC, (eds) Nitrates III. Cardiovascular effects. Springer, Berlin Heidelberg New York, pp 355–358
3. Rentrop P, Blanke H, Karsch KR, Kaiser H, Köstering H, Leitz K (1981) Selective intracoronary thrombolysis in acute myocardial infarction and unstable angina pectoris. Circulation 63:307–317
4. Rentrop P, De Vivie ER, Karsch KR, Kreuzer H (1978) Acute coronary occlusion with impending infarction as an angiographic complication releaved by a guide-wire recanalization. Clin Cardiol 1:101–106
5. Sigwart U, Essinger A, Sadeghi H, Rivier J-L (1982). Emergency reopening of right coronary artery occlusion with guide-wire and thrombolysis. In: Kaltenbach M, Grüntzig A, Rentrop P, Bussmann WD (eds) Coronary heart diesease. Springer, Berlin Heidelberg New York, pp 151–154
6. Grüntzig AR (1978) Transluminal dilatation of coronary stenosis. Lancet 1:263
7. Smith GT, Geari GG, Blanchard W, McNamara JJ (1981) Reduction of infarct size by synchronized selective coronary venous retro-perfusion of arterialized blood. Am J Cardiol 48:1071–1075
8. Baughman KL, Pasternak RC, Fallon JT, Block PC (1981) Transluminal coronary angioplasty of post mortem human hearts. Am J Cardiol 48:1044–1047
9. Heintzen PH, Moldenhauer K, Lange PE (1974) 3-dimensional computerized contraction pattern analysis. Eur J Cardiol 1/3:229
10. James TN (1961) Anatomy of the coronary arteries. Harper and Row, New York, p 16, Fig. 3 A

Combined Coronary and Peripheral Angiography

K. Bachmann, G. Raab, and W. Niederer

Medizinische Poliklinik, University of Erlangen-Nürnberg, FRG

Wherever atherosclerosis becomes symptomatic – in the coronary, peripheral, supra-aortic, or abdominal area – a generalized disease must be suspected, rather than a local one restricted to the site of symptoms. Thus, symptoms of peripheral arterial vascular disease may provide the chance of early angiographic diagnosis of coronary heart disease, and vice versa. This, together with complications such as stroke and myocardial infarction reported in patients who underwent coronary bypass or vascular surgery [6, 8, 9], was the reason why, in 1971, we extended coronary and left ventricular angiography to total cine angiography [1]. By total angiography, we mean combined arteriography of abdominal, peripheral and supra-aortic arteries. A similar diagnostic approach termed "total body angiography" was reported from the laboratory of Favoloro in 1974 [3, 4].

Combined angiography of coronary and peripheral arteries seems to be a rational diagnostic approach in vascular multimorbidity, which may be proposed if certain requirements are fulfilled, including that
a) the extension of selective coronary angiography to total angiography must be without additional risk to the patient with regard to the invasive procedure, contrast material, and X-ray exposure; and
b) total angiography must lead to therapeutic consequences concerning secondary prevention, medical treatment, vascular surgery and angioplasty. Furthermore, total angiography has been linked from the very beginning with the expectation that differentiation into isolated coronary heart disease and generalized atherosclerotic vascular disease may be of help in evaluating risk factors and thereby the epidemiology of atherosclerosis.

Subjects and Methods

In the decade from February 1971 to February 1981 we studied a total of 3328 patients, the vast majority of them males aged from 31 to 79 years, with a mean age of 53 years; 438, that is, 11.7%, of them were 60 years of age or above (Fig. 1). All of them had suspected or already diagnosed coronary heart disease, and in a small group coronary angiography was performed pre-operatively to valvular replacement.

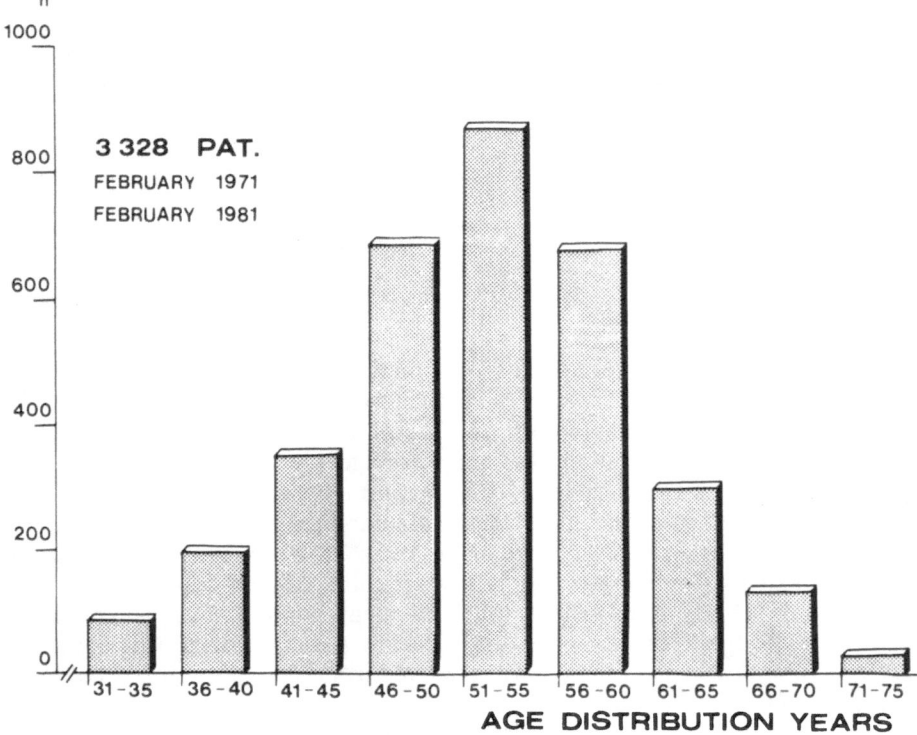

Fig. 1. Total cineangiography in 3328 patients: age distribution

The method employed has always been the transbrachial approach using the Sones technique. We start with left ventricular angiography. After completion of selective coronary angiography, the catheter can easily be advanced down to the right and left iliac artery for downstream opacification as far as the popliteal and tibial arteries. Then angiography of the pelvic arteries, the abdominal aorta, and the supra-aortic arteries is performed. In patients with arterial hypertension, selective renal arteriography is included (Fig. 2).

In more than 4000 studies so far, there have been only two serious complications. A 42-year-old patient with a history of cerebral attacks experienced blindness lasting 30 min after injection of 15 ml contrast material into the right vertebral artery. In a 41-year-old hypertensive patient, selective injection of 15 ml Urografin 76% into the left carotid artery provoked an epileptic seizure. Nausea or histamine-type reactions, such as flushing or urticaria, were seen in some rare cases.

Total angiography is performed using the same technique and procedure as are routinely employed in selective coronary angiography. Until 1981 all procedures were performed with a 7–9 image intensifier (Siemens). Cine radiography exposures were 400 ms, pulsed at 60 to 100 kV at 250 mA at 25 frames/s (Pandoros V). The film in use at present is Agfa scopic RP IC for cine. The

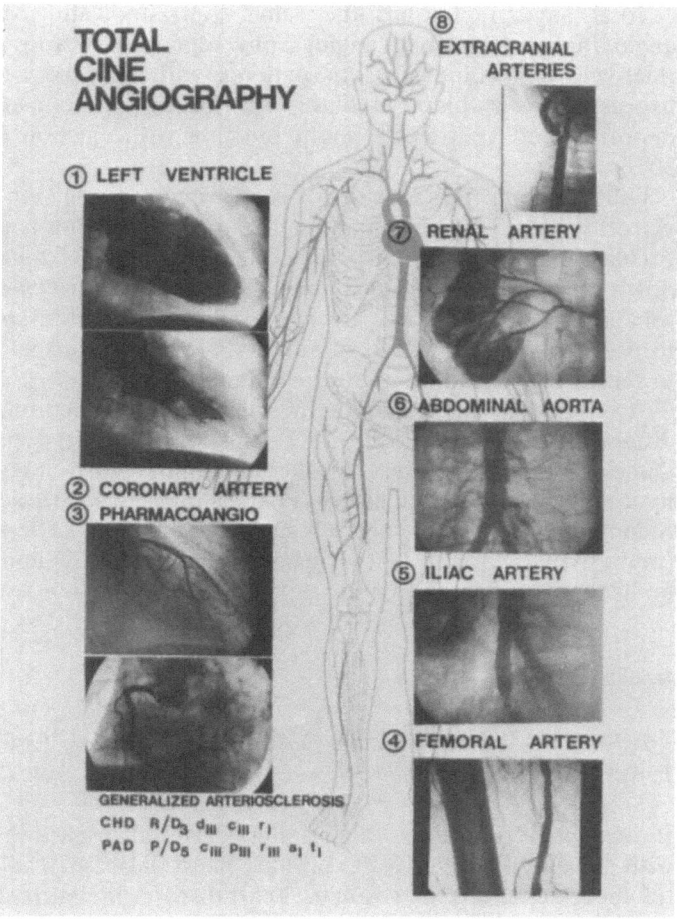

Fig. 2. Total cineangiography in a 59-year-old patient with arterial hypertension and generalized atherosclerosis: coronary heart disease (*CHD*) of type/ R/D 3, d III, c III, r I (3-vessel disease with severe stenosis of the left anterior descending artery and circumflex artery, wall irregularities in the dominant right coronary artery, non-stenotic atherosclerotic lesion of the left superficial femoral artery, severe segmental stenosis of the right common iliac artery, the right renal artery and the right internal carotic artery, and atherosclerotic plaques in the abdominal aorta)

cradle is mounted on the Coordinat and moved by hand according to the opacification of the area under investigation.

When comparing selective coronary angiography and left ventricular angiography with combined arteriography, fluoroscopic time increases from 2.8 to 8.6 min and X-ray dose from 6100 Rcm^2 to 15 300 Rcm^2, respectively. The contrast material used has always been renografin 76%. The total amount increases from 1.3 ml/kg body wt. to 3.1 ml/kg body wt. on average.

Total angiography has the same contra-indication as selective coronary angiography. Combined angiography of coronary and peripheral arteries is relatively contra-indicated in patients with reduced cardiac index, arterial hypotension with blood pressure of 100 mmHG systolic and below, or critically depressed left ventricular pump function with ejection fractions of less than 30%.

Our premedication consists of corticosteroids (8–12 mg dexamethasone) and glycosides (0.25 mg strophanthin); 20 ml 10% calcium is given before left ventricular angiography. When injecting more than 3.0 ml/kg body wt. we slow down the procedure and lengthen the intervals between opacification of different areas. Furthermore, we start infusion of saline solution and 10–20 mg furosemide i.v. in order to stimulate diuresis and thus avoid excessive increase in serum concentration of contrast material.

According to the angiographic classification of coronary heart disease we differentiate between diffuse (D) and localized (L) type of angiographically detectable atherosclerosis in the abdominal aorta (a), pelvic arteries (p), femoral artery (f), renal artery (r) and supra-aortic arteries (c). The severity of reduction in lumen diameter is classed as I (50% or less), II (51%–75%), III (more than 75%), and IV (occlusion). Only classes III and IV are considered to be haemodynamically effective.

Results

Incidence of Angiographically Documented Coronary heart Disease and Peripheral Atherosclerotic Vascular Disease

Basically, the incidence of peripheral arterial disease is positively correlated with age and the severity of coronary heart diesease. The older the patient and the more advanced the coronary heart disease, the more extracoronary arteries or the abdominal aorta will be documented as abnormal angiographically.

There is an *age-related* increase of incidence of class I to IV lesions of the abdominal, peripheral, and supra-aortic arteries of from 15% for patients aged 31–35 years, to 71.3% in patients aged 61–65 years; while the corresponding proportions for classes III and IV are 3.0% and 21.1%, respectively (Fig. 3). According to the *severity* of coronary heart disease, our patients can be divided into three groups:

Group 1. No angiographic evidence of coronary heart disease; 12.8% incidence of noncoronary lesions, 3.3% of them of class III or IV
Group 2. Hemodynamically noneffective coronary lesions of class I or II demonstrating a 44.5% incidence of peripheral atherosclerosis with 11.5% in class III or IV
Group 3. Severe coronary heart disease of class III or IV with a 69.9% incidence of the generalized type of atherosclerosis; 20.3% of them of class III or IV

Furthermore, the likelihood of combined coronary and peripheral artery disease increases with the *extent* of coronary atherosclerosis in terms of one-, two-,

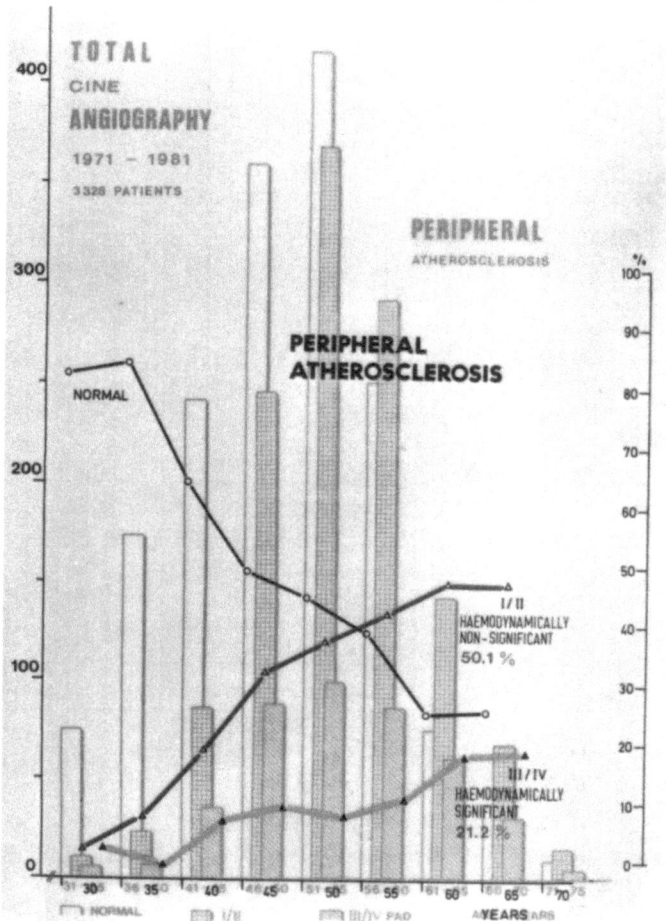

Fig. 3. Age-related incidence of angiographically documented peripheral, abdominal and supra-aortic arterial lesions in 3328 patients who underwent total angiography due to suspected or already diagnosed coronary heart disease

three-, and four-vessel disease. The incidence of combined coronary and peripheral atherosclerosis was as follows: one-vessel disease, 27.5%; two-vessel disease, 49.1%; three-vessel disease, 66.3%; and four-vessel disease, 77.1% (Fig. 4).

Thus, if we analyse a selected group of patients aged 60 years or above with coronary three- or four-vessel disease of class III or IV in at least two coronary arteries, the incidence of associated peripheral artery disease is as high as 82.8%: 57.4% in class I or II and 25.4% in class III or IV. This high probability of generalized atherosclerotic vascular disease as compared with isolated coronary heart diesease seems to be a strong argument for combined arteriography of coronary and peripheral vessels. Therefore, after an investigational period

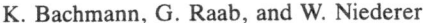
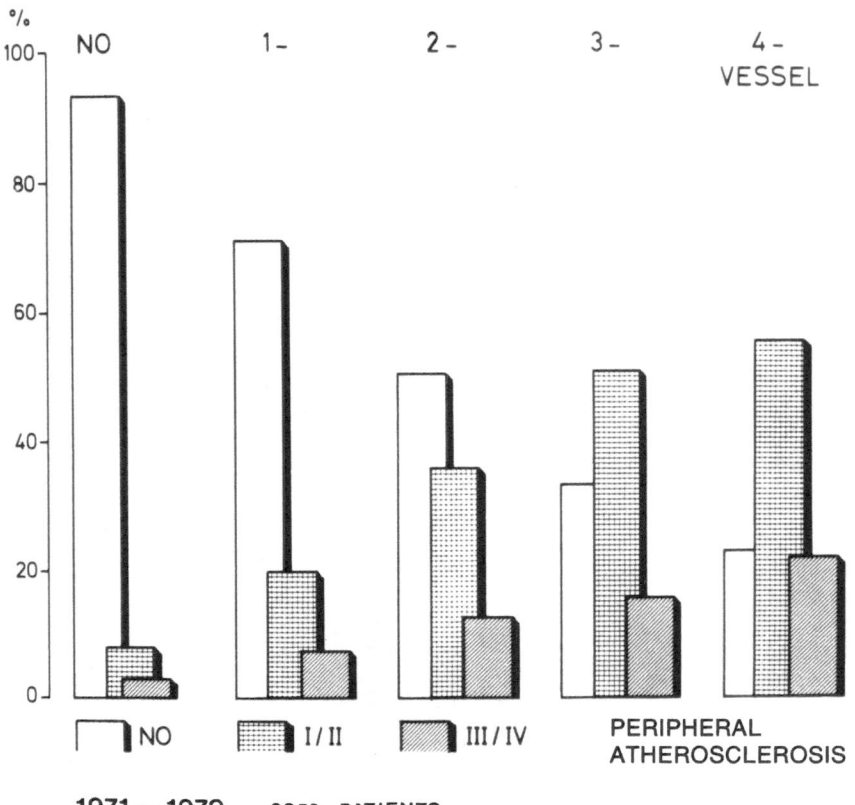

1971 — 1979   2852 **PATIENTS**

Fig. 4. Increase of the type of "generalized atherosclerosis" with the extent of coronary heart disease in terms of one-, two-, three- and four-vessel disease

these data may provide a basis for a rational approach to total angiography. It seems to be realistic to recommend this method

1. In coronary patients over the age of 60 with class III or IV coronary heart disease in at least two coronary arteries
2. In patients of all ages who are candidates for operative treatment, regardless of whether it will be bypass grafting or peripheral vascular surgery

Angiographic Findings and Risk Factors

On the basis of angiographic information on both coronary heart disease and peripheral artery disease it seems rational to differentiate into two groups patients with isolated coronary heart disease and those with a generalized atherosclerosis including the coronary arteries. In comparing potential risk

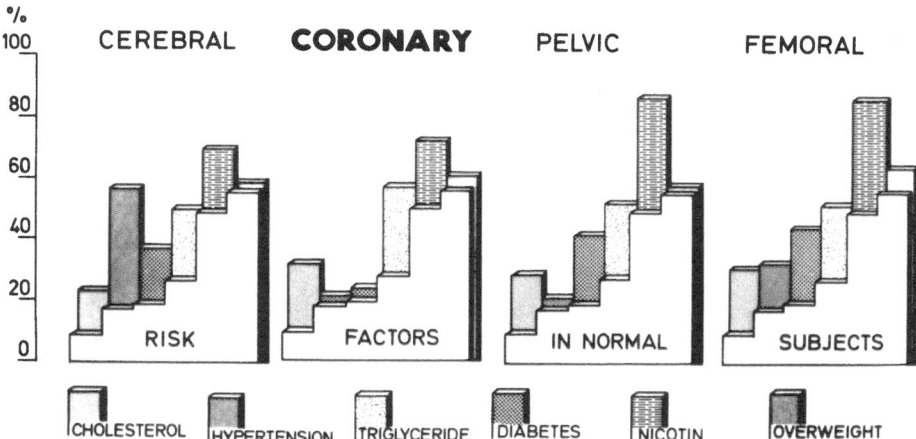

Fig. 5. Incidence of atherosclerotic risk factors in patients with angiographically documented cerebral, abdominal, and peripheral atherosclerotic lesions as compared to coronary heart disease

factors such as smoking, overweight, hypercholesterinaemia, hypertriglyceridaemia, diabetes and arterial hypertension, we expected to find some topography of these risk factors in regard to the manifestation of atherosclerosis.

Our findings are in line with the present state of epidemiological research. There is a high incidence of risk factors, especially smoking and overweight, in normal subjects. The profile as a whole in both patients with coronary heart disease and peripheral vascular disease is markedly above that of normal subjects (Fig. 5). As far as the topography of arterial lesions and the incidence of risk factors are concerned, however, the results are rather disappointing. One notes only the tendency of arterial hypertension to affect more the extracranial arteries, whereas smoking is linked with the occurrence of arteriosclerotic lesions in the abdominal and femoral regions. But we should not like to say that every risk factor has a specific influence on the topography as far as the manifestation of arteriosclerotic vascular lesions are concerned.

At the moment the discussion centres on HDL cholesterol as a preventive and LDL cholesterol as a risk factor in coronary heart disease. We therefore analysed the lipoproteins in three groups: 56 patients with coronary heart disease, 42 patients with generalized atherosclerotic vascular disease and 20 subjects in whom angiographically we had no evidence either of coronary or peripheral atherosclerosis.

Comparing the mean values for cholesterol, triglycerides, and HDL and LDL cholesterol in normal subjects and patients with either coronary or peripheral artery disease, the results show statistically significant differences for cholesterol and LDL cholesterol only (Figs. 6, 7). Comparing patients with coronary heart disease and those with peripheral arterial disease using a non-parametric test (Kruskal-Wallis, Mann-Whitney, Wilcoxon) no differences could be found.

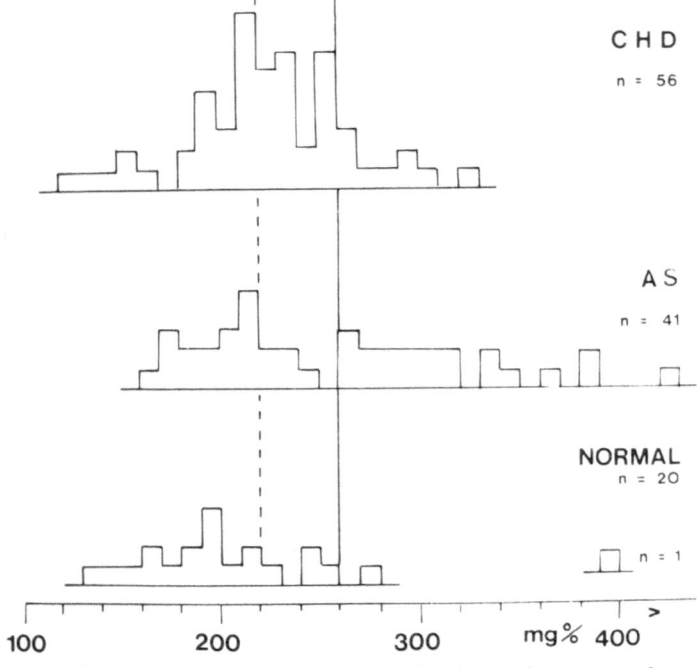

Fig. 6. Serum cholesterol in patients with isolated coronary heart disease (*CHD*) and generalized atherosclerosis (*AS*), compared with normal subjects

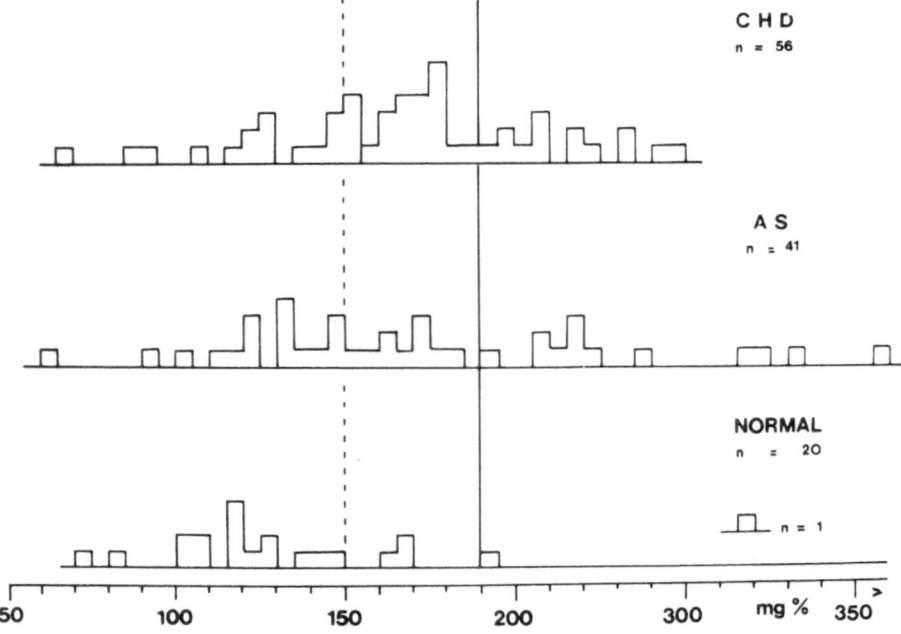

Fig. 7. LDL cholesterol in patients with isolated coronary heart disease (*CHD*) and generalized atherosclerosis (*AS*), compared with normal subjects

From these data one may reach three conclusions:
1. Abnormal findings in the lipid status are uncommon in subjects without angiographic evidence of atherosclerosis.
2. A significant increase in cholesterol or LDL cholesterol indicates a high probability of arterial vascular disease. On the other hand, normal values do not exclude severe generalized atherosclerosis.
3. No specific risk factor can predict the topography of potential atherosclerosis. Thus, from the type and degree of increase in risk factors we

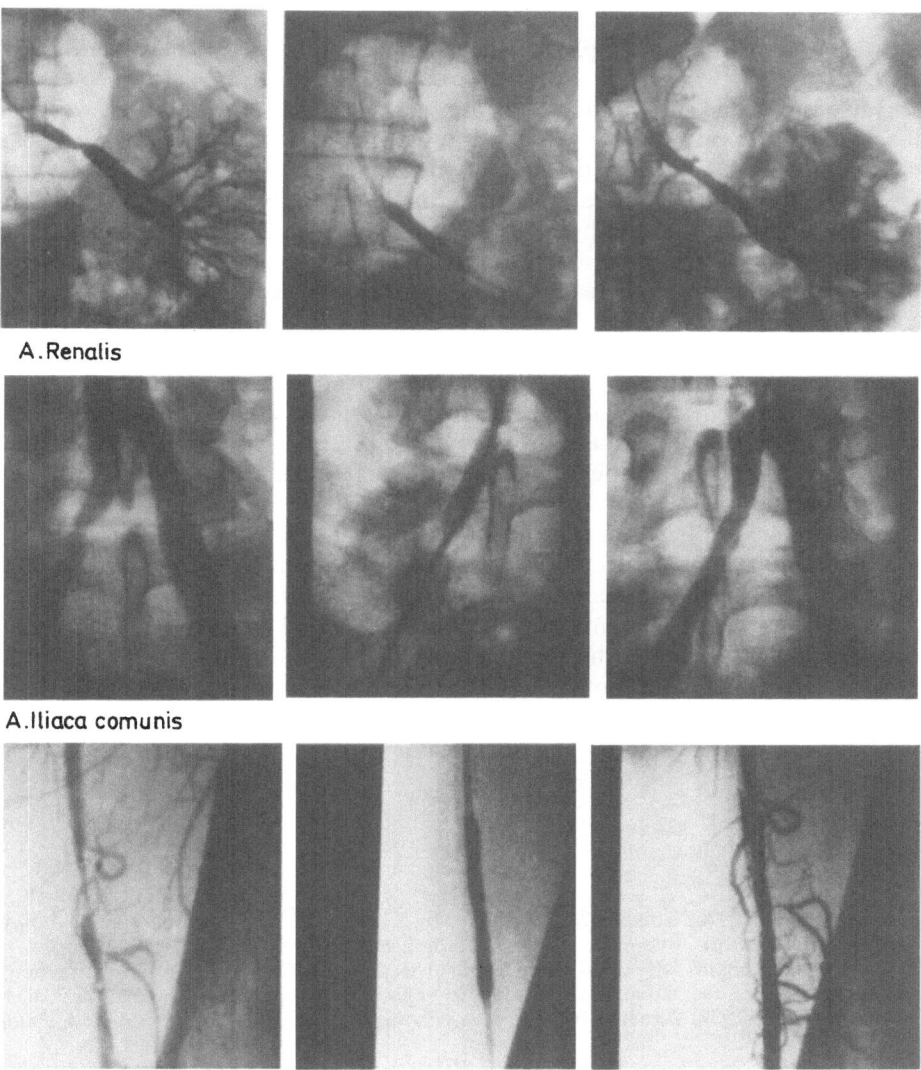

A.Renalis

A.Iliaca comunis

A.Femoralis superficialis

Fig. 8. Transbrachial transluminal dilatation (BTD) of severe segmental arterial stenosis in the renal artery, iliac artery and femoral artery

cannot decide whether atherosclerosis affects coronary or peripheral arteries or both.

Transbrachial Angioplasty as a Therapeutic Consequence of a Total Angiography

At least for the patient, every diagnostic procedure is qualified by therapeutic consequences. It has already been said that bypass surgery and operative treatment of peripheral arterial disease may be less risky after the surgeon has been informed by total angiography of the likelihood of severe atherosclerosis in other areas.

But besides this, as a practical consequence of total angiography, we performed angioplasty by the transbrachial route (BTD) using a modified Grüntzig catheter [5] (Fig. 8). This method was used for the first time in our laboratory in December 1978 in a 40-year-old patient with severe stenosis (class III) of the left common iliac artery. Since then we have performed BTD in 20 patients with 21 stenoses without a single complication: 17 stenoses were haemodynamically effectively dilated, which means a primary success rate of 81%.

As compared with the percutaneous transfemoral approach [9] the method has some advantages. The transbrachial approach avoids puncture of the femoral artery and thereby most of the complications encountered with percutaneous transfemoral dilatation. There is no need to stop anticoagulant treatment which may be continued throughout and after the procedure. Finally, the dilatation of stenosed peripheral arteries can be performed immediately following total angiography.

The method of transbrachial angioplasty should not be considered as an alternative to percutaneous transfemoral angioplasty. It is, rather, a substitute in patients who need coronary arteriography and who are known or suspected to have stenosis in the abdominal, peripheral, or renal arteries. Furthermore, transbrachial dilatation is the only method for patients with severe peripheral atherosclerosis including both femoral arteries. We should however point out that recanalisation of already occluded abdominal or peripheral arteries has not yet been attempted using the transbrachial approach.

References

1. Bachmann K (1976) Total cineangiography. In: Lichtlen PR (ed) Coronary angiography and angina pectoris. Symp. Europ. Soc. Cardiol. Hannover 1975, Thieme, Stuttgart
2. Dotter CT, Judkins MP (1964) Transluminal treatment of arteriosclerotic obstruction. Description of a technique and a preliminary report of its application. Circulation 30:654
3. Favoloro RG (1979) Direct myocardial revascularisation: a ten-year journey. Am J Cardiol 43:109
4. Grinfeld, LR, de la Fuente LM, Shinji K (1974) Total body angiography in patients with diffuse atherosclerosis (abstr.). Am J Cardiol 33:141
5. Grüntzig A, Hopff H (1974) Perkutane Rekanalisation chronischer arterieller Verschlüsse mit einem neuen Dilatationskatheter. Dtsch Med Wochenschr 99:2502

6. Rubio PA, Guinn GA (1975) Myocardial infarction following carotid endarterectomy. Cardiovasc Dis 2:402
7. Shore RT, Johnson WD (1974) Combined surgical treatment for coronary artery surgery complicated by extracranial carotid disease. Chest 66:336
8. Tomatis LA, Fierens EE, Verbrügge GP (1972) Evaluation of surgical risk in peripheral vascular disease by coronary arteriography: a series of 100 cases. Surgery 71:429
9. Zeitler E (1978) Complications in and after PTR. In: Zeitler E, Grüntzig A, Shoop W (eds) Percutaneous vascular recanalisation. Springer, Berlin Heidelberg New York

Optimal Visualization of Coronary and Collateral Blood Flow

H. E. ALDRIDGE

Cardiovascular Investigation Unit, Toronto General Hospital, Toronto, Canada, and Department of Medicine, University of Toronto, Canada

Two advances in the last decade have made a major impact on coronary arteriography, namely, the introduction of the caesium iodide image intensifiers and the routine use of caudo-cranial (cranial) and cranio-caudal (caudal) angled projections [1–11].

Caesium Iodide Image Intensifiers

The early caesium iodide image intensifiers almost doubled the previously best resolution obtained with the zinc cadmium sulphide screens of 2.5 line pairs/mm, to between 4 and 5 line pairs. Subsequent improvements with thin-glass screens to the current metal screens have improved resolution to over 7 line pairs.

Cranial/Caudal Angled Projections

Routine use of cranial/caudal angled projections permit all segments of the coronary arteries to be viewed perpendicularly and circumferentially, thus overcoming the problem of foreshortening, overlap, and the asymmetric lesion. These may be present singly or in combination. In the vertical heart, the major problem is overlap and in the horizontal heart, foreshortening.

The best method to obtain the projection is by mounting the X-ray equipment on a C-arm or a U-arm combined with a table top rotating horizontally through the isocentrically placed cardiac axis. These work best with the percutaneous femoral approach.

Basic Technique

The ideal anatomic display may be modified by radiological factors such as the spine, the diaphragm, or areas of greatly differing contrast such as occur at lung and heart borders. The cine film should have a low base fog and be processed to retain a wide latitude in the grey range. Overly contrasting film may obscure important data where vessels cross. The cine films should be studied on the best available cine analyser. The analyser should be selected by observing a projection alignment test film to pick the one with the highest resolution. So-called "routine" projections are only a rough guide and injections should not be recorded on cine film until test boluses of contrast, adjusting each of the angles, give optimal display of the anatomy. Hence, a high resolution video system and video recorder for replay are not only desirable, but a must for good arteriography.

Data from cranial/caudal projections in 100 consecutive studies led to upgrading of stenosis in 33.5% and unmasking of otherwise "hidden" lesions in a further 20.5%; an improved diagnosis in 54%.

In the left coronary artery, the areas of improved information were: the proximal left anterior descending artery (LAD) 32%, the origin of the first diagonal branch 32%, the origin of the first obtuse marginal branch (OM) 8%, and the proximal circumflex artery (CX) 7%. *In the right coronary artery,* it was the origin of the acute marginal branch (AM) 15%, the origin of the posterior intraventricular branch (PIV) 10%), the proximal right artery when there is a sharp, almost right-angle downturn in 4%. Often there was better visualization in more than one area [12–15].

Basic Projections

Left Coronary Artery

To overcome foreshortening in the proximal LAD and first diagonal branch, a 25°–30° cranial angle is added to the standard 60°–70° left anterior oblique (LAO) projection. The distal vessel will be overlapped by the diaphragm. The CX artery is best seen in the left lateral, or, better, in a 70° left posterior oblique (LPO). If foreshortening is present, a 30° cranial angle must be added. We use a routine 30° right anterior oblique (RAO) with a 30° caudal angle which opens up the take-off angles of the secondary branches. The caudal angle may have to be increased even further in some patients. In the heavy patient, the caudal angle is best omitted because of the diaphragm obscuring the distal vessel. With multiple small branch disease, a rotational projection setting a 30° cranial angle and rotating the RAO from 60° to 15° is most useful. In a heavy patient, a shallow 10°–15° RAO is useful but does not overcome foreshortening.

Right Coronary Artery

The addition of a 30° cranial angle and reduction of the LAO to 30° enables good visualization of the origin of the PIV, especially in the heavy patient. Each angle must be adjusted by viewing test doses of contrast on fluoroscopy to place the PIV in the apex of a triangle bounded by diaphragm and spine. This is especially useful in heavy patients. The right posterior oblique (RPO) 70° shows the origin of the acute marginal (AM) branch well. In heavy patients, a 30° cranial angle will move the diaphragm from off the distal vessel. The U-turn branches and proximal right segment can be well seen in a postero-anterior (PA) projection. The 30° cranial angle widens the take-off angle of the U-turn branches.

Visualization of Distal Vessels and Collaterals

The coronary arteries are under tone and change in size. This change is less, or absent when localized disease is present. Thus coronary arteriography is more like a "snapshot". It tells us *only* something about the lumen. Repeated contrast injections produce some vasodilation. The vessel distal to a severe obstruction is often difficult to demonstrate, and an underperfused vessel must be distinguished from a diffusely diseased one, sometimes an insoluble problem. Intracoronary nitroglycerin into the respective vessel or into the vessel supplying the collaterals may result in blood flow being shunted away into branches with a lower vascular resistance, thus giving a poorer visualization of the segment under study. Sometimes the presence of good segmental wall contraction in the distribution of a poorly visualized vessel will suggest an underperfused rather than distally diseased vessel. Manipulation of the circulation with nitroglycerin or ergonovine may be essential for a correct diagnosis.

All normal myocardium has a vascular supply. An apparently avascular area may appear so for one of the following reasons:
a) a super-selective injection,
b) collaterals present too faint to be seen on the fluoroscope,
c) a branch blocked flush at its origin from the parent vessel, or
d) an anomalous supply.

Despite all skills in using special angled projections diagnostic problems may persist. Here, the use of macro-aggregate studies at rest and with pacing may show an "apparent" 50% lesion to produce ischaemia in the absence of spasm.

Biplane Angiography

This is essential for congenital heart disease and perhaps desirable for ventriculography. Its place in coronary arteriography has not been fully defined. Usually, bulky 25/17 or 20/15 cm image intensifiers are used. These cannot be placed close to the chest wall without encroaching on the field of the second plane. When steep cranial/caudal angles are used, this problem is increased. The large image mode avoids panning but minifies the picture, while the small mode requires panning unless only a localized area is being studied. Panning in the one plane may not be optimal for the second plane. Lastly, the increased cost of a biplane C-arm system must be taken into consideration.

What Lies in the Future?

Digital vascular imaging offering contrast enhancement, fluoroscopy radiation factors, and perhaps venous contrast injections sound attractive. The resolution obtained at present with these techniques is not acceptable for coronary arteriography. Venous contrast injection complicates the problem of overlap and foreshortening. Tomoscopy techniques may solve this situation. Cardiac motion remains a problem and imposes gating or the use of sequential image subtraction. Venous contrast injection may enable patients to be screened for coronary artery disease or be of use in postcardiac surgery follow-up evaluation. Probably we will continue with selective coronary injections, but use more dilute and smaller quantities of contrast with these new imaging techniques.

In summary, the caesium iodide image intensifiers and routine use of cranial/caudal angled projections have made a significant improvement in coronary arteriography. Five injections each of the left and right coronary arteries will usually give basic optimal data (see Table 1). The angles are approximate and need to be individually adjusted using test injections of contrast observed using high resolution video system and playback equipment before recording on cine film. Visualization of the underperfused vessel distal to a severe block may remain an insoluble problem. Manipulation of the coronary circulation with intracoronary nitroglycerin or ergonovine may be necessary for diagnosis. The place of biplane coronary arteriography is not fully defined and may have some drawbacks. Digital vascular imaging techniques appear promising, especially when the resolution has been significantly improved. It is likely that selective coronary injections, but of dilute contrast material, will remain with us in the future.

Table 1. Basic cranial/caudal angled projections

Left coronary artery[a]	Right coronary artery[a]
LAO 70°	LAO 50°
LAO 70° + 30° cranial	LAO 30° + 30° cranial
Left lateral or LPO 70° +/− 30° cranial	RAO 30° +/−25° caudal
Cranial 30° rotating RAO from 60° to 15°	RPO 70° +/− 30° cranial
RAO 30° +/− 25° cranial	Posteroanterior +30° cranial

[a] All angles are approximate and must be adjusted to the individual case

References

1. Bunnell IL, Greene DG, Tandon RN, Arani DT (1973) The half axial projection. A new look at the proximal left coronary artery. Circulation 48:1151–1156
2. Aldridge HE, Taylor KW (1974) The Cardioskop-U. A report of the preliminary clinical experience. Electromedica 2:31–38
3. L'Esperance J, Saltiel J, Peticlerc R, Bourassa MG (1974) Angulated views in the sagittal plane for improved accuracy of cine coronary angiography. Am J Roentgenol 121:565–574

308　　H. E. Aldridge

4. Sos TA, Lee JG, Levin DG, Baltaxe HA (1974) New lordotic projection for improved visualization of the left coronary artery and its branches. Am J Roentgenol 121:575–582
5. Eldh P, Silverman JF (1974) Methods of studying the proximal left anterior descending coronary artery. Radiology 113:738–740
6. Ludwig JW (1975) Supplementary x-ray beam projections in coronary angiography. Medicamundi 20:59–71
7. DenBrinker JA (1975) A newly developed unit for cardiovascular radiography. The Poly Diagnost C. Medicamundi 20:72–73
8. Arani DT, Bunnel IL, Greene DG (1975) Lordotic right posterior oblique projection of the left coronary artery. A special view for anatomy. Circulation 52:504–508
9. Aldridge HE, McLoughlin MJ, Taylor KW (1975) Improved diagnosis in coronary arteriography with routine use of 110° oblique views and cranial and caudal angulations. Am J Cardiol 36:468–473
10. Eldh P (1976) Axial views. Cathet Cardiovasc Diagn 2:315–317
11. Bergman RF (1976) Oblique, caudal and cranial x-ray beam angulation with the Poly Diagnost C. A schematic approach to the optimum visualization of the coronary arteries. Medicamundi 21:114–120
12. Aldridge HE (1977) Better visualization of the asymmetric lesion in coronary arteriography utilizing cranial and caudal angulated projections. Chest 71:502–507
13. Aldridge HE, McLoughlin MJ, Taylor KW (1977) Special angulated projections in coronary arteriography. Confusion in terminology. Cathet Cardiovasc Diagn 3:335–359
14. Taylor KW, McLoughlin MJ, Aldridge HE (1977) Specifications of angulated projections in coronary arteriography. Cathet Cardiovasc Diagn 3:367–374
15. Aldridge HE (1980) Invasive diagnosis of coronary artery disease. Med N Am 4:421–437

Introduction to Morphometry and Roentgen Densitometry of Coronary Artery Stenosis

W. Rutishauser

Centre de Cardiologie, Hospital Cantonal, Geneva, Switzerland

One approach towards quantitation of a coronary stenosis could be characterization of its hemodynamic effect. We could do this in the same way as we calculate the surface of valvular stenoses, that is, by measuring the pressure drop while probing the stenosis and the blood flow through the stenosis (e.g., using roentgen densitometry). In conscious man, however, this is a procedure which will probably not have wide application.

If we do not want to probe the stenosed vessel, we can characterize the stenosis by trying to describe its morphology. The most widely used approach is to measure the percentage of diameter reduction. We have to be aware, however, that we should aim for the cross-sectional area of the stenoses, compared with the normal lumen (that means the percentage of lumen reduction). Ideally we should know the lumen and the length in absolute values. Only in the case of circular cross sections can we deduce the amount of lumen reduction from diameter measurements – bearing in mind that, e.g., a 50% diameter reduction means a 75% lumen reduction, while a 75% diameter reduction means a 94% lumen reduction (Fig. 1).

If the cross section of the stenosis is not circular, the true value of the lumen reduction cannot be obtained from "diameter" measurements.

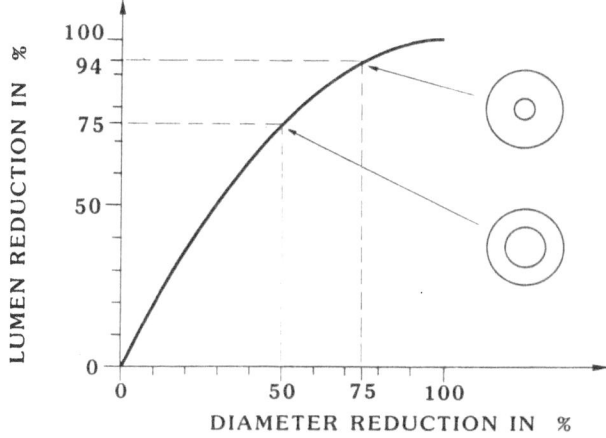

Fig. 1. Relation between diameter and lumen reduction in stenoses with circular cross sections

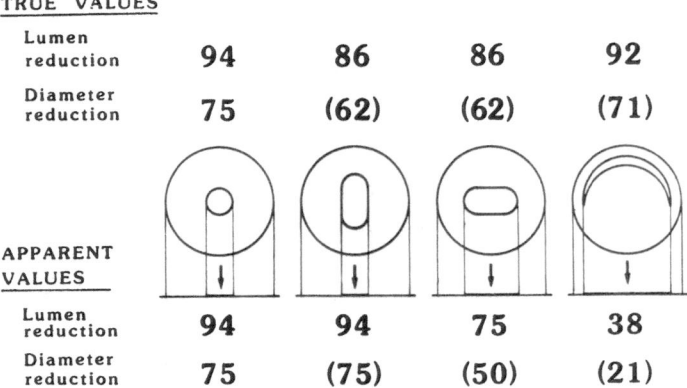

Fig. 2. Comparison of true and apparent values of lumen reduction, examples of stenoses of different forms. The apparent lumen reduction has been calculated assuming circular cross sections. The noncircular cross sections lead to considerable errors

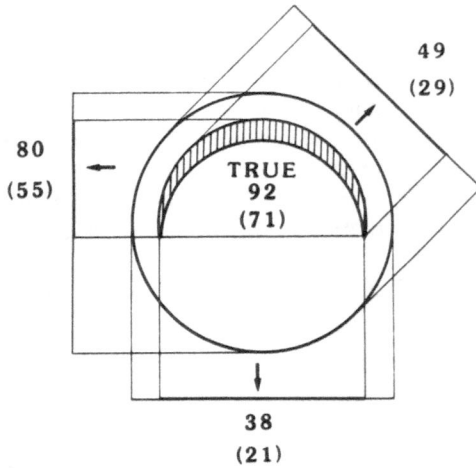

Fig. 3. If a crescent-shaped lumen is present, every projection will considerably underestimate the true lumen reduction, which in this example amounts to 92%

Figure 2 shows examples of slit-like and crescent-shaped lumens, demonstrating that the apparent lumen reduction calculated from a "diameter" is markedly in error in noncircular cross sections.

Figure 3 shows a situation in which the cross section of the subsistent lumen has a crescent shape, a situation which occurs, e.g., after complete obstruction and thrombus retraction. Even the clearest delineation of the edges in all different projections will severely underestimate the true lumen reduction. No morphometric approach, but only a densitometric approach will lead to a reasonably accurate evaluation of this type of lesion.

Quantitative Coronary Angiography with Automated Contour Detection and Densitometry: Technical Aspects *

J. H. C. Reiber,[1] J. J. Gerbrands,[2] C. J. Kooijman,[1] J. C. H. Schuurbiers,[1] C. J. Slager,[1] A. den Boer,[1] and P. W. Serruys[1]

[1] Laboratory for Clinical and Experimental Image Processing, Thoraxcenter,
 Erasmus University, Rotterdam, The Netherlands
[2] Information Theory Group, Delft University of Technology, Delft, The Netherlands

Introduction

The diagnostic value of coronary angiograms is severely limited by the usual visual and therefore subjective interpretation of the images. Inter- and intraobserver variations of from 8% to 37% in judging the location and severity of coronary obstructions from visual interpretations have been well documented in the literature (Detre et al. 1975; Zir et al. 1976; De Rouen et al. 1977). Also, visual inspection of the images does not allow accurate assessment of the hemodynamic effect of a narrowing in a coronary artery or bypass graft, since this requires detailed knowledge about the shape and absolute size of the obstruction. Moreover, the effects of short-term interventions, such as percutaneous transluminal coronary angioplasty (PTCA), intracoronary thrombolysis, and medical therapy, as well as of long-term interventions, such as surgical therapy, cannot be evaluated as accurately as would be desirable. Due to the limited value that can be attached to decisions based on the visual interpretation of the images, only coarse classifications can be used to distinguish patient groups; the same limitations apply to coronary research studies, particularly cooperative studies.

In view of the clinical need for optimal interpretation of these images, it has been attractive to develop an objective and reproducible quantitation method. Such a method should eliminate the imperfections mentioned above as much as possible and be particularly suitable for accurate classification of patients for coronary bypass surgery. Further developments of such a system could possibly lead to the implementation of a coronary data base. The main incentives for the design of such a data base are:
a) the need for reproducible and standardized reading and scoring of coronary angiograms, and
b) the possibility of computer storage and retrieval of these data with fast and accurate access for the benefit of scientific and clinical research.

This paper describes the procedures that we have developed for the computer-aided quantitative analysis of selected coronary lesions. These procedures have

* This work has been supported in part by the Dutch Heart Foundation under grant no. 80.129

been implemented at the Laboratory for Clinical and Experimental Image Processing of the Thoraxcenter in Rotterdam in close cooperation with the Information Theory Group of the Delft University of Technology.

After a brief overview of the pertinent literature on quantitative coronary angiography, the implemented coronary angiography analysis system (CAAS) will be discussed. The first quantitation procedure to be described deals with the assessment of the percentage diameter reduction of a coronary obstruction from single-view angiograms. This method requires the accurate delineation of the contours of the coronary artery at the obstruction. From these contours the diameter function is obtained. The percentage diameter reduction as well as the extent of the obstruction are computed from the diameter function. The mean diameter in absolute value (mm) of selected arterial segments can be determined as well. However, in cases with eccentric lesions, percentage diameter reduction in a single view poorly describes the true severity of the disease. To obtain the cross-sectional percentage area reduction, a densitometric procedure has been developed which uses the brightness information within the artery. Finally, we will discuss the feasibility of extending the densitometric procedure to the three-dimensional reconstruction of a coronary segment from two orthogonal views.

Overview of Pertinent Literature

Over the past decade various systems for the quantitation of the coronary arteries have been described in the literature. To manually measure absolute sizes of coronary arterial segments at a number of discrete positions, cross-hair measuring systems and vernier calipers have been used (Gensini et al. 1971; Rafflenbeul et al. 1976). A semiautomated computerized method for the analysis of biplane coronary cineangiograms has been described by Brown et al. (1977) and Bolson et al. (1977). This system requires manual tracing of the coronary lesions in two projected angiographic views. The contour data are transmitted to a digital computer. The two views are matched and a three-dimensional representation of the vessel is reconstructed assuming elliptical lumen, allowing the computation of various clinically significant parameters. A semiautomated computer-aided densitometry procedure for the evaluation of stenotic lesions in coronary angiograms requiring extensive operator interaction has been published by Sandor et al. (1979). In 1974, Starmer and Smith (1974, 1976) were the first to report on extensive computer processing methods for coronary angiograms. They developed algorithms for the efficient measurement, representation and storage of coronary trees by computer from biplane coronary arteriograms. Clinical results were not published after their initial publications. A semiautomated computer-based system was developed by Sanders et al. (1979). The boundaries of the artery are manually traced with a lightpen. Subsequently, a computer algorithm defines a more accurate delineation of the edges from video-converted cineangiograms. Selzer et al. (1976) and Ledbetter et al. (1978) have developed computer algorithms for the automated contour detection of selected coronary lesions. Required operator interaction consists of indicating a number of points along the approximate midline of the vessel with a sonic digitizer. The contours of the segment are then detected automatically from video-converted digital data. Various luminal measures are computed from the obtained contour data.

A digital densitometric procedure for the measurement of the degree of coronary stenosis as percentage area-reduction has been reported on by Doriot et al. (this volume). The region of interest of the coronary angiogram is converted into video format with a video camera. With a light-pen, the user defines rectangular windows at the stenotic and prestenotic segments. The video signal in these windows is digitized and stored in a computer, which computes the degree of area stenosis using the conventions of densitometry. For each window background subtraction is applied by using local background estimates or by searching for the corresponding image prior to the contrast injection.

The Coronary Angiography Analysis System

The coronary angiography analysis system (CAAS) is a PDP-11/34-based interactive image processing system developed and implemented in our labora-

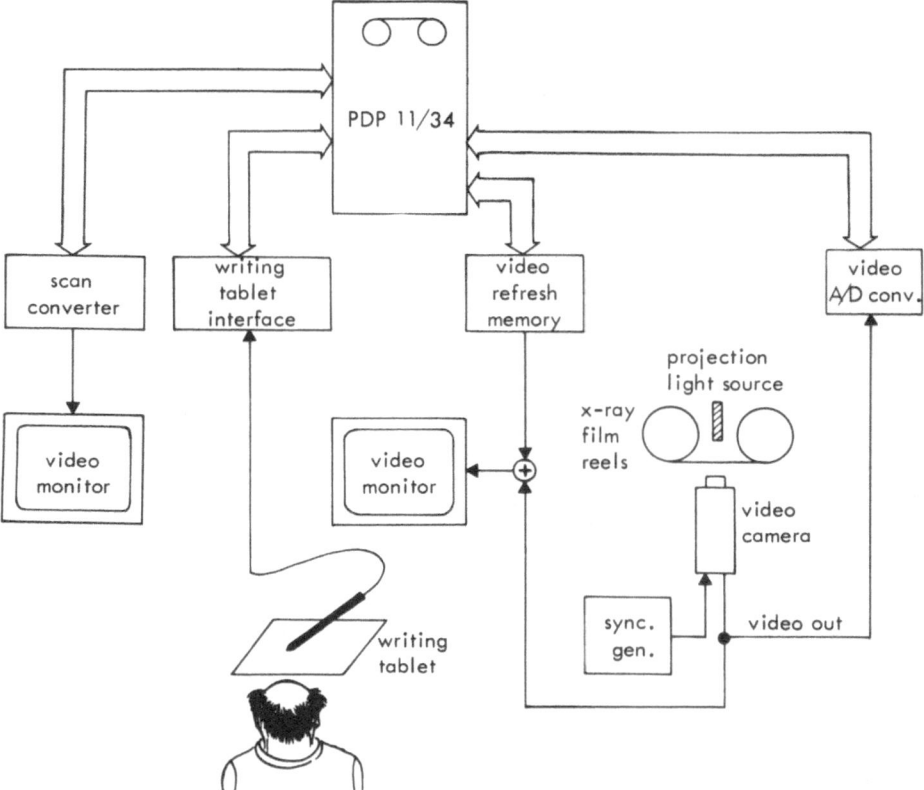

Fig. 1. Block diagram, coronary angiography analysis system

tory (Booman et al. 1979, Gerbrands et al. 1980; Reiber et al. 1981). A block diagram of the system is given in Fig. 1.

To analyze a selected frame, the image is converted into video format with a Tagarno cine film projector, which has been modified with a high-resolution transparent screen, and a high-resolution video camera (Sierra Scientific LSV-1.5 R). The video image is displayed on a video monitor. The video A/D converter identifies 800 picture elements (pixels) per video line, whereby both the even and odd lines of the 2:1 interlaced video system are utilized. The gray scale resolution of the digital data is 256 levels. A selected region is digitized column-by-column under program control through a DR11-C interlace. To reduce the effects of noise, the image may be digitized a number of times and averaged. The actual processing unit is the PDP-11/34 minicomputer with 96 K words of memory plus 2 K cache memory. The digital image can be visualized by writing the data onto the storage tube of a video scan-converter. Graphics and the contours of the analyzed arteries can be superimposed in the original video image with a video refresh memory organized as a 600×800 matrix with 1 bit information. Operator interaction is possible with a writing tablet.

Changes in the system in the near future include the replacement of the PDP 11/34 minicomputer by a PDP 11/44 minicomputer under the multi-user RSX-11M operating system and the use of a newly developed cine-video converter with greatly improved optical transmission characteristics. This cine-video converter is a mobile unit consisting of a standard 35-mm Vanguard projection head mounted on top of a cabinet (Fig. 2).

The image is projected downward into the cabinet onto the surface of the vidicon tube of our Sierra Scientific video camera via a drum with six different lens systems, which allows selection of the desired optical magnification factor from $\frac{1}{\sqrt{2}}$:1 to 4:1 in multiplicative steps of $\sqrt{2}$ with respect to a standard 35-mm cineframe.

The video camera is mounted on a movable x-y stage, which allows the selection of an area of interest in the 35-mm cineframe with the appropriate magnification factor. The cinefilm transport, the selection of the desired optical magnification and the x-y positioning will all be controlled by the PDP 11/44 minicomputer. At present the converter is being evaluated; the first results indicate greatly improved optical response as compared with the set-up used so far. The interfacing with the host computer still needs to be realized.

The improvement in the optical response can be demonstrated clearly with the following experiment. A 35-mm cineframe with homogeneous density over the entire field was digitized with both the present set-up (Fig. 1) with the Tagarno projector, the transparent screen and the video camera, and with the newly developed cine-video converter. The total digitized image of 504 vertical pixels and 672 horizontal pixels is divided into matrices of 28×28 pixels. This results in 18 of these submatrices in the vertical direction and 24 in the horizontal direction. For each submatrix the average brightness value of the 28×28 pixels is computed and the results are displayed in a pseudo-three-dimensional representation. Figure 3a shows the results for the present set-up. The length of a particular bar represents the average brightness level for the corresponding area of 28×28 pixels. A hot spot in the center of the image from the light

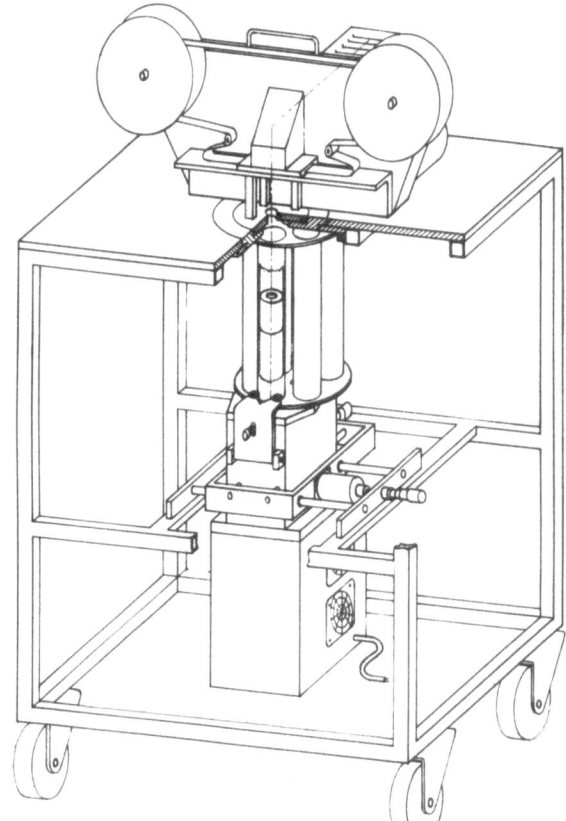

Fig. 2. Schematic drawing of newly developed cine-video converter

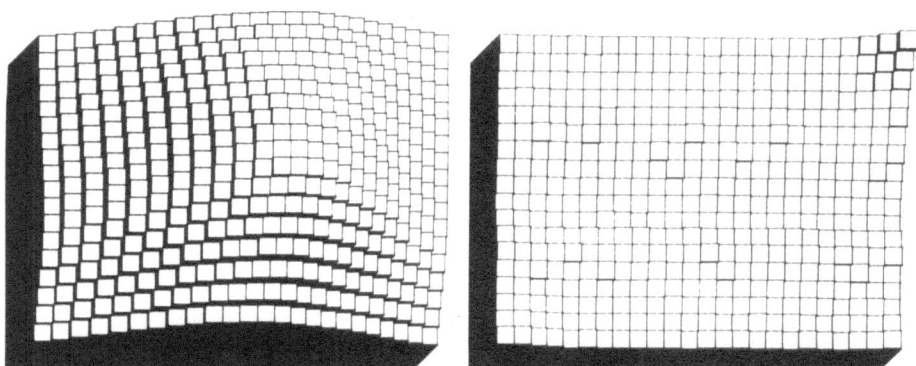

Fig. 3. *a* Pseudo-three-dimensional representation of the optical response of the present cine projector-transparent screen-video camera set-up and *b* the newly developed cine-video converter

source can be clearly distinguished. This shows that the optical transfer function for this part of the total image chain is rather inhomogeneous. The results for the new cine-video converter are shown in Fig. 3b. The greatly improved optical response is very clear; there is only a small hot spot in the right upper corner due to a shading effect from the video camera.

Contour Detection

The algorithm developed for the detection of the contours of an arterial segment will only be concisely described, as it has been reported elsewhere (Booman et al. 1979; Gerbrands et al. 1980). Since we have no facilities for the real-time digitization of an entire video image, regions of interest of 96 × 96 pixels encompassing the arterial segment are digitized sequentially and stored in the computer for subsequent processing. As a first step, the user indicates a number of center positions with the writing tablet, such that the straight line segments connecting consecutive pairs of these points are within the artery (Fig. 4a).

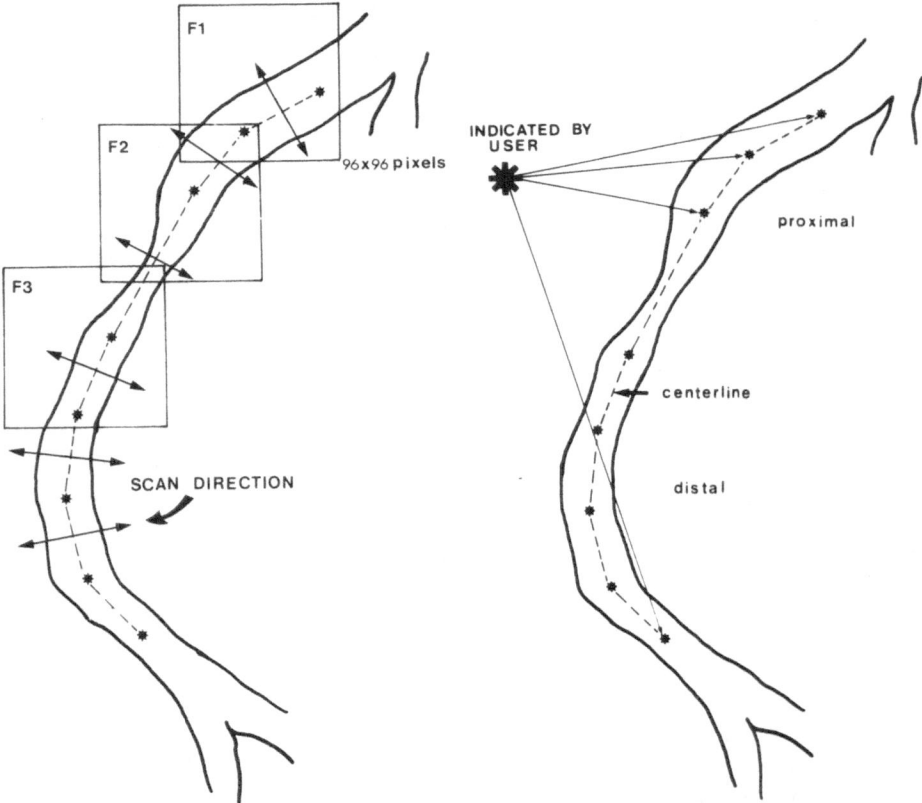

Fig. 4. *a* To analyze a selected coronary arterial segment the user indicates a number of center positions. The interpolated straight line segments form the tentative centerline. *b* The locations of the 96 × 96 pixel digitization matrices are determined by the tentative centerline. The scan directions are defined perpendicular to the corresponding centerline segments

These line segments form the tentative centerline for the lesion. The first part of this centerline is used to define the first 96 × 96 pixel region to be digitized. After the contours within this region have been detected, the next region to be digitized is defined by the last centerline segment of the current region and the next centerline segment. The overlap of consecutive regions is taken such that connectivity of the contours is assured (Fig. 4b). Each region is digitized three times and averaged for noise reduction. For the same reason, the digital data are smoothed with an unweighted 3 × 3 operator prior to detection of the edge points.

For each part of the piece-wise linear tentative centerline, the direction perpendicular to the part is defined as the local search or scan direction to determine the position of the edge points. The straight lines through the matrix in the scan direction are called the scanlines. On a specific scanline, the edge position at the left side of the artery is detected by applying the following one-dimensional averaging first-derivative operator to the brightness values.

$$[\frac{-2}{12} \quad \frac{-5}{12} \quad \frac{-5}{12} \quad \frac{+5}{12} \quad \frac{+5}{12} \quad \frac{+2}{12}]$$

The operator with the inverse weights is used for the right-sided edge position. The extreme values of the resulting first-derivative functions left and right of the tentative centerline are detected. From the positions of the extrema the edge positions are computed by applying a specific correction factor.

To prevent discontinuities in the detected contours due to disturbing sources such as noise or intervening structures, expectation windows with a width of five pixels are defined for each contour side. The center of the expectation window on the current scanline is the pixel with minimum chessboard distance to the detected edge point on the previous scanline. The possible positions of the new edge point are restricted to the expectation window. If the algorithm detects the edge outside the window, the outer position of the window closest to the detected position is defined to be the new edge point.

At the transitions of tentative centerline segments with different direction coefficients, discontinuities in the detected edges occur at one side and clusters of edge points at the other side. The missing edge points are obtained by interpolation with a straight line, whereas a thinning operator is applied to the clusters. Finally, for each edge a smoothing procedure is applied which consists of a least-squared error second-order polynomial fit. The results of this procedure are the final contours of the artery.

Figure 5 gives an example for the obtuse marginal branch in the RAO projection with the detected contours superimposed on the original video image. Administrative data are displayed in the administrative block at the top.

Percentage Diameter-Stenosis

From the detected contours the diameter function D(i) is determined by computing the shortest distances between the left and right contour positions. For the example of the obtuse marginal branch, the diameter function is shown at the right side of the image in Fig. 6.

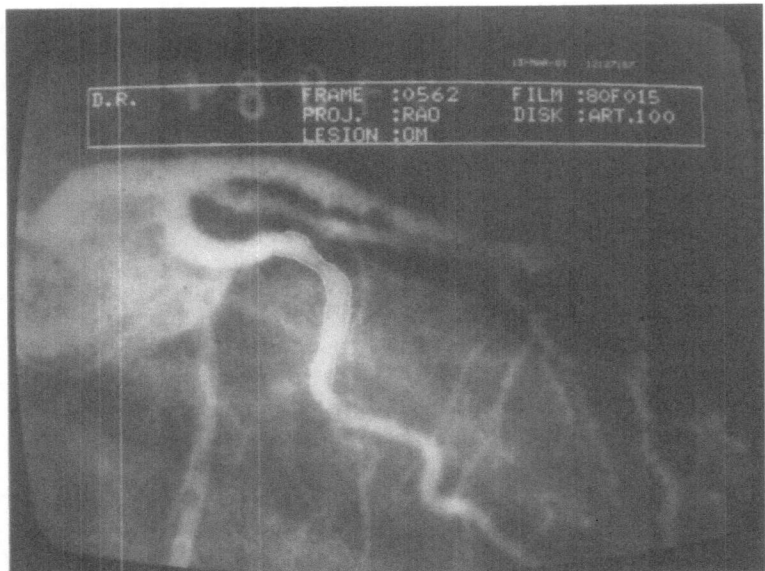

Fig. 5. Detected contours for obtuse marginal branch superimposed in original video image

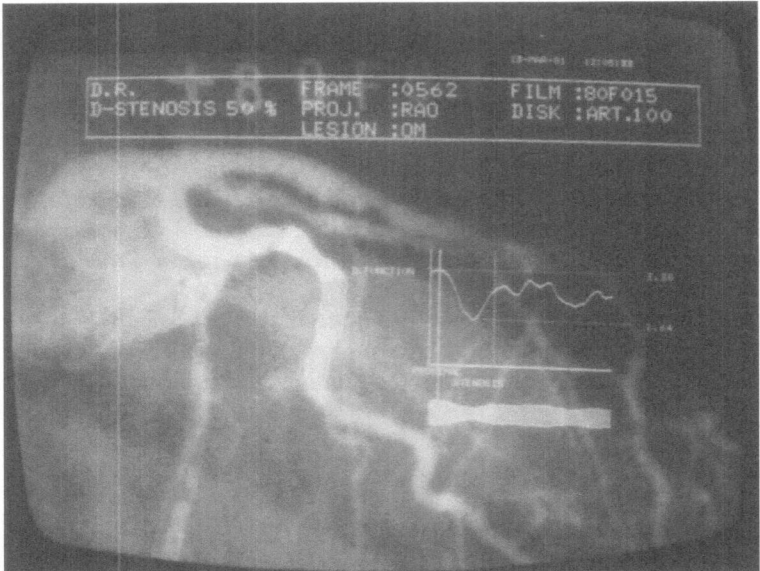

Fig. 6. Computer output of analyzed lesion in obtuse marginal branch. A percentage diameter reduction of 50% with respect to the user-defined reference region is found

The calibrated diameter values in mm are plotted along the ordinate and the centerline positions from the proximal to the distal part along the abscissa. From the minimum D_m of the diameter function and the mean diameter D_r at a user-indicated reference position, the percentage diameter reduction is computed as:

D-STENOSIS: $(1 - \frac{D_m}{D_r}) \times 100\%$ \hfill (1)

The mean diameter D_r is computed as the average of 11 diameter values in a symmetric region with center at the indicated reference position.

For this particular case the reference position was defined at the left side of the obstructive lesion as indicated in the diameter function by the extended vertical line. For this obstruction we find a percentage diameter reduction of 50%. Usually, the reference position is also marked in the artery by a straight line connecting the opposing contour sides. However, in the example of Fig. 6 the reference position was defined at the boundary of the computed lesion and as a result the reference marker is overwritten by the shaded obstructive area.

Calibration of the diameter data is achieved by using the intracardiac catheter as a scaling device. To this end, the contours of part of the projected catheter are detected automatically in a way similar to that described above for the arterial segment. A mean diameter value is determined in pixels, so that the calibration factor can be computed from the known size of the catheter. Particularly for intervention studies the absolute dimensions of pre-, post-, and stenotic segments are of great clinical importance.

Presently, the extent of the obstruction is determined by applying an averaging first-derivative operator to the diameter function $D(i)$. Starting from the minimal diameter position, this operator is applied in the proximal and distal directions separately. The proximal and distal boundaries of the obstruction are determined by the first zero-crossing of the output of the derivative function for which the value of the diameter function exceeds 75% of the average diameter value of the complete segment that is being analyzed. This threshold of 75% has been arrived at empirically. The extent of the stenotic lesion is indicated in the diameter function by the two dotted lines and is represented by the shaded area superimposed on the artery.

It is clear from the above that the computed percentage diameter narrowing of an obstruction depends heavily on the selected reference position. In arteries with a focal obstructive lesion and a clearly normal proximal arterial segment, the choise of the reference region is straightforward, and simple. However, in cases where the proximal part of the arterial segment shows combinations of stenotic and ectatic areas, the choice may be very difficult. To circumvent these problems as much as possible, we have implemented an alternative method to express the severity of a coronary obstruction, which is not dependent on a user-defined reference region. First, the extent of the obstruction is determined from the diameter function as described above. Then, for both the proximal and the distal segment, a reference diameter value is defined by the 90th percentile of the corresponding diameter values. The diameter values of a possibly present poststenotic dilation are automatically excluded in these calculations. These two reference diameter values are then assumed to be a measure for the normal size

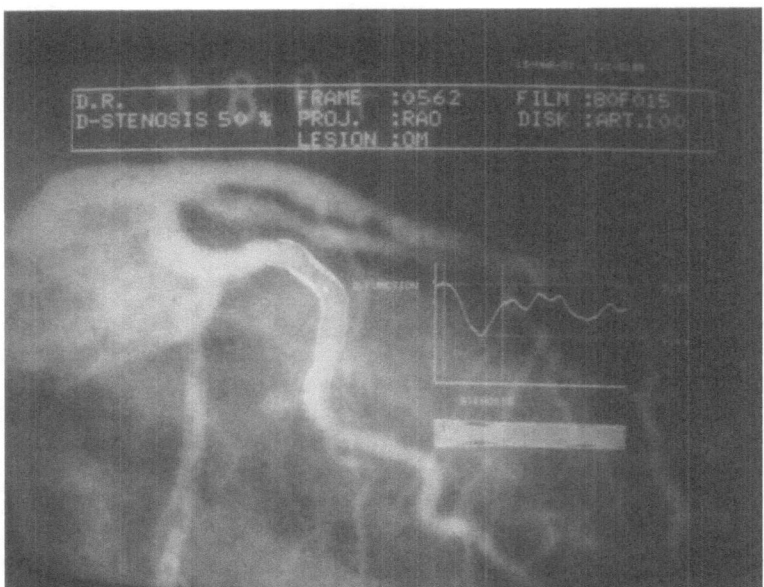

Fig. 7. For the lesion of Fig. 5 the normal size of the artery has been estimated from the normal proximal and distal diameter values (90th percentile). The marked area is a measure for the atherosclerotic plaque. An interpolated percentage diameter-stenosis of 50% results

of the proximal and distal segments, respectively. Similarly, normal sizes over the obstructive lesion can be obtained by interpolation between the proximal and distal reference values. The resulting normal size of the arterial segment of Fig. 5 is shown in Fig. 7, with the difference area between this boundary and the detected contours marked, being a measure for the atherosclerotic plaque. The interpolated percentage diameter-stenosis is then computed by comparing the minimal diameter value at the obstruction with the corresponding interpolated diameter value. For Fig. 7 an interpolated diameter-stenosis of 50% results. Further evaluation of this method is necessary to determine its diagnostic value.

The system also allows the computation of the mean diameter (in mm) of a selected arterial segment. The user indicates with the writing tablet in the artery the two boundaries of the segment to be analyzed. These two positions are also marked in the diameter function and the average diameter value is computed. The mean diameter of the selected segment of the circumflex artery in the RAO projection of Fig. 8 is 2.40 mm.

The accuracy of the quantitation method has been validated from ten copper models of obstructed coronary arteries with circular cross sections. The percentage diameter narrowing for the set of models ranges from 0 through 90 in steps of approximately 10%. The proximal and distal diameters of the models is 4.0 mm and all diameters are produced with an accuracy of 0.01 mm. Cine films were made of the models immersed in a water basin with 10 cm of water, with the same X-ray system settings as during coronary angiography. The cine films

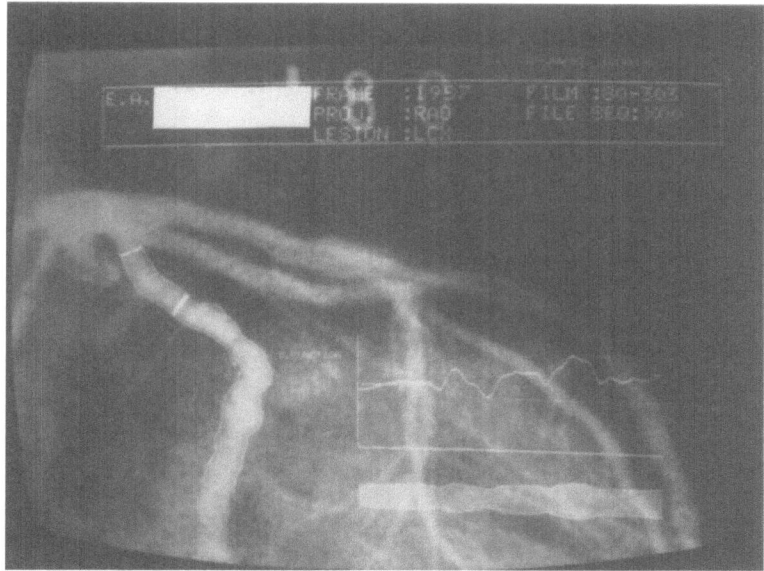

Fig. 8. The straight lines within the detected contours of the circumflex artery denote the boundary positions of the selected arterial segment; mean diameter, 2.40 mm

were analyzed as described above. The computer measurements in terms of diameter-stenosis were compared with the known true percentages in a linear regression analysis. The accuracy was found to be 1.9% and the precision 1.6%.

Densitometric Procedure

Since the luminal cross section at a coronary obstruction is frequently irregular in shape, percentage diameter reduction measured in a single projection is of limited diagnostic value. The hemodynamic resistance of an obstruction is determined to a great extent by the changes in the cross-sectional areas of the lumen. Computation of the cross-sectional area reduction from the percentage diameter reduction measured in a single view requires the assumption of, e.g., circular cross sections, an assumption which hardly ever holds. The resulting error may be reduced by incorporating two orthogonal projections and computing elliptical cross sections. However, with the often occurring eccentric lesions even this last approach provides poor results, as can be shown with the following example. Figure 9 diagrammatically depicts the complex problems stemming from a slit-like stenosis having a crescent shape. In cases such as this, even three or more views will not "provide a faithful portrayal of their severity" (Gensini 1975). A "lateral" view of the crescent would suggest a 10% reduction in lumen diameter, a "left oblique" would yield a 25% narrowing, and an "anteroposterior" would imply a 60% stenosis. Even a technique of quantitating area

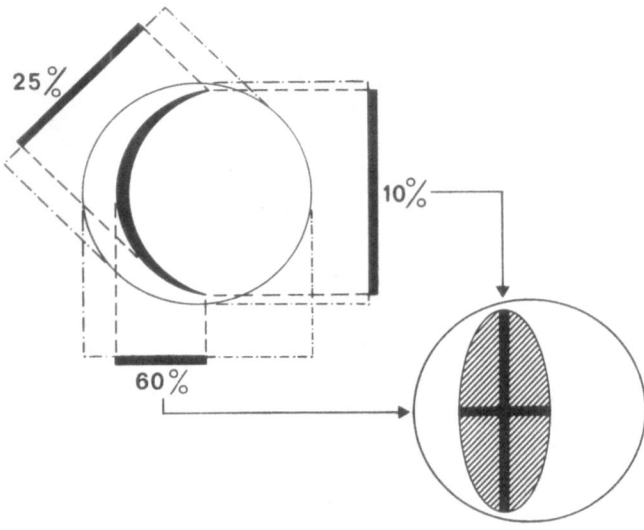

elliptical cross section

Fig. 9. Potential errors in the evaluation of the severity of a crescent-like lesion from single and orthogonal views

DENSITY

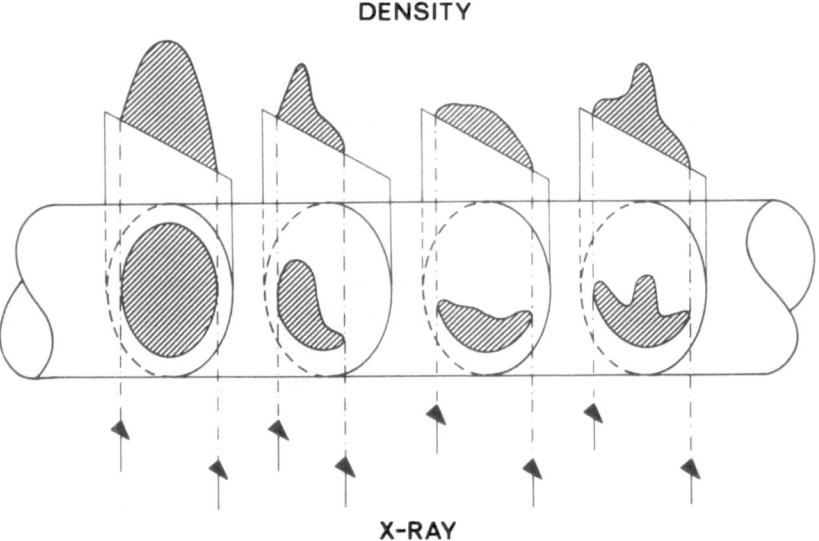

X-RAY

Fig. 10. Schematic illustration of the relationship between the irradiated object thickness and the density in the angiographic image

stenosis from two orthogonal measurements and computing area based on an elliptical model would fail to describe accurately the severity of this lesion.

However, some clue to the presence of this grossly asymmetrical lesion will exist, because the density of contrast medium is markedly reduced in that area, even though the caliber seems normal. Unexplained diminution of the opacity of a contrast-filled lumen (density changes) should alert the angiographer to the severity of the luminal narrowing. If one could constitute the relationship between the path length of the X-rays through the artery and the brightness values in the digital image, one would obtain the information required to compute the cross-sectional areas from a single view (Fig. 10).

The block diagram of the complete X-ray/video chain is given in Fig. 11. Constitution of the relationship between path length and brightness values requires detailed analysis of the complete imaging system. In a simplified approach, we are only interested in the static properties of the system. Analysis of the static transfer function of each link in the chain reveals that computation of the complete transfer function is very difficult. There is a large number of parameters involved, many of which are spatially variant. For the time being, we have settled for the following compromise. For the first part of the chain from the X-ray source to the output of the image intensifier we use a simple model. From the output of the image intensifier up to the brightness values in the digital image we measure the transfer function on a point-by-point basis.

Let p denote a position in the plane of the digital image which lies within the contours as detected with the method described in the previous section, and let p_b denote a background position just outside the contours. Let $I(p)$ be the intensity at the output of the image intensifier at a position corresponding with p in the image plane. The background intensity $I(p_b)$ is defined similarly. A simplified argument, involving a model of the X-ray source, the Lambert-Beer law for X-ray absorption, and a model of the image intensifier, yields that

$$d(p) = c_1 [\log I(p_b) - \log I(p)] \tag{2}$$

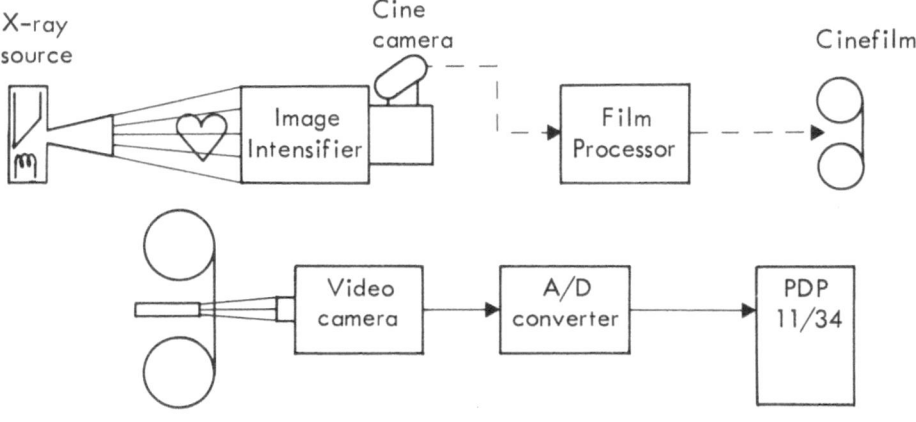

Fig. 11. Block diagram of X-ray/video imaging system

where d(p) is the path length through the contrast agent in the artery which results in the intensity $I(p)$. In this simple model all parameters of the source, the absorption process, and the image intensifier are mapped into the single unknown constant c_1.

The mapping T from intensities at the output of the image intensifier to brightness values in the digital image is measured on a point-by-point basis. The inverse T^{-1} of this mapping must exist to be able to compute the intensities $I(p)$ and $I(p_b)$ from the brightness values f(p) and f(p_b). For position p we have

$$\log I(p) = c_2 T^{-1}[\mathrm{f}(p), p] + c_3 \tag{3}$$

A similar equation can be defined for the background position p_b.

The mapping T is measured in the following way. The first 10 frames of the cine film are exposed homogeneously at different density levels. These frames are photographically processed simultaneously with the rest of the coronary cineangiogram. In the computer each test frame is divided into 432 subimages of size 28 × 28; in each subimage the average brightness level is computed. By using all 10 frames this results in a total of 432 local mapping functions, each of which is represented by its 10 sample points. Intermediate function values are obtained by linear interpolation. Each of the 432 mapping functions is assigned to the center position of the corresponding 28 × 28 subimage. The mapping for intermediate positions is obtained by spatial bilinear interpolation.

The brightness values f(p) and f(p_b), in the projected artery and the background, respectively, are now used to compute the length of the absorption path at position p by combining Eqs. (2) and (3) into

$$\mathrm{d}(p) = c_4 \{ T^{-1}[\mathrm{f}(p_b), p_b] - T^{-1}[\mathrm{f}(p), p] \} \tag{4}$$

where c_4 is an unknown spatially independent constant. In this way the brightness values in the projected artery can be calibrated in terms of the amount of X-ray absorption. By means of this calibration procedure many nonlinear and spatially variant effects in the film processing and the film/video system are taken into account.

The percentage cross-sectional area reduction of a selected lesion is then obtained as follows. When selecting the cineframe for the densitometric analysis of a particular arterial segment, we make sure that the main axis of the segment in three-dimensional space is reasonably parallel to the projection plane. The contours of the artery are detected as described in the previous section. On every scanline perpendicular to the centerline, a profile of brightness values is measured. This profile is transformed into an absorption profile by means of Eq. (4). The background contribution is estimated by computing the linear regression line through the background points directly left and right of the detected contours. Subtraction of this background portion from the absorption profile within the arterial contours yields the net cross-sectional absorption profile. Integration of this function results in a measure for the cross-sectional area at the particular scanline. This procedure is illustrated in Fig. 12.

By repeating this procedure for all the scanlines, the cross-sectional area function $A(i)$ is obtained. It is clear that a homogeneous mixing of the contrast agent with the blood must be assumed for the measurements to be correct.

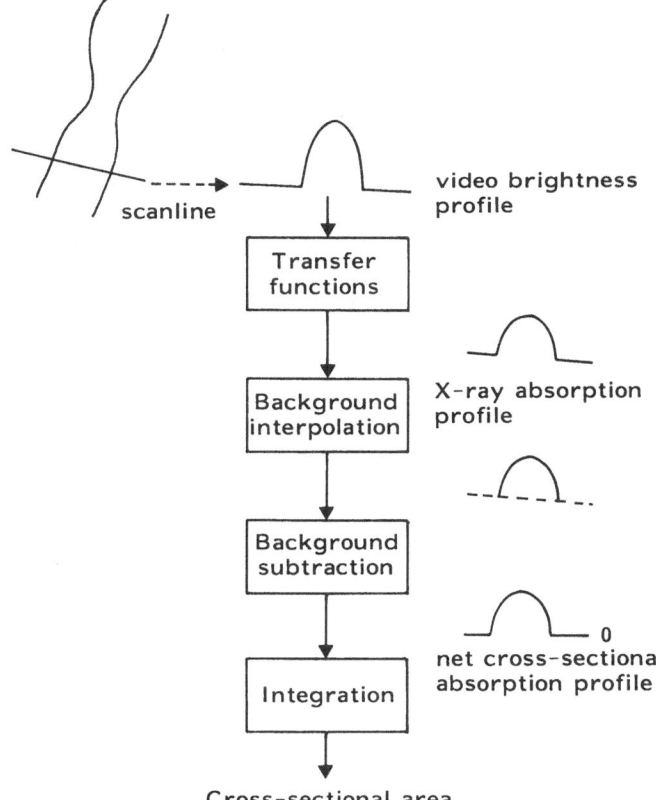

Fig. 12. Schematic drawing for determining the cross-sectional area data from the densitometric information within the arterial segment

Figure 13 shows the clinical case of Fig. 5 with the computed diameter function (upper curve) and area function (lower curve). The severity of the obstruction can now be expressed as a percentage area reduction, by comparing the minimal area value at the obstruction with the mean value at the selected reference position. For this particular obstruction we found a percentage area reduction of 81%. Assuming a model with circular cross sections, a percentage area reduction of 75% would have resulted, thus underestimating the true severity of the obstruction.

The complete procedure has been evaluated with cine films of four perspex models of coronary obstructions. These models have circular cross sections and were filled with contrast medium. The area reduction percentages were measured for various settings of the X-ray system and with different concentrations of the contrast agent (Table 1).

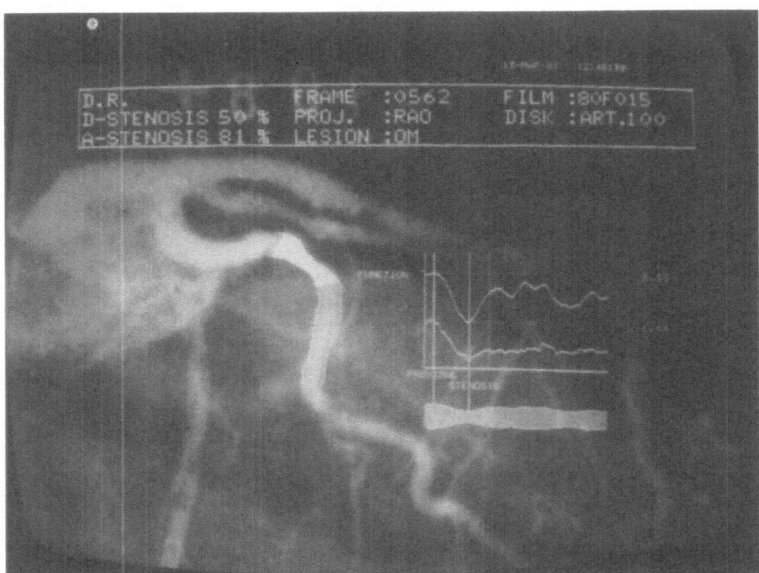

Fig. 13. For the obstruction of Fig. 5 the densitometric area function (lower curve) and the diameter function (upper curve) have been computed. A percentage densitometric area reduction of 81% is found

Table 1. Area reduction percentages measured for various settings of the X-ray system and with different concentrations of contrast agent

True percentage-area stenosis	Measured percentage-area stenosis		
	Film 1	Film 2	Film 3
86	85	87	85
75	78	72	73
44	44	41	39
0	8	8	4

Extension of the evaluation studies to noncircular models and to postmortem casts is currently being carried out. Also, studying the effects of dynamic flow of blood and contrast agent through the models is being anticipated.

Three-Dimensional Reconstruction Arterial Segment

As a next step we have looked at the feasibility to extend the densitometric procedure to the three-dimensional reconstruction of a coronary segment from two orthogonal views. Such a development is clinically of great importance, since it may allow the computation of several hemodynamic parameters, such as the hemodynamic resistance of the arterial segment and the blood flow through the artery after selective administration of a contrast bolus. These parameters may augment our knowledge in searching for the definition of the so-called "critical" stenosis. Furthermore, these three-dimensional data may provide us with detailed information about the development and presence of atherosclerotic plaque, e.g., insight into the possibly positive correlation between the location of the obstruction and the structure of the coronary arterial system, and in the influence of local blood flow profiles on the atherosclerotic process. Finally, the cardiologist and thorax surgeon may benefit from studying the three-dimensional representation of coronary arterial segments of a candidate for coronary bypass surgery prior to the operation.

The approach to the binary reconstruction problem from two orthogonal projections was originally developed by Slump and Gerbrands (1982) for the reconstruction of the left ventricle from biplane left ventricular angiograms. Since the two applications are basically identical, the algorithms actually implemented for the coronary arteries are very similar to those proposed for the reconstruction of the left ventricle. It should be mentioned here that the method can also handle the case where the projections are corrupted by noise. Details may be found in the references (Slump and Gerbrands 1982; Ford and Fulkerson 1962). In the remainder of this paper we will describe only briefly the applied principles. An example of the results obtained so far will be given.

If two orthogonal projections are available, the three-dimensional shape of the selected arterial segment can be reconstructed slice-by-slice in the following way. The two projections are analyzed sequentially in the way described, providing two densitometric absorption profiles for each cross section.

Under the assumption of complete and homogeneous filling of the artery with contrast agent and of the X-rays to be parallel at the structure of interest, we adopt the following discrete model. A slice of the artery is represented by a binary matrix. The matrix elements are "1" for positions that lie within the arterial cross section, and "0" for positions outside of it. In this discrete model the two absorption profiles obtained from the cineangiograms represent the row and column sums of the matrix. Therefore, we state our problem of reconstructing one slice as the reconstruction of a binary matrix from its row and column sums. From combinatorial mathematics the conditions are known for the existence of no, one, or more than one solution of this problem. Usually, there are many solutions, and other information has to be used to reduce the ambiguity. On physiological grounds, there must be a strong resemblance between two adjacent cross sections of the artery. We therefore reformulate our problem as the search for a binary matrix satisfying the projections with maximum resemblance to the previously reconstructed adjacent slice. It is attractive to incorporate a resemblance criterion in the reconstruction process directly, which we have achieved by introducing a cost coefficient $c(i, j)$ for every element (i, j) of the matrix, which represents the penalty for assigning that element the value "1" in the reconstruction. A simple example is to set $c(i, j)$ equal to zero if the matrix element (i, j) was an element of the arterial cross section in the previously reconstructed slice and equal to one otherwise. The minimum cost solution of the reconstruction problem will then show a high degree of similarity to the previous cross section. We have adapted algorithms from the operations research literature to find this minimum cost solution.

The two orthogonal frames required for the reconstruction are selected manually and the analyzed arterial segments in the two projections are aligned interactively by indicating two corresponding landmarks in the two frames. By this procedure the scales of both projections are matched as well. The first slice to be reconstructed is at the user-indicated reference region where the cross section of the artery is assumed to be elliptical in shape. A plot of an obstructed right coronary arterial segment, reconstructed slice-by-slice from two orthogonal arteriograms, is given in Fig. 14. Notice that similar plots can be displayed for any viewing angle, independent of the original projection angles. For this particular example a total of 155 slices were reconstructed. The two original coronary angiograms of the right coronary artery in the LAO and RAO projections with the detected contours superimposed are shown in Fig. 15a and b.

Concluding Remarks

The diameter analysis procedure has been evaluated extensively and is clinically used as a diagnostic tool. Also, different studies on the effects of interventions on coronary morphology, such as drug administration during cardiac catheterization, the percutaneous transluminal coronary angioplasty procedure (PTCA),

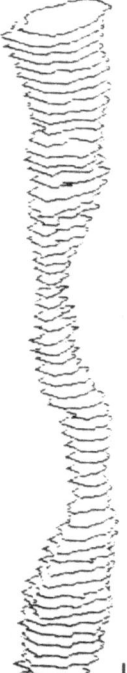

LAO 60   **Fig. 14.** Three-dimensional representation of obstructed arterial segment reconstructed from two orthogonal projections

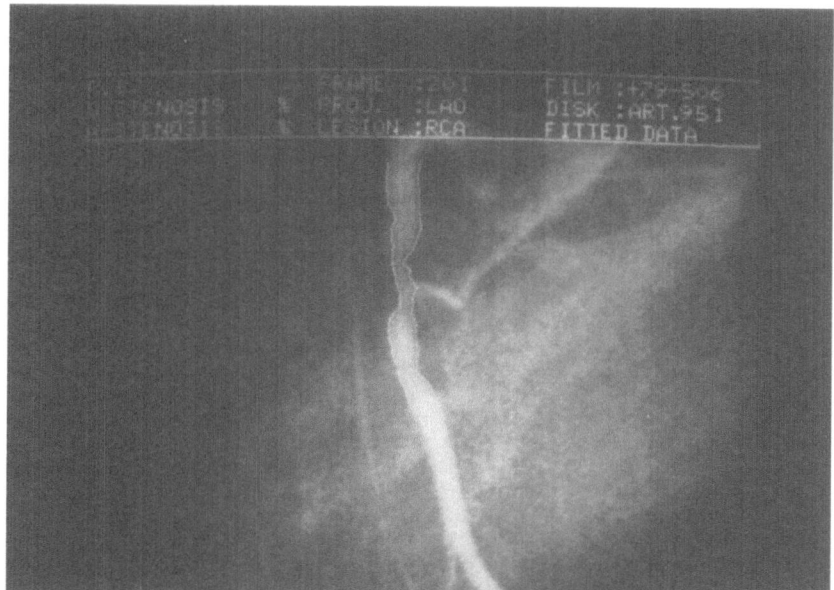

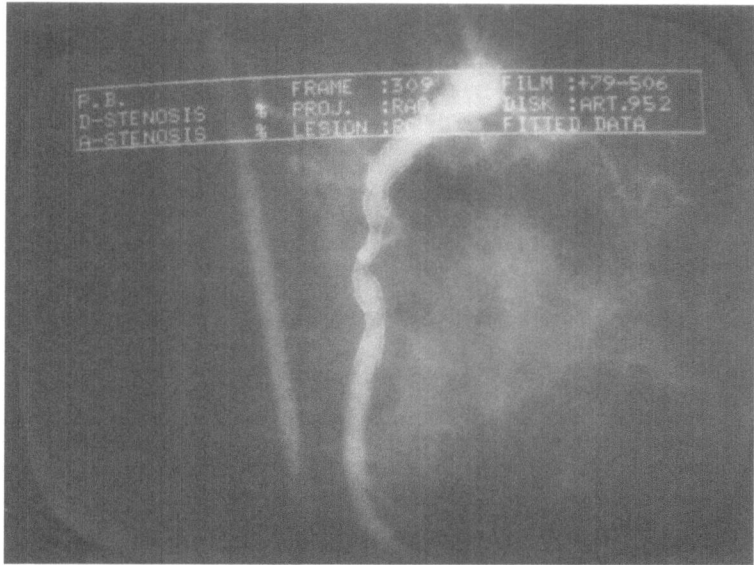

Fig. 15. The two orthogonal angiograms of a right coronary artery with the detected contours superimposed from which the three-dimensional presentation of Fig. 14 was reconstructed. *a* LAO projection, *b* RAO projection

and intracoronary thrombolysis have been or are being carried out (Serruys et al. 1980, 1981). The densitometric area reduction analysis procedure is currently being applied to the PTCA films. The first results from these clinical evaluations are certainly very promising. Three-dimensional reconstruction of coronary obstructions has not yet emerged from the research state.

Acknowledgements. The authors wish to acknowledge the support given by the Central Research Workshop of the Medical Faculty Rotterdam, which resulted in the implementation of the cinevideo converter. They also wish to thank Ria Kanters-Stam for preparing the manuscript.

References

Bolson EL, Brown BG, Dodge HT, Frimer M (1977) Computer analysis of coronary lesions. Proceedings of the Digital Equipment Computer Users Society, San Diego, pp 453–458

Booman F, Reiber JHC, Gerbrands JJ, Slager CJ, Schuurbiers JCH, Meesters GT (1979) Quantitative analysis of coronary occlusions from coronary cineangiograms. Proceedings computers in cardiology. IEEE Computer Society, Long Beach, pp 177–181

Brown BG, Bolson E, Frimer M, Dodge HT (1977) Quantitative coronary arteriography. Estimation of dimensions, hemodynamic resistance, and atheroma mass of coronary artery lesions using the arteriogram and digital computation. Circulation 55:329–337

De Rouen TA, Murray JA, Owen W (1977) Variability in the analysis of coronary arteriograms. Circulation 55:324–328

Detre KM, Wright E, Murphy ML, Takaro T (1975) Observer agreement in evaluating coronary angiograms. Circulation 52:979–986

Ford LR, Fulkerson DR (1962) Flows in networks. Princeton University Press, Princeton

Gensini GG (1975) Coronary angiography. Futura, New York

Gensini GG, Kelly AE, Da Costa BCB, Huntington PP (1971) Quantitative angiography: the measurement of coronary vasomobility in the intact animal and man. Chest 60:522–530

Gerbrands JJ, Reiber JHC, Booman F (1980) Computer processing and classification of coronary occlusions. In: Gelsema ES, Kanal LN (eds) Pattern recognition in practice. North-Holland, Amsterdam, pp 223–233

Ledbetter DC, Selzer RH, Gordon RM, Blankenhorn DH, Sanmarco ME (1978) Computer quantitation of coronary angiograms. In: Miller HA, Schmidt EV, Harrison DC (eds) Noninvasive cardiovascular measurements. SPIE 167:17–20

Rafflenbeul W, Heim R, Dzuiba M, Henkel B, Lichtlen P (1976) Morphometric analysis of coronary arteries. In: Lichtlen PR (ed) Coronary angiography and angina pectoris. Thieme, Stuttgart, pp 255–265

Reiber JHC, Troost GJ, Gerbrands JJ, Booman F, den Boer A, Serruys PW (1981) Densitometric assessment severity of coronary obstruction from monoplane views; three-dimensional reconstruction arterial segment from two orthogonal views. Proceedings computers in cardiology. IEEE Computer Society, Long Beach, pp 333–336

Sanders WJ, Alderman EL, Harrison DC (1979) Coronary artery quantitation using digital image processing techniques. Computers in cardiology. IEEE Computer Society, Long Beach, pp 15–20

Sandor T, Als AV, Paulin S (1979) Cine-densitometric measurement of coronary arterial stenoses. Cathet Cardiovasc Diagn 5:229–245

Selzer RH, Blankenhorn DH, Crawford DW, Brooks SH, Barndt R (1976) Computer analysis of cardiovascular imagery. Proceedings of the Caltech/JPL conference on image processing technology, data sources and software for commercial and scientific applications. Pasadena, pp 1–20

Serruys PW, Steward R, Booman F, Michels R, Reiber JHC, Hugenholtz PG (1980) Can unstable angina pectoris be due to increased coronary vasomotor tone? Eur Heart J 1 [Suppl B]:71–85

Serruys PW, Booman F, Troost GJ, Reiber JHC, Gerbrands JJ, Brand M, v. d. Cherrier F, Hugenholtz PG (1981) Computerized quantitative coronary angiography applied to the PTCA-procedure; advantages and limitations. Proceedings IVth symposium on coronary heart disease, Frankfurt, May 18–20

Slump Ch, Gerbrands JJ (1982) A network flow approach to reconstruction of the left ventricle from two projections. Comput Graphics and Image Proc 18:18–36

Smith WM, Starmer CF (1976) Computer representation of coronary arterial trees. Comput Biom Res 9:187–201

Starmer CF, Smith WM (1974) Problems in acquisition and representation of coronary arterial trees. Proceedings Computers in Cardiology. IEEE Computer Society, Long Beach, pp 143–147

Zir LM, Miller SW, Dinsmore RE, Gilbert JP, Harthorne JW (1976) Interobserver variability in coronary angiography. Circulation 53:627–632

Pressure Gradient and Cross-Sectional Area of Coronary Stenosis in Patients With and Without Exertional Angina

P. W. Serruys, J. H. C. Reiber, J. M. Lablanche, W. Wijns, M. v. d. Brand, P. G. Hugenholtz

Thoraxcenter, Erasmus University, P.O. 1738, DR 3000-Rotterdam, The Netherlands

Introduction

How "dynamic" is a coronary obstruction? What is a "critical" coronary stenosis? We do not pretend to bring a definitive answer to these two essential questions; however, we would like to demonstrate how quantitative coronary angiography has helped us to clarify these issues a little further.

Over the past few years we have developed and implemented a computer-based coronary angiography analysis system (CAAS) that allows accurate assessment of the percentage diameter narrowing of coronary lesions by means of automated contour detection principles [1–5]. Further developments over the past year have been directed towards the quantitative analysis of the density changes in coronary vessels, due to luminal narrowing, thus allowing the computation of percentage area stenosis of the analyzed lesion from a single projection (see also Reiber et al., this volume) [3].

How "Dynamic" Is a Coronary Obstruction?

In a highly selective group of 18 patients, known to have complaints of exertional and resting angina, we tried to explore the entire spectrum of coronary vasomotor tone by measuring the maximal changes in coronary arterial diameter, induced by a provocative test – bolus i.v. of 0.4 mg methylergobasine (Methergine) followed by an intracoronary injection of 3 mg isosorbide dinitrate (Risordan). A total of 20 stenotic coronary segments were selected for quantitative angiographic analysis. Before the pharmacologic intervention, a baseline coronary angiogram (control) was performed. Five minutes later, 0.4 mg Methergine was injected intravenously.

A second arteriogram was obtained 5 min after the i.v. injection of Methergine, or as soon as the patient developed chest pain and/or ST-T changes showed on his electrocardiogram. The third coronary angiogram was recorded 2 min after an intracoronary injection of isosorbide dinitrate (3 mg Risordan).

The quantitative analysis of selected coronary segments was carried out with the help of a computer-based coronary angiography analysis system (CAAS), developed and implemented at the Thoraxcenter [3–5] (see also Reiber et al., this volume). The basic principles of the system have been described in detail in

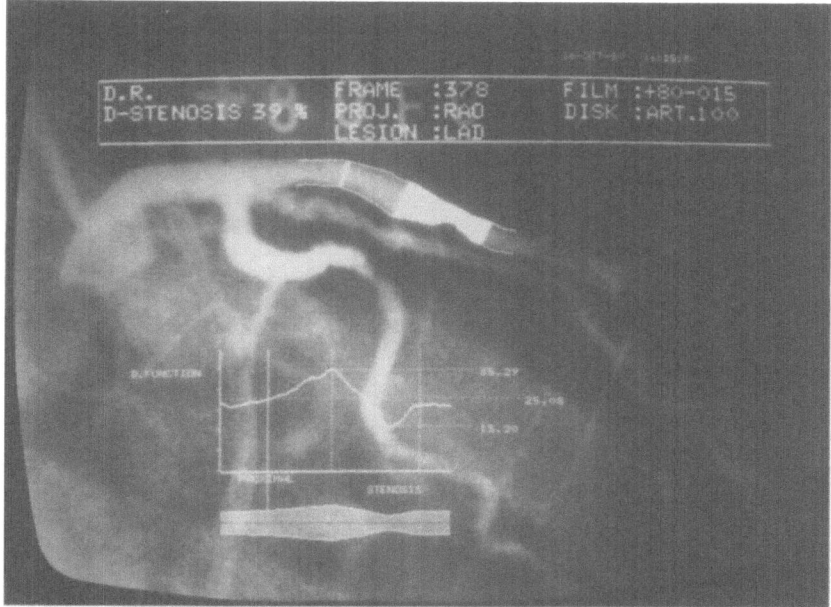

Fig. 1. Computer output of analyzed lesion in left anterior descending artery. A percentage diameter reduction of 50% with respect to the user-defined reference region is found

these proceedings and elsewhere. The final output of the system for a segment of the left anterior descending artery in the right anterior oblique projection is shown in Fig. 1. From the detected contour positions a diameter function is computed which is also shown in Fig. 1. Calibration of the diameter data is achieved by using the intracardiac catheter as a scaling device. The diameter values are plotted along the ordinate in mm and the positions along the centerline of the arterial segment from proximal to distal along the abscissa. From the minimum value Dm of the diameter function at the obstruction and the mean proximal diameter Dr at a user-indicated reference position, the percentage diameter reduction is computed as:

D-stenosis: $(1 - \dfrac{Dm}{Dr}) \times 100\%$

To determine the mean diameter of part of the processed arterial segment the boundaries of the segment in question must be indicated with a writing tablet.

It is emphasized that the X-ray system settings were not changed during consecutive filming after drug administration.

Results

The effects of Methergine i.v. and isosorbide dinitrate i.c. on the mean proximal diameter (Dr) and on the minimal obstruction diameter (Dm) are shown in Fig. 2.

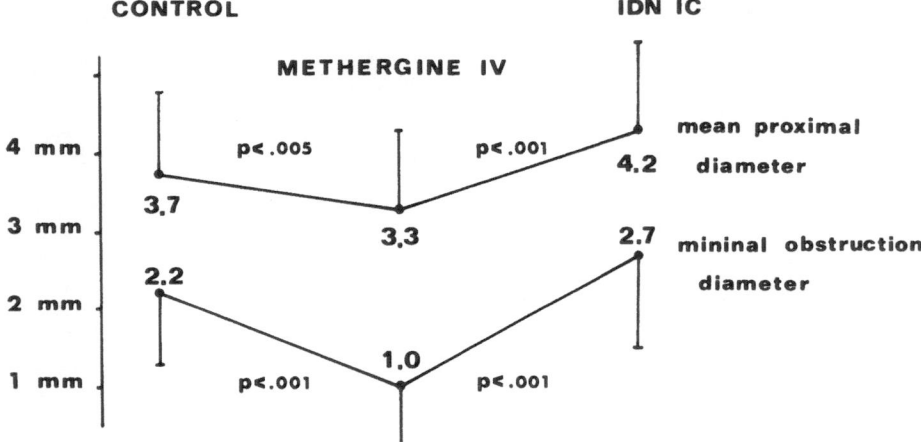

Fig. 2. Effects of Methergine i.v. and isosorbide dinitrate i.c. on the mean proximal diameter and on the minimal obstruction diameter

During the provocative test the mean proximal diameter decreases significantly ($P < 0.005$) by 10%, with respect to the basal condition, from 3.7 to 3.3 mm, whereas the minimal obstruction diameter is reduced by more than 50% from 2.2 to 1.0 mm ($P < 10^{-7}$). The intracoronary injection of isosorbide dinitrate provokes a very significant vasodilation of the obstructive lesion from 1.0 mm to 2.7 mm ($P < 10^{-8}$), as well as a significant increase in mean proximal diameter from 3.3 mm to 4.2 mm ($P < 10^{-6}$).

The individual changes in absolute stenosis diameter are given in Fig. 3. After Methergine six of the twenty analyzed stenotic lesions became transiently occluded, whereas isosorbide dinitrate i.c. increased the luminal diameters of all the obstructive lesions, which were vasoconstricted during the provocative test.

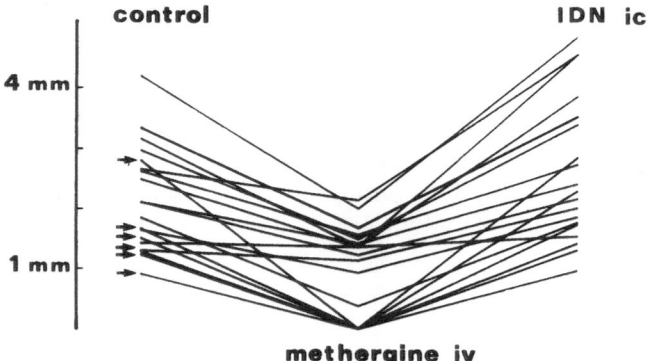

Fig. 3. Individual changes in absolute stenosis diameter after Methergine i.v. and isosorbide dinitrate i.c. Six (marked with *arrows*) of the 20 stenotic lesions analyzed are transiently occluded during the provocative test

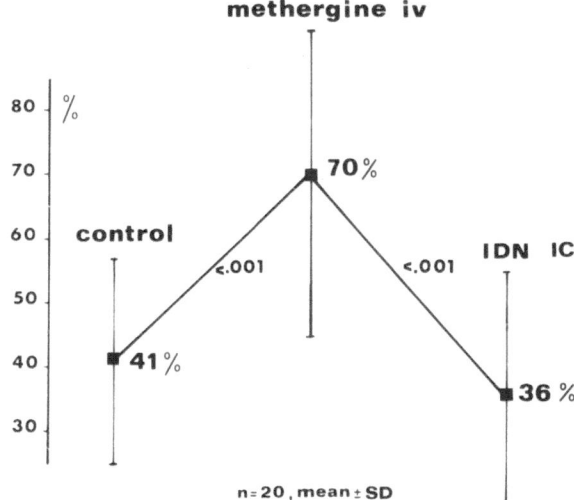

Fig. 4. Changes in percentage diameter stenosis during the provocative test and after the intracoronary injection of isosorbide dinitrate

In terms of percentage diameter stenosis, the severity of the obstructive lesions increased on average from 41% to 70% (P < 0.0001) during the provocative test and returned to an average value of 36% after the intracoronary injection of isosorbide dinitrate (Fig. 4).

Quantitation of vasomotion observed by angiography is limited to comparing the luminal diameter in two or more states of vasomotion. Because we cannot see the arterial wall itself, we do not always appreciate the changes occurring in it that produce the variations in luminal dimensions, which we call vasomotion.

Let us take a normal coronary artery segment with an outer diameter of 2.4 mm and an inner diameter of 2.0 mm (Fig. 5). If we assume that there is no change in the length of the artery as the result of changes in its diameter, then at any point of the artery the area of the arterial wall on a transverse cross section of the vessel will be constant regardless of the state of its contraction or dilatation. As vasoconstriction occurs, the luminal diameter decreases proportionately more than the outer diameter of the vessel and the wall thickness increases.

At the top of Fig. 5, we see a coronary stenotic lesion with a 30% diameter stenosis in the basal condition. Now let us assume that a 10% decrease in the outer diameter occurs as a result of vasoconstriction, that is, the outer diameter becomes 2.16 mm (bottom drawing of Fig. 5). Under the assumption of constant transverse cross section it can be derived from single geometric principles that a 15% decrease occurs in the luminal diameter of the prestenotic segment. At the stenotic site, because of the modest mural thickening due to disease, the luminal diameter decreases in greater proportion; in the present case a 34% decrease in obstruction diameter can be predicted. As suggested by MacAlpin, "a modest mural thickening due to disease may act as a 'lever' in translating physiologic degrees of medial smooth muscle shortening into critical luminal obstruction . . ." [6]. Therefore, using these elementary geometric principles, we calcu-

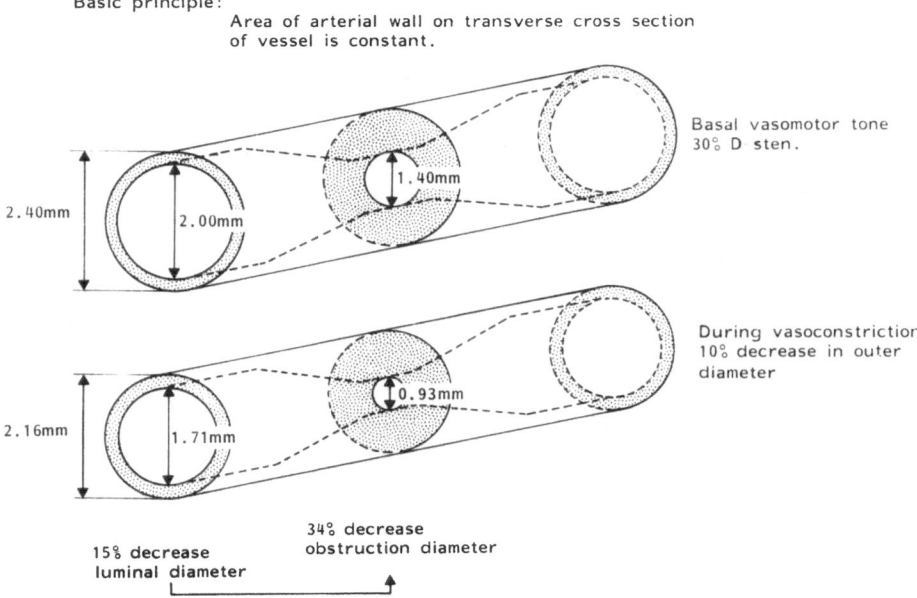

Basic principle:
Area of arterial wall on transverse cross section
of vessel is constant.

Basal vasomotor tone
30% D sten.

During vasoconstriction
10% decrease in outer
diameter

2.40mm   2.00mm   1.40mm

2.16mm   1.71mm   0.93mm

15% decrease
luminal diameter

34% decrease
obstruction diameter

Fig. 5. Contribution of dynamic vascular wall thickening to luminal narrowing during coronary arterial constriction

lated and reconstructed the changes that might occur at the stenotic sites as the result of vasomotion acting on the entire coronary segment (see Appendix). In Fig. 6, the decrease in luminal diameter of a normal prestenotic segment is plotted against the expected decrease in luminal diameter of the stenotic segment for a stenosis with a 20% diameter reduction. For this example a 20% decrease in luminal diameter of the normal segment causes a 33% decrease in diamter of the stenotic segment. When applying this theoretical relationship to the different states of vasomotion measured in our group of 18 patients, we found that the behavior of the stenotic lesions during vasoconstriction deviated considerably from this theoretical relationship, some stenotic lesions being hypercontractile and others being hypocontractile (Fig. 7).

As a matter of fact, only four stenotic lesions did react as predicted by the theory and we can conclude that their decrease in luminal diameter at the stenotic sites was simply the result of an increase in vasomotor tone superimposed on an organically narrowed vessel. Six stenotic lesions were hypocontractile and the vessel wall at the site of the lesion actually constricted less than suggested by the theoretical model. In five cases we even had predicted a total occlusion which was not observed. As for the 12 remaining lesions, they all showed arterial hypercontractility and four of them, unexpectedly, became totally occluded during vasoconstriction.

These results demonstrate how unpredictable the effects of changes in vasomotor tone can be on the large coronary artery. Understanding of these changes is essential before a rational definition of a critical stenosis can be made.

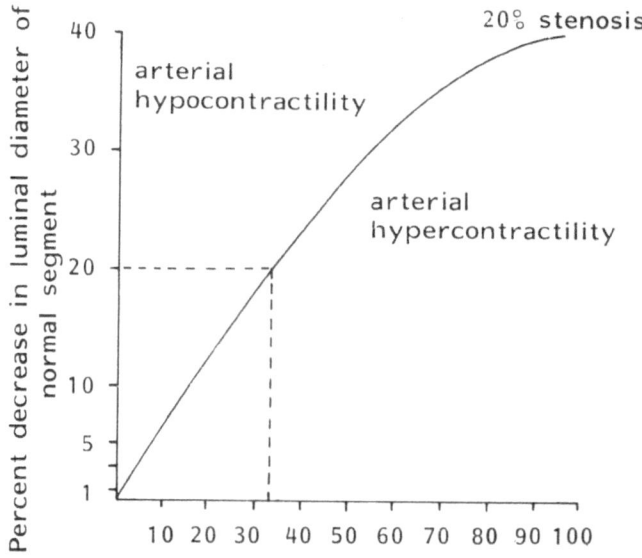

Fig. 6. Percentage decrease in luminal diameter in a normal segment of artery adjacent to a stenosis (*ordinate*) and percentage decrease in diameter at the stenosis, expected to result from the same degree of outer wall circumferential shortening that caused the observed decrease in lumen in the adjacent normal segment of vessel (*abscissa*). The curve is plotted for a stenosis of 20%

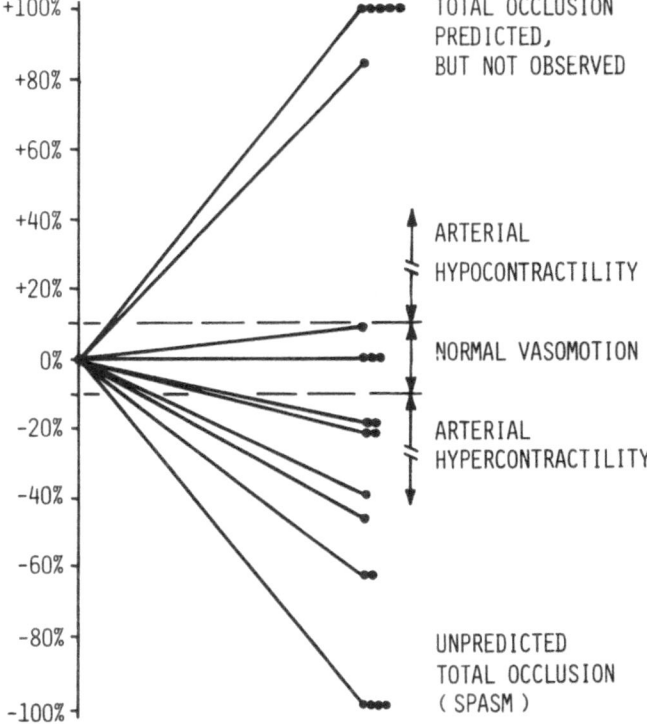

Fig. 7. Percentage deviation of the obstruction diameters from predicted values after Methergine

When trying to evaluate what constitutes a physiologically significant obstruction to blood flow during exercise, we implicitly assume that the pathogenesis of exertional angina pectoris is based primarily on the concept of a "fixed" stenosis [2]. Therefore in order to prevent any significant active vasomotion occurring and to "fix" the lesion, we decided to study our patients in a state of complete coronary vasodilation.

What Is a "Critical" Stenosis?

Study Population and Methods

Transstenotic pressure gradient and cross-sectional area stenosis were correlated in 43 individuals with an isolated obstruction in the left anterior descending artery. Of these 43 patients, 26 had undergone a successful transluminal angioplasty and the measurements obtained corresponded thus to the anatomical situation resulting from the procedure. In these patients the transstenotic gradient was measured with a variety of catheters: 2F (Ganz-Edwards coronary infusion catheter; Edwards Laboratories, Santa Ana, Calif.), 3F (Grüntzig coronary perfusion catheter; Schneider Medintag, Zürich), and 4F (Grüntzig dilatation catheter; Schneider). In the remaining 16 patients, the measurements were obtained during the procedure by measuring the transstenotic gradient with the dilating catheter (4.5F Grüntzig). Coronary angiography was performed systematically after an intracoronary injection of 0.2 mg nifedipine [7]. The day before catheterization, early and late postexercise thallium scintigraphy was carried out, 60 min after an oral administration of 10 or 20 mg nifedipine. Early postexercise scintigrams were acquired following the intravenous injection of 2 mCi thallium-201, 1 min before the end of a maximal or symptom-limited exercise test on the bicycle ergometer. Imaging was started within 10 min and 400 000 counts were collected in each of three views (anterior, LAO 45°, LAO 65°). Late postexercise scintigrams were obtained 3–4 h after the exercise test.

Early and late postexercise thallium-201 scintigrams were processed on a DEC gamma-11 computer system with a quantification procedure developed in our institute [8]. Basically, the procedure consists of computing circumferential profiles in the early and late postexercise images to quantitate the relative radionuclide activity in the myocardium. Corresponding early and late images are registered in the computer using external markers (Co-57 point sources) which were taped to the patient's chest. Circumferential profile analysis is facilitated by automated contour detection of the thallium-201 activity distribution in the images. Background activity is corrected using a method similar to the one developed by Watson et al. [9].

The circumferential profiles and the original images were interpreted by three independent observers. The myocardial thallium-201 uptake patterns of each view were divided into segments and the severity of a defect in both early and late postexercise images was scored as follows: 0, no thallium uptake; 1, severely abnormal; 2, definitely abnormal; 3, doubtfully abnormal; 4, normal.

In the three specific views, the scores of all segments for a given artery [10] (the LAD, in our study) were added and the difference between early and late postexercise values was taken as a measure for the amount of redistribution. Using this semiquantitative approach, the three independent observers decided on an area being ischemic or not.

Results

The principal determinants of the pressure gradient across a stenosis are the blood flow through the stenosis and the length and diameter of the stenosis. However, most studies on the hemodynamic effect of arterial stenosis have demonstrated that the most important determinant of pressure gradient across a stenosis is the diameter of the stenosis [11, 12].

In general, these studies have also shown that absolute dimensions and not percentage diameter stenosis determine the hemodynamic severity. The relationship between the mean pressure gradient normalized for the mean aortic pressure and the absolute dimension of the minimal obstruction diameter for our group of patients is shown in Fig. 8. The relationship is nonlinear and the curve which best fits (minimal residual error, maximal coefficient of correlation) the measured pressure gradient-diameter values is given by the equation $\triangle P/\overline{AOP} = a + b \log (Dm)$. In other words, a steep increase in pressure gradient with increasing severity of the stenosis appears only after a "critical stenosis" is reached. Obviously this approach to assessing the significance of a stenosis needs further validation and many problems, such as the influence of irregular geometric features of a stenosis on the pressure gradient, need to be solved.

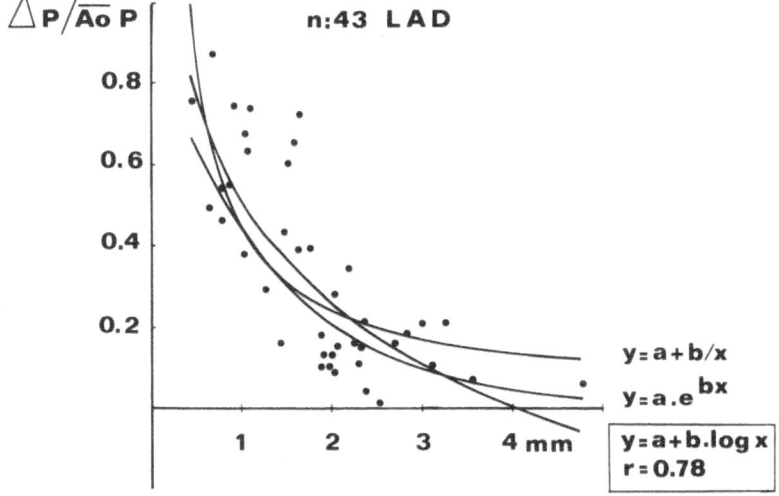

Fig. 8. Relationship between the mean pressure gradient normalized from the mean aortic pressure and the absolute dimension of the minimal obstruction diameter

In addition, measurement of luminal diameter for quantitation of lumen narrowing is subject to criticism, as we have demonstrated previously [3, 13] (see also Reiber et al., this volume).

Since the luminal cross section at a coronary obstruction is frequently irregular in shape, percentage diameter reduction measured in a single projection is of limited diagnostic value. The hemodynamic resistance of an obstruction is determined to a great extent by changes in the cross-sectional areas of the lumen. Computation of the cross-sectional area reduction from the percentage diameter reduction measured in a single view requires the assumption of, e.g., circular cross sections, an assumption which hardly ever holds.

To circumvent these limitations we have developed a densitometric procedure to determine the changes in cross-sectional areas of a coronary segment by using the density information within the artery [3] so that the severity can be expressed as a true percentage area reduction, by comparing the minimal area value at the obstruction site with the mean area value at the selected reference position. That ist the reason why, on Fig. 9, the degree of obstruction is now expressed in percentage area stenosis.

When analyzing the relationship between pressure drop ($\triangle P/\overline{AOP}$) and percentage area stenosis (% – A sten), minimal residual error and maximal coefficient of correlation ($r = 0.76$) were obtained by an exponential equation ($y = 0.036e^{0.028x}$). It must be emphasized that this exponential relationship gives a curve closely resembling the data experimentally obtained in isolated human coronary arteries when the hydraulic effects of actual human coronary stenoses on pressure gradient are investigated [14]. Moreover, diverse experimental work has shown that the critical point, for an adequate resting blood flow is reached when cross-sectional area has been reduced to approximately 10% of the preexisting lumen [15].

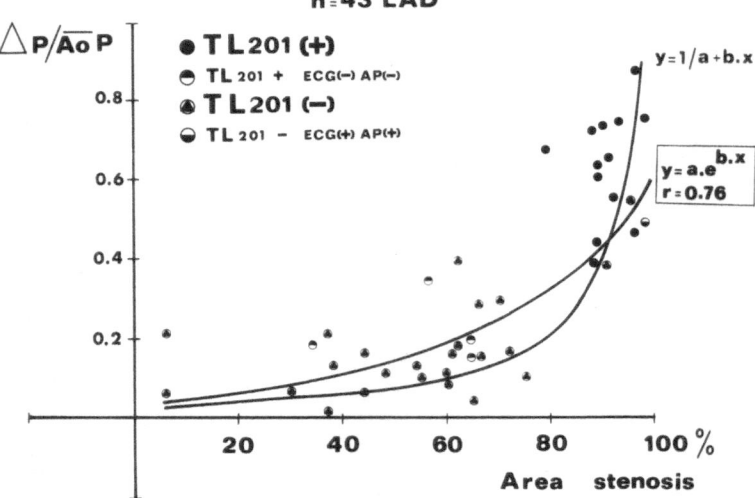

Fig. 9. Relationship between the mean pressure gradient normalized for the mean aortic pressure and the percentage area stenosis. Positive and negative stress thallium scintigraphies are indicated

In Fig. 9, the dots indicate positive stress thallium scintigraphies, whereas the triangles correspond to negative thallium scintigraphies. In our patients, a value of 0.4 normalized mean pressure gradient as well as a percentage area stenosis of 80% seems to constitute under resting conditions two critical thresholds beyond which stress thallium scintigraphy is mostly positive. However, three cases must be considered as false negatives; two of them had an important collateral network which could explain the negativity of the test. Conversely, four patients must be considered as having false positive thallium scintigrams, although they were asymptomatic and without ECG changes during maximal exercise.

In summary,

1. Based on the present study, we conclude that the geometric changes that occur at the stenotic sites as a result of vasomotion are unpredictable for individual patients.

2. When studying our patients in a state of complete coronary vasodilation, we found that a cross-sectional area obstruction of 80% constitutes a physiologically significant obstruction to blood flow during exercise.

Appendix: Geometric Considerations: Dynamic Vascular Wall Thickening

Let us assume a coronary artery that is circular in cross section when distended by a normal blood pressure and has an outer radius R_o (including the media but excluding the adventitia). Furthermore, there is a coronary obstruction in the segment under consideration with a minimal (luminal) obstruction diameter r_i; the luminal reference diameter in the normal prestenotic segment equals R_i.

Figure 10 shows the cross sections at the reference position and at the site of the obstruction with the definitions of the different radii. The area A_R of the arterial wall at the reference cross section equals $A_R = \pi (R_0{}^2 - R_i{}^2)$ and the area A_0 at the obstruction $A_0 = \pi (R_0{}^2 - r_i{}^2)$. These diameter values define the control situation. A new situation is created as vasoconstriction occurs. For practical purposes, the material of the arterial wall is plastic but incompressible. If we assume that there is no change in the length of the artery as the result of changes in its diameter, and no extrusion of tissue from the constricted area into nonconstricted, adjacent parts of the artery, then at any point of the artery the area of the arterial wall on a transverse cross section of the vessel will be constant regardless of the state of its contraction or dilation.

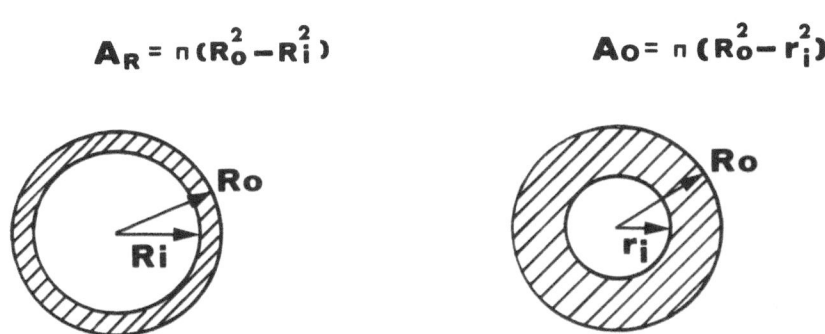

REFERENCE CROSS SECTION   OBSTRUCTION CROSS SECTION

Fig. 10. A hypothetical coronary artery with circular cross sections at a prestenotic reference position and at the site of a coronary obstruction

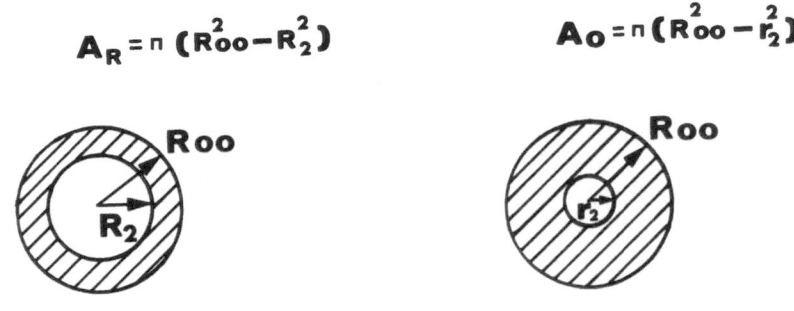

REFERENCE CROSS SECTION   OBSTRUCTION CROSS SECTION

Fig. 11. Cross sections of artery in Fig. 10 after vasoconstriction

If we denote the new outer diameter R_{00}, the luminal obstruction diameter r_2, and the reference diameter R_2 in the state of vasoconstriction, then the following equations hold (Fig. 11):

$$A_R = \pi \ (R_{00}^2 - R_2^2) = \pi \ (R_0^2 - R_i^2) \tag{1}$$
$$\text{or} \quad R_0^2 - R_{00}^2 = R_i^2 - R_2^2 \tag{2}$$
$$\text{and } A_0 = \pi \ (R_{00}^2 - r_2^2) = \pi \ (R_0^2 - r_i^2) \tag{3}$$
$$\text{or} \quad R_0^2 - R_{00}^2 = r_i^2 - r_2^2 \tag{4}$$

Then Eqs. (2) and (4) yield:

$$r_2^2 = r_i^2 - R_i^2 + R_2^2 \tag{5}$$

Thus, if we know the reference diameter in the control state (R_i) and after vasoconstriction (R_2) and the obstruction diameter r_i in the control state, then we can predict the minimal obstruction diameter r_2 after vasoconstriction from Eq. (5).

It should be clear that Eqs. (1)–(5) are equally valid for vasoconstriction and vasodilation.

References

1. Serruys PW, Steward R, Booman F, Michels R, Reiber JHC, Hugenholtz PG (1980) Can unstable angina pectoris be due to increased coronary vasomotor tone? Eur Heart J 1 [Suppl B]: 71–85
2. Epstein SE, Talbot TL (1981) Dynamic coronary tone in precipitation, exacerbation and relief of angina pectoris. Am J Cardiol 48:797–803
3. Reiber JHC, Troost GJ, Gerbrands JJ, Booman F, den Boer A, Serruys PW (1981) Densitometric assessment severity of coronary obstruction from monoplane views; three-dimensional reconstruction arterial segment from two orthogonal views. Proceedings computers in cardiology. IEEE Computer Society, Long Beach
4. Booman F, Reiber JHC, Gerbrands JJ, Slager CJ, Schuurbiers JCH, Meester GT (1979) Quantitative analysis of coronary occlusions from coronary cineangiograms. Proceedings computers in cardiology. IEEE Computer Society, Long Beach, pp 177–181
5. Gerbrands JJ, Reiber JHC, Booman F (1980) Computer processing and classification of coronary occlusions. In: Gelsema ES, Kanal LN (eds) Pattern recognition in practice. North-Holland, Amsterdam, pp 223–233
6. MacAlpin RN (1980) Contribution of dynamic vascular wall thickening to luminal narrowing during coronary arterial constriction. Circulation 60:296–301

7. Serruys PW, Steward R, Booman F, van den Brand M, Reiber JHC (1980) Effects of intracoronary nifedipine on coronary vasomobility and left ventricular hemodynamics. Circulation 62 [Suppl III]:87
8. Lie SP, Reiber JHC, Simoons ML, Gerbrands JJ, Kooy PPM, Bakker WH (1981) Computer processing of thallium-201 myocardial scintigrams. Proceedings 2nd International Conference on Visual Psychophysics and Medical Imaging. IEEE CH 16 766, pp 19–26
9. Watson DD, Campell NP, Read EK, Gibson RS, Teates CD, Beller GA (1981) Special and temporal quantitation of plane thallium myocardial images. J Nucl Med 22:577–584
10. Rigo P, Bailey IK, Griffith LSC, Pitt B, Burow RD, Wagner HN, Becker LC (1980) Value and limitation of segmental analysis of stress thallium myocardial imaging for localization of coronary artery disease. Circulation 61:973–981.
11. Fiddian RV, Byar D, Edwards EA (1964) Factors affecting flow through a stenosed vessel. Arch Surg 88:105–112
12. Gould L, Lipscomb K, Hamilton GW (1974) Physiologic basis for assessing critical coronary stenosis. Am J Cardiol 33:89–94
13. Serruys PW, Booman F, Troost GJ, Reiber JHC, Gerbrands JJ, van den Brand M, Cherrier F, Hugenholtz PG (1981) Computerized quantitative coronary angiography applied to the PTCA-procedure; advantages and limitations. Proceedings IVth symposium on coronary heart disease, Frankfurt, pp 18–20
14. Logan SE (1975) On the fluid mechanics of human coronary artery stenosis. IEEE Trans Biomed Eng 22:327–334
15. Mates RE, Gupta RL, Bell AC, Klocke FJ (1978) Fluid dynamics of coronary stenosis. Circ Res 42:152

Measurement of the Degree of Coronary Stenosis Using Digital Densitometry

P. A. DORIOT,[1] L. RASOAMANAMBELO,[1] Y. POCHON,[2] and W. RUTISHAUSER[1]

[1] Center of Cardiology, University Hospital, Geneva, Switzerland
[2] Institute of Applied Physics, EPF, Lausanne, Switzerland

Introduction

Experimental studies have shown that the demarcation between hemodynamically irrelevant and significant stenoses of a vessel is quite sharp. Accurate evaluation of the degree of stenosis of a coronary artery (or, indirectly, of the cross-sectional area of the subsistent lumen) is therefore an important aspect in many clinical studies.

The various methods which have been proposed to improve accuracy can be classified into two groups: those which use morphologic information only, and those based upon densitometry [1–6].

We have chosen the second approach because of the inherent limitation set on any morphologic method by the noncircular shape of the stenotic cross section.

Basic Principle

The basic principle of our method is illustrated in Fig. 1. It consists in establishing the quotient M_s/M_p of the quantities of contrast medium M_s and M_p contained in two thin vessel slices of the same width. The degree of stenosis is then

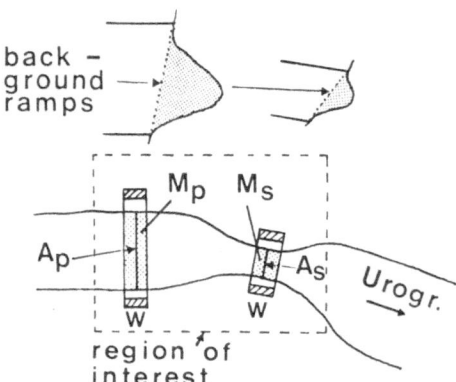

Fig. 1. Principle of measurement of the degree of stenosis

$1 - M_s/M_p$. (M_s/M_p is equal to the quotient A_s/A_p of the cross-sectional areas A_s and A_p if constant concentration of the contrast medium in the vessel segment is realized in the analyzed cine frames.)

The information necessary to compute M_s/M_p is obtained from the optical density of the film measured on scans perpendicular to the vessel axis, under application of corrections for the nonlinearity of the film and for the nonapplicability of the Lambert-Beer absorption law for polychromatic X-ray radiation.

This approach has two essential advantages. First, one is independent of the shape of the stenotic cross section. Secondly, if, instead of diameters, cross sections are measured with the same percentual accuracy, the error of the calculated degree of stenosis is reduced by a factor of two.

Since in reality we measure volumes, namely, the volumes of the two thin slices, this methodological aspect is even more favorable (M_s and M_p are also proportional to the slice volumes).

Measurement System

The measurement system consists of a cine projector, a TV camera with TV monitor to visualize the diseased artery segment with great magnification, a video-analog-to-digital converter, a computer PDP-11/10 with digital disk and a light-pen for interaction of the operator with the program (for instance, to define measurement windows onto the vessel).

Measurements of the reduction of the degree of stenosis achieved by transluminal dilatation and studies of the effect of 1.6 mg nitroglycerin sublingual on isolated coronary stenosis performed with this system have shown that densitometry provides quite reasonable results [3].

Accuracy Considerations

However, the accuracy of densitometric (and morphologic) methods cannot be assessed in vivo only. In vitro experiments are necessary to clarify some fundamental aspects.

Since accuracy is the decisive advantage that densitometry is expected to offer, it is helpful to establish first a comparison base with the morphologic approach.

Let us consider an ideal case of stenosis with perfectly circular stenotic and prestenotic cross sections. The respective diameters shall be 1.34 mm and 3.00 mm, which yields a degree of stenosis of 80% (area reduction). If we assume that the four vessel walls involved can be delineated with an accuracy of $\pm$ 0.15 mm (which from our experience is not always achievable [2,6]), we obtain two "worst-case" erroneous degrees of stenosis of 63% and 90%. This means that the stenosis can be evaluated as hemodynamically irrelevant just as well as severe. Even if we assume an accuracy of $\pm$ 0.1 mm, the correct evaluation remains problematic, since we obtain 70% and 87% respectively for the degree of stenosis.

Model Experiments

A primordial step in assessing the accuracy in vitro is to investigate the quality of the information on the film. At this level, the characteristic curve of the film (Hunter-Driffield, or H-D, function) plays an important role. Densitometry indeed involves differences between logarithms of the local film exposure, but in cine densitometry only the resulting optical densities are readily measurable. If the densities of interest are not restricted to the rectilinear part of the H-D curve, the influence of the film nonlinearity must be assessed.

To this purpose, and to investigate the achievable accuracy at film level, a model consisting of nine test sections drilled in a Plexiglas plate and filled with Urografin 76% was used. This phantom was filmed under similar conditions as by routine coronarograms and analyzed with the help of a microdensitometer.

By combining the nine cross-sectional areas obtained densitometrically (Fig. 2, top left panel) in pairs, the 36 degrees of stenosis shown in the right panel can be calculated.

The data were obtained from a single image, so that the impact of quantum noise can also be appreciated. The scanning width on each test section was 8 mm in order to reduce the effect of film grain (the same reduction could be obtained by averaging eight images with a scanning width of 1 mm).

As can be seen from the two middle panels of Fig. 2, the correction of the film nonlinearity does not remove the strong deviation from linearity of the densitometric cross sections, nor does ist improve the accuracy of the derived degrees of stenosis. (The scales of the ordinates are freely chosen for ease of comparison. The figure does not allow for quantification of the deviation from the identity line.)

Importance of the Correction for Polychromasy

If the correction for the nonapplicability of the Lambert-Beer law as described by Pochon et al. (this volume) is applied, the cross sections are forced to the identity line (Fig. 2, bottom left panel) and the 36 measured degrees of stenosis improve markedly (bottom right panel), the greatest error being inferior to 6% (SEE 2.7%). These results demonstrate that the information contained in the optical density of the film has a potential accuracy far beyond the accuracy that could be obtained using the best morphologic method.

The maximum error of 6% is not quite independent of the model chosen, and it is possible to design a specially sensitive case where it would be a few percent larger. On the other hand, one must consider first that the "true" values for the degrees of our stenosis drilled in Plexiglas are themselves only accurate to ± 3%, and, secondly, that only one image of the cine film was used, so that the greatest errors could be further compressed by averaging, for instance, five images.

The necessity of a correction for the polychromasy effect can be evidenced in a still more striking manner by the experiment depicted in Fig. 3 under A and B. Two 50% stenoses were created by introducing two identical pieces of Plexiglas

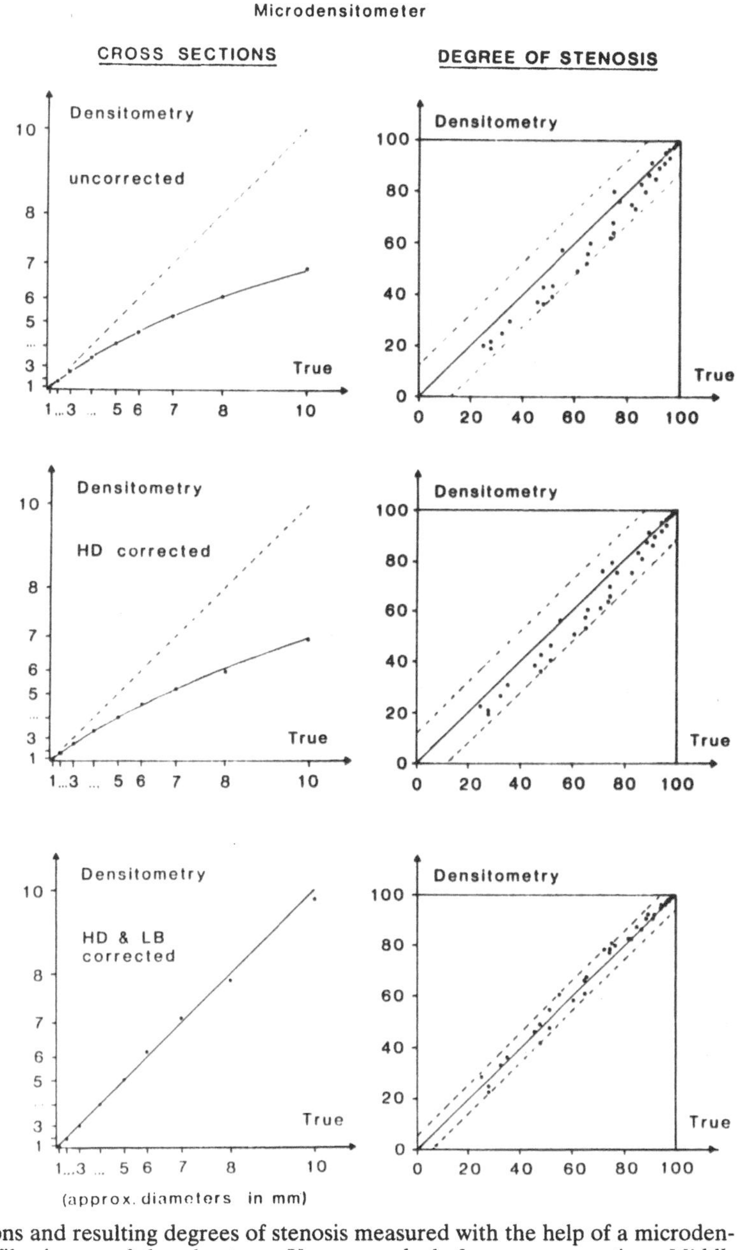

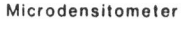

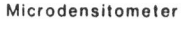

Fig. 2. Cross sections and resulting degrees of stenosis measured with the help of a microdensitometer on one film image of the phantom. *Upper panels:* before any correction. *Middle panels:* after correction of the film nonlinearity. *Bottom panels:* after correction for the film nonlinearity and for the X-ray beam polychromasy

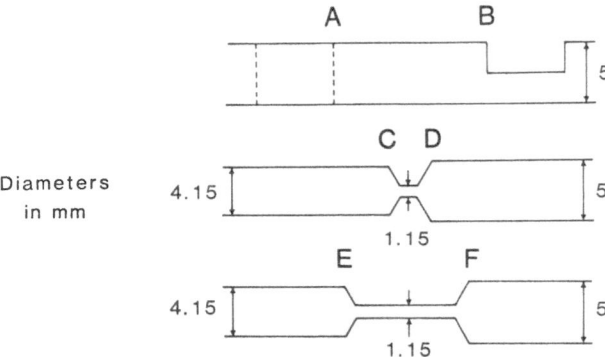

Diameters in mm

DEGREE OF STENOSIS
(Area reduction in %)

	A	B	C	D	E	F
True	50	50	92	95	92	95
Uncorrected	28	58	89	92	90	93
HD corrected	37	55	91	93	93	95
HD & LB corrected	49	51	92	96	95	97

Fig. 3a–f. Identical stenosis of 50% seen frontally (*A*) and from the side (*B*). The particular shape of the stenotic cross-sectional area (*half-moon*) and the large nonstenotic diameter (5 mm) chosen allow demonstration of the necessity of a correction for polychromy of the X-ray beam. *C, D, E, F:* Experiment showing that the light diffusion of the prestenotic and poststenotic segments does not appreciably influence the measured 4 degrees of stenosis shown here

with half-moon shaped cross sections into a hole of 5 mm in diameter drilled into a Plexiglas plate. The first one is seen frontally and the second one from the side. The model is filled with Urografin 76%. As can be seen from the degrees of stenosis (columns A and B, second and third line), correction of the film nonlinearity improves the accuracy slightly, but a correction of the polychromacy effect is indispensable to obtain accurate values (third line). Note that the degree of stenosis in column B, which one would expect to be always close to 50%, is also forced to the expected value.

To correct for the nonlinearity of the film, a gray scale step wedge registered several weeks before the experiment was used. This allows the consideration that a sample H-D curve, or, better, an average one, might be included into the computer program and used as long as the film type and the development parameters are not changed.

Figure 3 shows also in C, D, E, and F an experiment performed simultaneously to test whether the pre- and poststenotic segments influence the optical

System

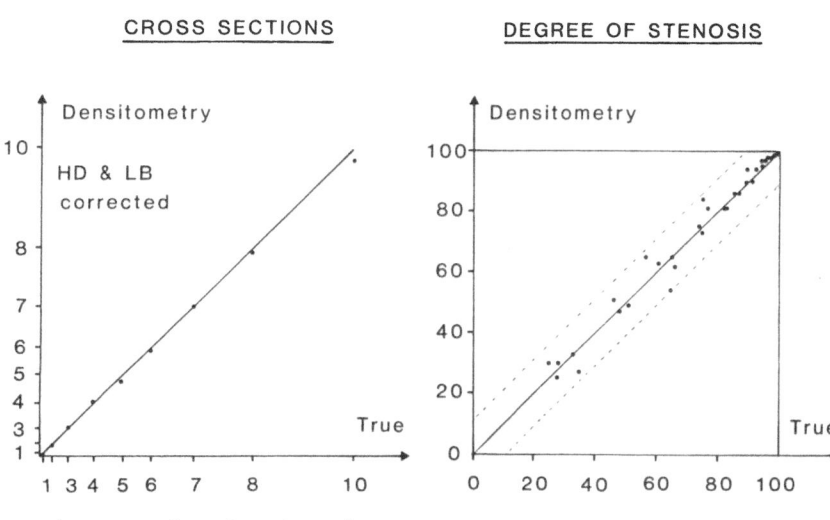

CROSS SECTIONS   DEGREE OF STENOSIS

Fig. 4. Results of measurements performed on the test sections phantom with help of the system under particularly severe conditions

density of the stenotic segment by light diffusion. The densitometric cross-sectional area of the short stenosis was indeed slightly greater (10%), but this had no influence on the degree of stenosis measured.

Robustness of the Method

Figure 4 shows the degrees of stenosis obtained by averaging five images of the nine test sections modeled by using the measurement system under very severe conditions. In this test, the nine cross sections were measured with the same settings, the smallest tube being buried in noise. The inverse transformation of the H-D function was not explicitly performed. Instead we used intermediate coefficients A_{1phot} and A_{3phot} obtained from the wedge experiment described by Pochon et al. (this volume). These coefficients correct for monochromaticity and, to a certain extent, for the film nonlinearity, but they are not so accurate as the coefficients A_1 and A_3 obtained by explicit inverse transformation of the H-D function. Under these extreme conditions, the greatest error dit not exceed 11%.

Figure 5 shows the corresponding standard deviations of the nine densitometric cross sections. At 2 mm diameter, it has already dropped to under 5%.

Standard deviation in %

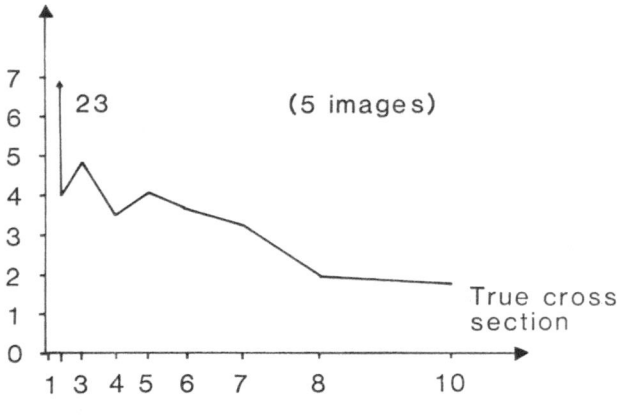

(approximate diameters in mm)

Fig. 5. Standard deviation of each cross section measured on five images

Conclusion

This basic study shows that the information content of the optical density of the film has the potential for very accurate evaluation of degrees of stenosis (and also for assessment of the subsistent cross-sectional area of the stenotic segment in mm^2 by calibration on an intact artery segment with circular cross section). In vivo measurements, however, require care during the contrast medium injection into the coronaries to achieve momentary constant concentration of the dye in the vessel segments investigated.

References

1. Booman F, Reiber J, Gerbrands J, Slager C, Schuurbiers J, Meester G (1979) Quantitative analysis of coronary occlusions from coronary cine-angiograms. Computers in cardiology. IEEE Computer Society, Long Beach, pp 177–180
2. Brown B, Bolson E, Frimer M, Dodge H (1977) Estimation of dimensions, hemodynamic resistance and atheroma mass of coronary artery lesions using the arteriogram and digital computation. Circulation 55:329–337
3. Doriot P, Rasoamanambelo L, Honegger H, Mérier G, Bopp P, Rutishauser W (1981) Measurement of the degree of coronary stenosis by digital densitometry. Computers in cardiology. IEEE Computer Society, Long Beach, pp 329–332
4. Reiber J, Troost G, Gerbrands J, Booman F, Den Boer A, Serruys P (1981) Densitometric assessment severity of coronary obstruction from monoplane views; three-dimensional reconstruction arterial segment from two orthogonal views. Computers in cardiology. IEEE Computer Society, Long Beach pp 333–336
5. Sandor T, Als A, Paulin S (1979) Cinedensitometric measurement of coronary arterial stenosis. Cathet Cardiovasc Diagn 6:229–245
6. Hoornstra K, Hanselman J, Holland W, De Wey Peters G, Zwamborn A (1980) Videodensitometry for measuring blood vessel diameter. Acta Radiol Diagn 21 [2A]:155–164

Clinical Implications and Results of Quantitative Coronary Angiography

W. Rafflenbeul and P. R. Lichtlen

Hannover Medical School, Division of Cardiology, Hannover, FRG

Introduction

Quantitative coronary angiography involves in the first place an accurate analysis of the severity of coronary artery stenosis. This objective assessment using different measuring techniques (Rafflenbeul et al. 1975; Brown et al. 1977; Reiber et al 1979) is mandatory, predominantly for of the following reasons:

1. Estimation of coronary stenosis severity solely by guessing by eye too often carries substantial under- and overestimation (Björk et al. 1975; Detre et al. 1975; Zir et al. 1976; Sanmarco et al. 1978).
2. Several investigations gave convincing evidence that coronary stenosis severity may be reduced either after administration of vasodilator drugs (Rafflenbeul et al. 1980b) or with balloon dilation (Grüntzig et al. 1977). In addition, repeated coronary angiography after an interval of specific drug therapy may reveal changes in stenosis severity only detectable with quantitative measurements (Rafflenbeul et al. 1979).

Therefore, quantitative analysis of coronary artery stenosis, particularly in intervention studies, in order to accurately assess changes in stenosis severity constitutes a major clinical implication of quantitative coronary angiography. Furthermore, the morphological configuration of coronary stenosis may be evaluated more precisely with quantitative measurements.

According to these criteria results of clinically relevant studies using quantitative coronary angiography will be presented in this paper.

Precise Assessment of Coronary Artery Vasomobility

Various interventions, primarily pharmacologic, have been developed to provoke coronary artery vasoconstriction. Generalized coronary artery constriction in normal coronary arteries and reduction of stenosis diameter as well as its reversion have been quantitatively demonstrated by Raizner et al. 1980. In another quantitative study Curry et al. (1977) showed an overall 18% coronary artery diameter reduction in response to i.v. ergonovine.

Coronary vasodilation following nitroglycerin was quantitatively demonstrated by Gensini et al. as early as 1971. In our own study (Rafflenbeul et al.

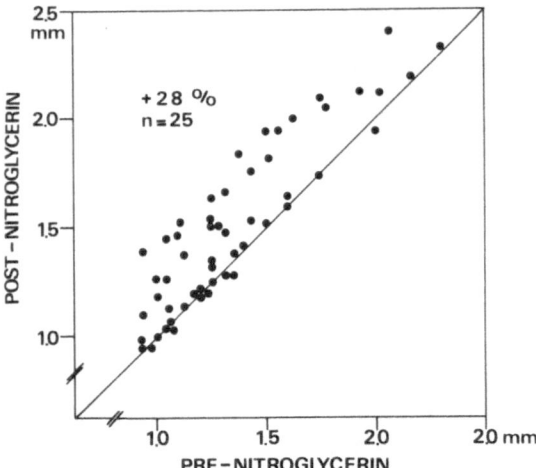

Fig. 1. Vasodilatory effect of 0.8 mg nitroglycerin sublingually on the smallest diameter measured in 54 coronary artery stenoses of different severity; 25 stenoses increased their smallest diameter significantly, averaging +28%

1980) using 0.8 mg nitroglycerin sublingually we measured a significant increase of the narrowest diameter in 25 out of 54 coronary stenoses with an average increase of +28% (Fig. 1). These data were strikingly reconfirmed by Brown et al. (1981) only recently.

A similar dilatory effect on the most obstructed segment of coronary stenoses was demonstrated with nifedipine (Leutenegger et al. 1980). As depicted in Fig. 2, again in about 47% of lesions, i.e., 20 out of 42 stenoses, the smallest

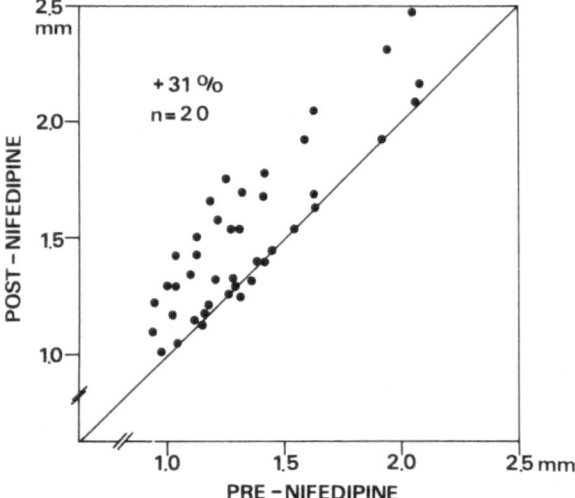

Fig. 2. Vasodilatory effect of 20 mg nifedipine sublingually on the smallest diameter measured in 42 coronary artery stenoses of different severity; 20 stenoses increased their smallest diameter significantly, averaging +31%

diameter (D_{STEN}) dilated with a mean +31% increase after application of 20 mg nifedipine sublingually.

This relaxation of a residual vascular tone elicited with both nitroglycerin and nifedipine may be regarded as an additional factor contributing to the antianginal properties of both vasodilator drugs.

Prerequisites and Follow Up of Transluminal Coronary Angioplasty

Another relevant application of quantitative coronary angiography is to define accurately some of the anatomical requirements for transluminal coronary angioplasty (PTCA) and to objectivize the outcome of PTCA on coronary stenoses.

With regard to the minimum diameter of coronary stenoses passable with the deflated balloon catheter, we measured a significant difference of the smallest diameter between stenoses which could be crossed and stenoses which could not be crossed with the balloon catheter (Fig. 3). From these comparative data it is evident that in coronary stenosis a diameter measuring less than 1.0 mm after application of vasodilator drugs represents a major cause of unsuccessful PTCA.

Fig. 3. The smallest diameter (±SD) measured in coronary artery stenoses before PTCA; *left,* 34 stenoses which could be crossed, and *right,* 12 stenoses which could not be crossed with the balloon catheter

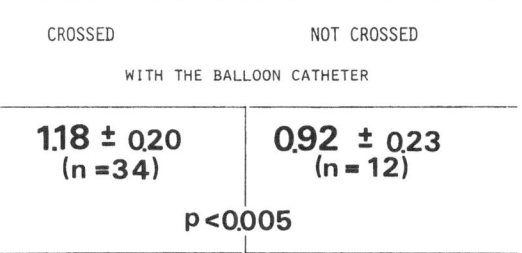

Furthermore, the morphology of coronary stenosis seems to influence the results of PTCA as demonstrated in Fig. 4 (Rafflenbeul et al. 1981). We subdivided 50 coronary obstructions before PTCA according to the following criteria: lesion with similar smallest diameters, i.e., less than 25% difference, measured in different angiographic projections was defined as stenosis with a *circular* residual lumen (left panel in Fig. 4), whereas a stenosis with a difference in the smallest diameters of more than 25% measured in different projections was called a lesion with an *elliptical* residual lumen (right panel in Fig. 4). With PTCA, 17 out of 18 circular stenoses were successfully dilated. In contrast, the response of the elliptical stenoses was less uniform: in 10 out of 32, i.e., 31% of measured obstructions, PTCA left the smallest diameter nearly unchanged. The open triangle on the right panel points to the average smallest diameter increase of the same 32 obstructions after application of 0.8 mg nitroglycerin plus 20 mg nifedipine, indicating a similar vasodilation in coronary stenoses already triggered by smooth muscle cell relaxants. Therefore, to assess the definite success

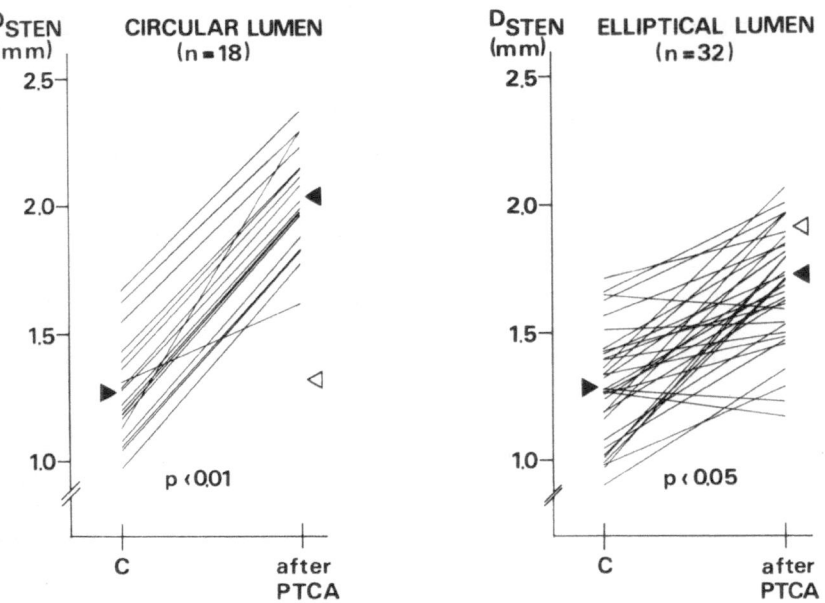

Fig. 4. The effect of balloon dilatation (PTCA) on the smallest diameter (D_{STEN}) in coronary stenoses with different morphology

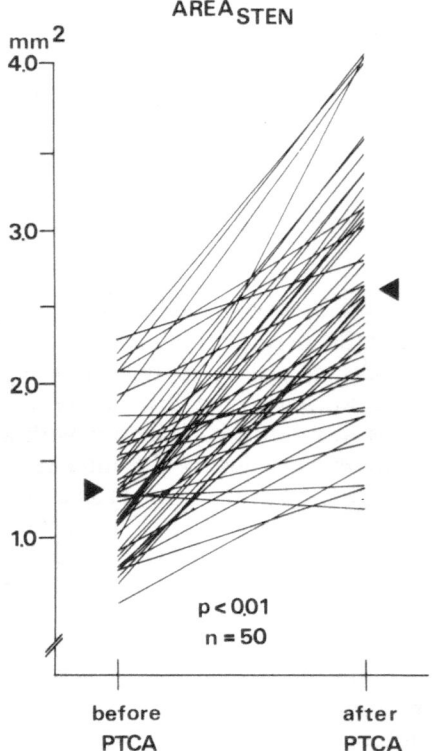

Fig. 5. Effect of balloon dilatation (PTCA) on the cross-sectional area ($Area_{STEN}$) in a series of 50 consecutive coronary stenoses

of PTCA, reangiography should be performed some weeks after the procedure (Engel et al. 1980).

The overall results of PTCA, analysed with quantitative coronary angiography in the same series of 50 consecutive stenoses, is depicted in Fig. 5. The mean value of the cross-sectional area calculated from the diameter measurements (Rafflenbeul and Lichtlen, 1979) increased significantly after the procedure.

Evaluation of Interval Studies

Subjective evaluation of repeated coronary angiography is insufficient and often misleading, particularly with different laboratories involved. Quantitative analysis objectivizes interpretation of interval angiograms and is particularly sensitive in assessing the devolutionary pattern of coronary artery disease in the individual patient. Data from our own study (Rafflenbeul et al. 1979) of 25 patients with unstable angina pectoris initially show strong evidence that in most of these patients the disease is stationary, with only an insignificant amount of progression in coronary stenoses over 1-year period. We found no significant difference in the mean degree of obstruction between the first and second angiogram in any vessel under scrutiny (Table 1). Only about 25% of obstructed vessels demonstrated a marked increase in the degree of obstruction (Table 2).

Table 1. Average degree of stenoses (%) measured in the initial (Study A) and the repeated (Study B) angiograms of 25 patients with unstable angina restudied after a 1-year interval

	Study A (%)	Study B (%)
RCA	79	84
LAD	78	77
LCX	73	83

RCA, right coronary artery; LAD, left anterior descending coronary artery; LCX, left circumflex coronary artery

Table 2. Total number of obstructed vessels, number of vessels with no change, with progressive and regressive degree of stenosis in 25 patients with unstable angina initially restudied after 1 year

	Obstructed vessels n	No change	Progressive ($n = 11$)	Regressive ($n = 5$)
RCA	20	15	4	1
LAD	22	14	5	3
LCX	16	10	5	1

Table 3. Quantitatively evaluated degree of coronary artery stenosis in five patients with regressive degree of obstruction (data from same study as Table 2)

| | Degree of stenosis in | |
	Study A (%)	Study B (%)
RCA	80	49
LAD	82	44
LAD	88	65
LAD	88	69
LCX	70	49

Thus, the rate of progression was found to be slower in this group of patients with unstable angina than the rate reported in more qualitative studies of patients with stable angina (Bemis et al. 1973; Kimbiris et al. 1974; Gensini et al. 1974; Roesch et al. 1976).

On the other hand, we found in five stenoses a distinct regression of stenosis severity, i.e., more than 20% decrease of area stenosis (Table 3).

In another interval study we evaluated quantitatively the effect of aortocoronary venous bypass (ACVB) on the luminal size of poststenotic coronary arteries in 73 vessels with a high degree of proximal obstruction (mean area stenosis, 82%) (group I) and in 19 vessels with a total proximal occlusion (group II). In group II the vessel under scrutiny was adequately filled by collaterals preoperatively.

In the arterial segments proximal at and distal to the graft implantation, identical cross sections were measured and compared before and after surgery (Table 4). In group I the proximal segment showed a decrease in the average

Table 4. Effect of an aortocoronary venous bypass (ACVB) on poststenotic coronary artery diameters in 73 vessels with high-degree proximal stenosis (group I) and 19 vessels with a proximal occlusion (group II) but adequate filling via collaterals preoperatively

| | Group I ($n = 73$) | | Group II ($n = 19$) | |
	Pre-ACVB (mm)	Post-ACVB (mm)	Pre-ACVB (mm)	Post-ACVB (mm)
2 cm proximal to ACVB implantation	2.56	2.02 $P < 0.05$	1.54	2.23 $P < 0.05$
At implantation site of ACVB	2.34	2.20 NS	1.72	2.34 $P < 0.05$
2 cm distal to ACVB implantation	1.64	1.76 NS	1.54	1.98 $P < 0.05$

diameter, whereas the distal segment including its immediate vicinity to graft implantation remained essentially unchanged. The diameter decrease in the proximal segment could be caused both by further diminished antegrade flow across the high grade stenosis after grafting with additional thrombotic narrowing, and by the suction effect due to enhanced flow provided by the graft. In contrast, in group II with complete obstruction but adequate retrograde filling via collaterals, a significant increase of the mean diameter at all three measuring points occurred after surgery. Postoperatively reestablished systemic blood pressure could be the cause of this increase in diameters.

New Insights into Pathophysiology of the Coronary Circulation

Systematic engagement with quantitative analysis of coronary angiograms offers a great variety of new aspects of coronary circulation, some of which are outlined here.

Quantitative Difference in the Degree of "Critical" Stenosis Between the Left and the Right Coronary Artery

Measuring the degree of proximal stenoses in an unselected group of 74 patients who underwent coronary angiography because of exertional angina (NYHA classes II and III) we found a significant difference between the average degree of area stenosis in the left anterior descending coronary artery (LAD) and the

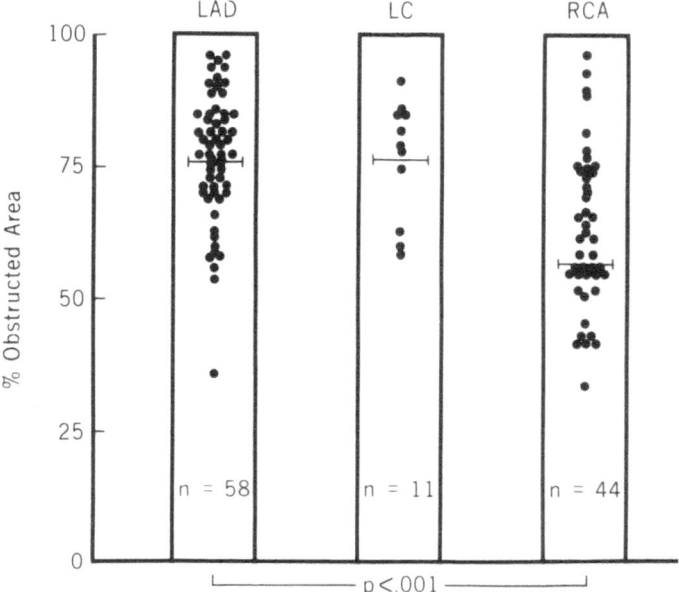

Fig. 6. Quantitatively evaluated degree of proximal obstructions in 74 patients with exertional angina pectoris NYHA class II and III

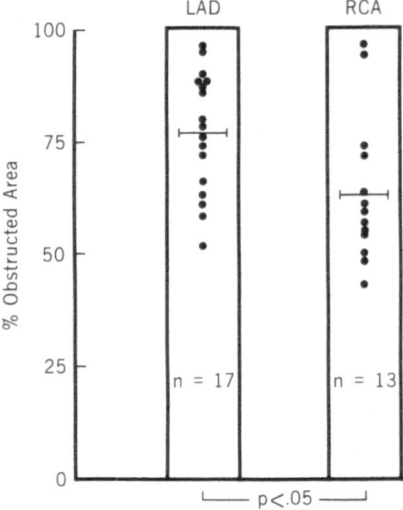

Fig. 7. The quantitatively evaluated degree of obstruction in 30 patients with an isolated proximal stenosis either of the proximal LAD ($n = 17$) or of the proximal RCA ($n = 13$).

right coronary artery (RCA), with a mean value of 75% and 56%, respectively (Fig. 6). In order to pursue this trend, we investigated whether the same degree of stenosis in either the proximal LAD or the proximal RCA causes critical flow reduction in a more selected group of symptomatic patients with isolated stenosis (Rafflenbeul et al. 1980). Measurements of the degree of stenosis were correlated with different manifestations of critical flow reduction, i.e., angina pectoris, development of collaterals, and segmental wall motion abnormalities.

As shown in Fig. 7, in 13 patients with anginal pain and isolated RCA stenosis the mean degree of obstruction was 63% area stenosis, which was significantly lower than the one measured in 17 symptomatic patients having an isolated obstruction of the LAD (77%). In patients with an identical degree of obstruction (78%) in either LAD or RCA, collateral vessels were angiographically demonstrable in 53% of the RCA stenoses but only in 29% of the LAD stenoses. Furthermore, when the stenoses were less than 63% in the LAD and the RCA, regional wall motion abnormalities were more frequently associated with RCA than with LAD stenoses (Table 5). These quantitative data indicate that a significantly lesser degree of stenosis is critical in the RCA than in the LAD.

Table 5. Number and location of hypo- or akinetic ventricular wall segments and their distribution with regard to the degree of obstruction in the nutrient coronary artery

Coronary artery	Number and location of hypo- or akinetic wall segments		*Degree of stenosis*	
			$\leq 63\%$	$\geq 63\%$
LAD	33	Anterior wall	5	28
RCA	23	Posterior wall	11	12

$X^2 = 7.09$
$P < 0.01$

Evidence for a Differential Segmental Behavior of Proximal and Distal Coronary Arteries

As we have learned from experimental studies with isolated strips of animal coronary arteries, large and small coronary arteries react differently to various stimuli including vasoactive drugs, metabolic changes, and autonomic nervous discharge. In man this variable response of large and small coronary arteries may play an important role in the adjustment of epicardial coronary arteries to atherosclerotic lesions. Therefore, we used quantitative analysis of coronary angiograms to test a different responsiveness between large and small coronary arteries.

First, the effect of isosorbide dinitrate (ISDN) on proximal vs distal epicardial coronary artery segments was studied. Coronary angiography before and 5 min after 5 mg ISDN sublingually was performed in 18 patients with angiographically normal coronary arteries (Table 6). In the proximal third of the LAD, the LCX, and the RCA ISDN dilated the diameters by 0.4 to 0.6 mm, which is equivalent to a percentage increase of $+15\%$ to $+19\%$ of the initial diameter. The diameters of the distal thirds of the same arteries dilated by similar absolute values. In these small arterial segments, however, the percentage increase of the diameters was significantly higher than in the proximal segments, amounting to 25%, 26%, and even 31% of the initial diameters.

Table 6. Effect of 5 mg isosorbide dinitrate (ISDN) sublingually on proximal vs distal coronary artery segments in 18 patients with angiographically normal coronary arteries

	Proximal segments		Distal segments	
	(mm)	(%)	(mm)	(%)
LAD	3.0——→3.5	+17	1.6——→2.0	+25
LCX	2.7——→3.1	+15	1.9——→2.4	+26
RCA	3.2——→3.8	+19	1.8——→2.4	+33

$P<0.05$ $P<0.05$
$P<0.05$

Secondly, to assess the progression rate of proximal vs distal coronary artery stenoses, coronary angiography was repeated after approx. a 1-year interval in 33 patients with optimal antianginal medical therapy. In both the initial and the repeated angiograms, stenoses of the proximal third and the distal third of the LAD, the LCX, and the RCA were measured. Only obstructions which showed a more than 20% decrease in the stenotic diameter were classified as progressive stenoses (Table 7). Considering these criteria, 5 out of 11 proximal LAD stenoses progressed over the 1-year interval, as did 5 out of 16 LCX stenoses but only 4 out of 27 RCA stenoses. Overall, 14 out of 54 proximal stenoses, i.e., 26%, showed a substantial progression. Out of 15 stenoses in the distal third of

Table 7. Progression rate of proximal vs distal coronary artery stenoses in 33 patients who underwent reangiography approx. 1 year after optimal medical treatment

	Proximal stenoses		Distal stenoses	
	Initially	Progressive	Initially	Progressive
LAD	11	5	15	2
LCX	16	5	14	0
RCA	27	4	10	1
Total	54	14	39	3

$X^2 = 3.893$ $P<0.05$

the LAD, only two progressed, while this was the case for none of the 14 LCX stenoses and only one of the 10 RCA stenoses. The chi-square test for the difference between progressive and nonprogressive stenoses of the proximal and distal vessel segments was significant. It has to be emphasized that proximal and distal stenoses were of similar severity, ranging from 28% to 95% and from 35% to 89%, respectively.

Thirdly, to test the response of proximal vs distal epicardial coronary arteries to aortocoronary venous bypass (ACVB) implantation in 55 coronary arteries with high degree proximal stenosis (on average, 88% area stenosis), identical poststenotic arterial segments were measured before and after ACVB implantation. As depicted on Table 8, for each major coronary branch the vessel diameters proximal to the graft decreased significantly, whereas the distal diameters remained virtually unchanged.

Compared with proximal coronary artery segments by quantitative means, distal coronary artery segments demonstrate
1. A more distinctive dilation after administration of ISDN
2. A lower progression rate of obstructions with comparable severity
3. Minor diameter changes after bypass implantation

Despite the fact that the exact reason for this segmentally different behavior is still to be defined, we would suggest some of the possibly important factors. The variations in response to different stimuli may be due to differences in

Table 8. Response of proximal vs distal coronary artery segments to aortocoronary venous bypass implantation in 55 coronary arteries with a proximal high-degree stenosis

	Proximal segments	Distal segments
LAD	2.87——→2.19	1.73——→1.59
LCX	2.53——→2.35	1.62——→1.75
RCA	2.25——→1.83	1.94——→2.17
	$P<0.05$	NS

a) basal tone of vascular smooth muscle,
b) metabolism of the arterial wall, and
c) impact of mechanical forces like phasic perfusion pressure or myocardial contraction.

Although there is no conclusive evidence that the amount of smooth muscle cells is different between proximal and distal epicardial coronary arteries, the ability to relax may be different due to differences in pharmacologic behavior as pointed out by Norton and Detar (1970) and/or competitive neurogenic vaso-constrictor influence as demonstrated by Zuberbühler and Bohr as early as 1965. Recent experimental studies have demonstrated differences in the metabolic activity of the arterial wall between large and small coronary arteries which in turn may affect the tone of vascular smooth muscle. Particular emphasis has been directed towards the differences in catabolism of vasoactive drugs like adenosine or serotonin metabolism (Winbury et al. 1969; Rubio and Berne 1969).

Conclusions

Quantitative analysis of coronary angiograms, particularly of coronary artery stenosis severity, eliminates the subjective element in detecting and grading of coronary artery stenosis which leads to a wide range of intra- and interobserver variability. Accurate assessment of the degree of coronary artery stenosis is predominantly important in interventions which are known to change the degree of obstruction, i.e., the administration of vasodilator drugs like nitrogly-cerin or nifedipine, or transluminal balloon dilatation (PTCA). The decision on PTCA is further influenced by exact information about the morphological configuration and the minimum diameter of the stenosis under scrutiny pro-vided with quantitative measurements. In addition, the long-term results of PTCA are documented precisely by quantitative means. Quantitatively ana-lysed interval studies establish either the effectiveness of a specific treatment or the natural history of coronary artery disease over a certain period of time. Particular emphasis was directed towards new insights into the pathophysiology of the coronary circulation offered by quantitative coronary angiography, i.e., the difference in the degree of "critical" stenosis between left and right coronary artery or the segmentally different behavior of epicardial coronary arteries. These new aspects, together with the finding of pharmacologically induced decrease in the degree of coronary artery stenosis, demonstrate convincingly the clinical relevance of quantitative analysis of coronary arteriograms in patients with coronary artery disease.

References

Bemis CE, Gorlin R, Kemp HG, Herman MV (1973) Progression of coronary artery disease. Circ Res 47:455

Björk L, Spindola-Franco H, van Houten FX, Cohn PF, Adams DF (1975) Comparison of observer performance with 16 mm cine-fluorography and 70 mm camera fluorography in coronary arteriography. Am J Cardiol 36:474

Brown BG, Bolson E, Frimer M, Dodge HT (1977) Quantitative coronary arteriography: estimation of dimensions, hemodynamic resistance, and atheroma mass of coronary artery lesions using the arteriogram and digital computation. Circulation 55:329

Brown BG, Bolson E, Petersen RB, Pierce CD, Dodge HT (1981) The mechanism of nitroglycerin action: stenosis vasodilation as a major component of the drug response. Circulation 64:1089

Curry RC, Pepine CJ, Sabom MB, Feldman RL, Chriestie LG, Conti CR (1977) Effects of ergonovine in patients with and without coronary artery disease. Circulation 56:803

Detre KM, Wright E, Murphy ML, Takaro J (1975) Observer agreement in evaluating coronary angiograms. Circulation 52:979

Engel H-J, Kaltenbach M, Kober G, Scherer D, Lichtlen P (1980) Spontaneous regression of coronary obstructions after transluminal dilatation. Circulation 62 [Suppl III]:159

Gensini GG, Kelly AE, DaCosta BCB, Huntington PP (1971) Quantitative angiography: the measurement of coronary vasomobility in the intact animal and man. Chest 60:522

Gensini GG, Esenti P, Kelly AE (1974) Natural history of coronary disease in patients with and without coronary bypass graft surgery. Circulation 50 [Suppl II]:98

Grüntzig AR, Myler RK, Hanna ES, Turina MI (1977) Coronary transluminal angioplasty. Circulation 55/56 [Suppl III]:84

Kimbiris D, Lavine P, Broek H, Najmi M, Likoff W (1974) Devolutionary pattern of coronary atherosclerosis in patients with angina pectoris. Am J Cardiol 33:7

Leutenegger F, Rafflenbeul W, Gahl K, Walpurger G, Engel H-J, Lichtlen P (1980) Quantitative Koronarangiographie: Dilatation von Koronarstenosen nach Nifedipin. Schweiz Med Wochenschr 110[45]:1703

Norton JM, Detar R (1970) Adenosine and isolated coronary vascular smooth muscle. Physiologist 13:273

Rafflenbeul W, Lichtlen P (1979) Intravitale Morphometrie. In: Lichtlen P (ed), Koronarangiographie. perimed, Erlangen

Rafflenbeul W, Dziuba M, Henkel B, Lichtlen P (1975) Morphometric analysis of coronary obstructions during life. Circulation 52 [Suppl II]:27

Rafflenbeul W, Smith LR, Rogers WJ, Mantle JA, Rackley CE, Russell RO (1979) Quantitative coronary arteriography: coronary anatomy of unstable angina pectoris one year after optimal medical therapy. Am J Cardiol 43:699

Rafflenbeul W, Urthaler F, Lichtlen P, James TN (1980a) Quantitative difference in "critical" stenosis between right and left coronary artery in man. Circulation 62:1188

Rafflenbeul W, Urthaler F, Russell RO, Lichtlen P, James TN (1980b) Dilatation of coronary artery stenoses after isosorbide dinitrate in man. Br Heart J 43:546

Rafflenbeul W, Kaltenbach M, Engel H-J, Scherer D, Kober G, Lichtlen P (1981) Morphological and functional criteria for a successful coronary angioplasty (PTCA). Circulation 63/64 [Suppl IV]:253

Raizner AE, Chahine RA, Ishimori T, Verani MS, Zacca N, Jamal N, Miller RR, Luchi RJ (1980) Provocation of coronary artery spasm by the cold pressor test. Circulation 62:925

Reiber JHC, Booman F, Tan HS, Gerbrands JJ (1979) Computer processing of coronary occlusions from X-ray arteriograms. Inserm 88:79

Roesch J, Antonovic R, Trenouth RS, Rahimtoola SH, Sim DN, Dotter CT (1976) The natural history of coronary artery stenosis. Diagn Radiol 119:513

Rubio R, Berne RM (1969) Release of adenosine by the normal myocardium and its relationship to the regulation of coronary resistance. Circ Res 25:407

Sanmarco ME, Brooks SH, Blankenhorn DH (1978) Reproducibility of a consensus panel in the interpretation of coronary angiograms. Am Heart J 96:430

Winbury MM, Howe BB, Hefner MA (1969) Effect of nitrates and other coronary dilators on large and small coronary vessels: an hypothesis for the mechanism of action of nitrates. J Pharmacol Exp Ther 168:70

Zir LM, Miller SW, Dinsmore RE, Gilbert JP, Harthorne JW (1976) Interobserver variability in coronary angiography. Circulation 53:627

Zuberbühler RC, Bohr DF (1965) Responses of coronary smooth muscle to catecholamines. Circ Res 16:431

Introduction to Angiographic Quantitation of Coronary Flow

P. H. HEINTZEN

Department of Pediatric Cardiology, University of Kiel, Kiel, FRG

The high spatial and temporal resolution of coronary angiograms – obtained using modern single and biplane X-ray image intensifier systems – provide information for the assessment of the severity of coronary artery disease. Indication for bypass surgery is primarily based on subjective viewing of these high-quality image series, and in particular on the detection and gradation of stenotic lesions.

Standard diagnostic procedures, however, reflect primarily the *gross morphological* aspects of the disease. Although the anatomy of the arteries is a major determinant of the "specific function," i.e., the maintenance of the myocardial blood supply by an adequate flow, there is *no constant relationship between the anatomy and the functional consequences* of the stenosis, i.e., the blood flow through it so long there is no adaequate quantitation of the anatomy and fluid dynamics. A first attempt to establish this relationship more quantitatively sought an objective and precise definition of the structural anomaly by making a densitometric or videometric analysis of the stenotic region, as outlined in the preceding session; the clinical relevance of these efforts, however, remains a matter of discussion.

The principal goal of quantitative coronary angiography and left ventriculography remains the *characterization of the functional state of the myocardium* and in particular its dependence on coronary artery blood flow or myocardial perfusion. The quality of the coronary circulation is indirectly reflected by the global or regional left ventricular wall motion. How far the analysis of the dynamic geometry of the left ventricle, as obtained from angiocardiography, can reliably help to quantify the extent and localization of myocardial damage due to coronary artery lesions, is the topic of another symposium (held in Lausanne [1]) and will therefore not be discussed here.

The following papers deal with direct *densitometric* approaches for the evaluation of the functional aspects of coronary circulation which go back to the early studies of Rutishauser [2].

Attempts to quantify coronary circulation with the main goal of quantifying coronary blood *flow* always came close to overtaxing the capacities of the densitometric method. Nevertheless, continuous efforts have been made to improve these techniques. The present stage of the various concepts for flow or flow-velocity measurements in the coronary arteries and some experimental and clinical applications will be outlined in the following contributions. The two basic approaches try to measure the progress of the contrast bolus in the central coronary arteries by either (a) evaluating time parameters from the contrast bolus with two densitometric windows between which the distance (and therefore the length of the segment of the coronary artery) is known, or (b) measuring the progress of the front of the bolus within a fixed time interval. Digital subtraction techniques facilitate the dimensional measurements required using the second method.

With the advent of digital video image processing techniques there have been promising new developments which allow visualization of the myocardial wall by contrast enhancement during the phase of capillary perfusion by the injected dye. By this means not only can the wall thickness, systolic thickening, and wall motion be detected, but there is also some evidence that perfusion disturbances or defects become recognizable.

In conclusion, it is obvious to me from the contributions which follow, that there is much progress being made in the technological developments as well as in the physiological conceptualizations. However, we should not try to be always (or only) at the "front" or "leading edge" of the bolus. It might be worthwhile to also study its "body" and even the "tail" may contain fruitful information (e.g., clearance from the contrast bolus).

References

1. Sigwart U, Heintzen PH (1983) Ventricular wall motion. Int Symposium, Lausanne 20–22 May 1982, Thieme, Stuttgart
2. Rutishauser W (1969) Kreislaufanalyse mittels Röntgendensitometrie. Huber, Bern

Assessment of Myocardial Perfusion Using Digital Angiocardiography*

J. H. Bürsch, W. Radtke, R. Brennecke, J. Hahne, and P. H. Heintzen

Departments of Pediatric Cardiology and Bioengineering, University of Kiel, FRG

Introduction

Digital processing of coronary angiocardiograms provides the capability for visualizing myocardial opacification by applying contrast enhancement techniques. Smith et al. (1978) described roentgen scanning densitometry as a new method for the analysis of the spatial distribution as well as the movement of radiopaque indicators through the coronary microcirculation. The basic procedure in these studies was the subtraction of the natural image background (without contrast material) from images of the myocardial opacification period on a picture element basis. Previous work from this laboratory has similarly demonstrated the potential enhancement of angiographic contrast by digital subtraction, integration, and rescaling techniques (Brennecke et al. 1976, 1977; Heintzen et al. 1978). It was noticed that not only coronary but likewise aortic root or left ventricular injections of contrast medium could successfully be applied for the visualization of the perfused myocardium (Radtke 1982; Radtke et al. 1981a). It was the immediate goal of this experimental study to systematically examine the needs and performance of digitized myocardiography with regard to both normal and pathologic perfusion conditions of the coronary circulation.

Angiographic Studies

Left heart catheterization was performed in 20 closed-chest pigs weighing 15–21 kg. Biplane video angiocardiograms (Siemens, Gigantos) were obtained in the 45° X-ray projections and stored on video tape (Sirecord) for subsequent analysis. Following angiocardiography in the control state, experimental infarction was produced in the animals by complete embolization of the circumflex coronary artery or one of its branches. Comparable volumes of Urografin 76% were injected under both circulatory conditions applying aortic root as well as left ventricular injections. At the end of the experiment, the heart was dissected

* This investigation was supported by research grants from the Deutsche Forschungsgemeinschaft

following infusion of blue dye into the aortic root. By this means the extent of nonperfused myocardial muscle mass could be well estimated and utilized for the determination of myocardial infarction.

Processing Methods

Our digital processing system has recently been described in detail (Brennecke et al. 1978). A matrix buffer (256 × 256 picture elements, 256 gray level resolution) was used for the transfer of on-line digitized image data from video tape to the minicomputer PDP 11/40. The images were semiautomatically selected by means of an R-wave trigger (ECG), which thus provided a certain number of digitized images from identical cardiac phases for further analysis. At least four end-diastolic images were taken from the preinjection period (image background) as well as the myocardial perfusion phase. In case of left ventricular injections, in addition, two images were selected from the phase of contrast material washout from the ventricle (Fig. 1).

Angiograms obtained by making aortic root injections were preferably analyzed for studies of the spatial distribution of the contrast medium by visual inspection and densitometric analysis. The processing steps included

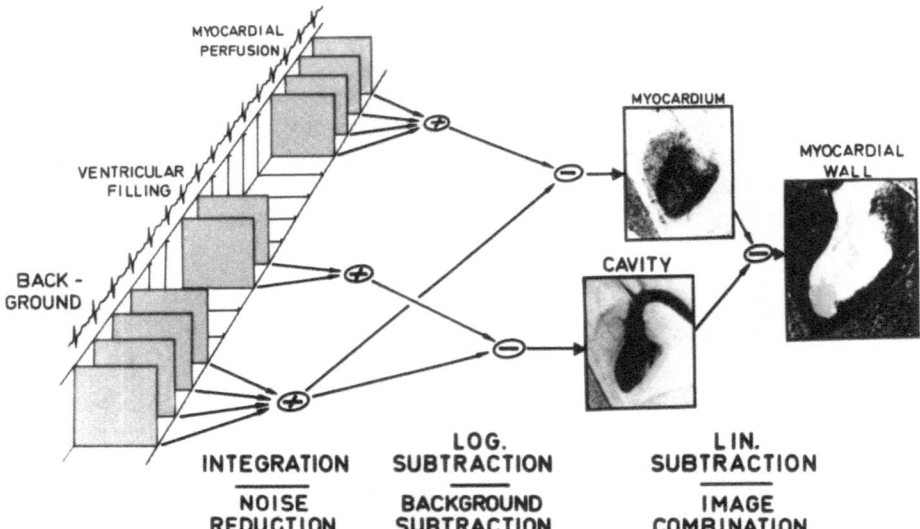

Fig. 1. Schematic drawing of the basic processing steps for myocardial imaging. ECG-gated images are selected from the preinjection period, the late ventricular filling phase, and the myocardial perfusion period. Several images from each of the phases are summed up in order to generate a new representative image with reduced image noise. The method applied for imaging contrast distribution of the total myocardium is based on logarithmic image subtraction only (myocardium, *upper middle*). The technique used for contour detection of the left ventricular wall additionally implies the combination of the myocardial image with the cavity image (myocardial wall, *mid-right*)

1. Integration of (four) images from the preinjection and myocardial perfusion period in order to generate representative images from these two phases with minimal image noise
2. Logarithmic data conversion from the resulting two images to account for the exponential attenuation of X-ray intensities and thereby provide potentially regional mass measurements of the contrast medium
3. Logarithmic subtraction of the converted images from each other in order to eliminate nonopacified cardiac and thoracic structures (image background)

Angiograms performed by left ventricular injections were likewise processed. In addition, a subtraction image from the left ventricular injection period was calculated.

This latter image was linearly subtracted from the myocardial subtraction image providing a composed image with contour information of both the inner and outer myocardial wall as far as the myocardium had been opacified. The two processing techniques described were principally applied to test the feasibility of regional myocardial perfusion studies as well as to estimate the extent of myocardial infarction.

Myocardial Imaging

The success of digital image processing for visualizing the left ventricular myocardium was dependent on controlled conditions in angiocardiography and data analysis. Adequate volumes of Urografin 76% injected into the aortic root were about 15 ml, equivalent to 0.75 ml per kg body weight. The tip of the end-closed catheter was positioned just above the aortic valve, providing maximal contrast concentration in the coronary arteries. Injection flow rates of more than 15 ml/s were necessary, resulting in about 1-s duration for injection. This high injection flow rate provided sufficient mixing (during diastole) and comparable flow of dye to the left as well as the right coronary artery. The bolus type of injection was also a prerequisite to provide maximal concentrations during the time course of myocardial perfusion before contrast medium was expected to run off the coronary veins into the right heart chambers, thereby potentially affecting the homogeneity of contrast during the microcirculatory phase. The optimal period for digitizing myocardial perfusion images was equivalent to the fifth, sixth, seventh, eighth, and ninth cardiac cycles following the onset of injection (heart rate about 80/min). A typical example for the control study is given in Fig. 2. It was noticed that the circumferential portions of the opacified myocardium appeared to be more contrasted than the central parts, which is in accordance with the model of an ellipsoidal thick-wall shell (myocardium) being transradiated. The lateral projection of the heart (Fig. 2, left) demonstrates a rather symmetrical gray level distribution with respect to the long axis (apex valves) of the left ventricle. This mostly homogeneous gray distribution was visibly broken up in experimental infarction studies (Fig. 3). Even the smallest infarction (8% of left ventricular mass) was recognized, at least by comparing the infarction image with that of the control state of the animal. In order to

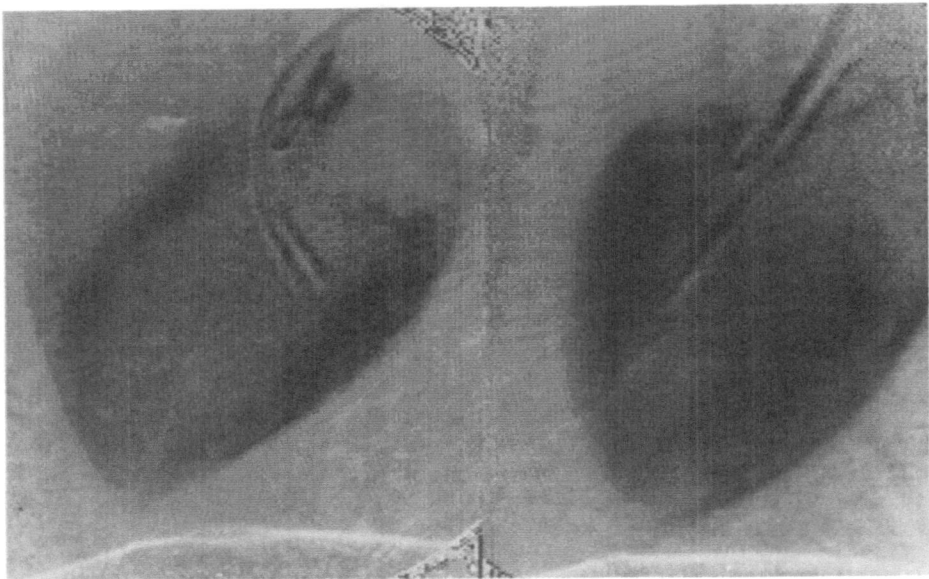

Fig. 2. Computer-processed pictures of monitor screen of the normal pig heart in biplane projection indicating the distribution of contrast material during the myocardial perfusion phase. Aortic root injections were performed just above the aortic valves. A second catheter was placed into the cavity for simultaneous pressure measurements. Double contouring of this catheter is caused by motion and associated subtraction artifacts

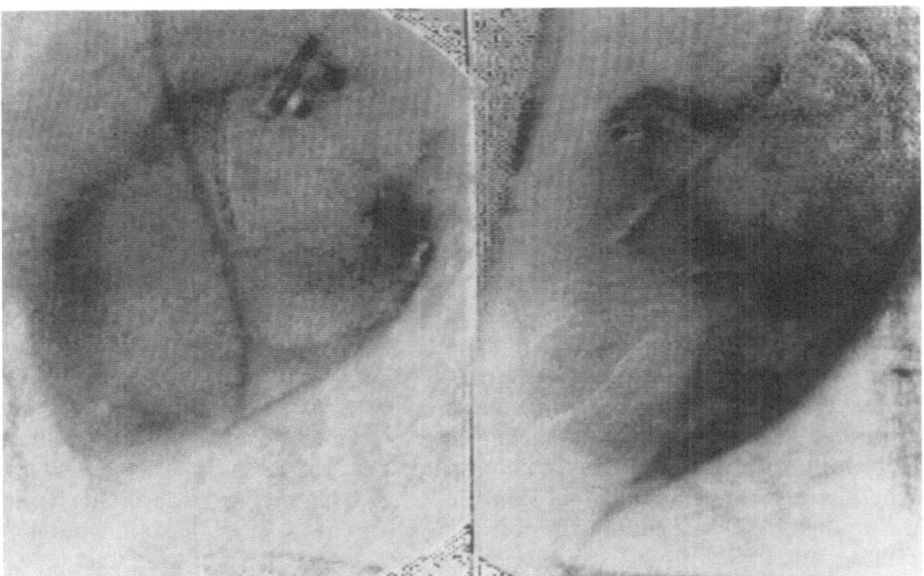

Fig. 3. Myocardial image of the pigs heart depicted in Fig. 2 as obtained after myocardial infarction by embolization of the peripheral circumflex coronary artery. Comparing these images with the appropriate control images (Fig. 2), the nonhomogeneous opacification becomes visible

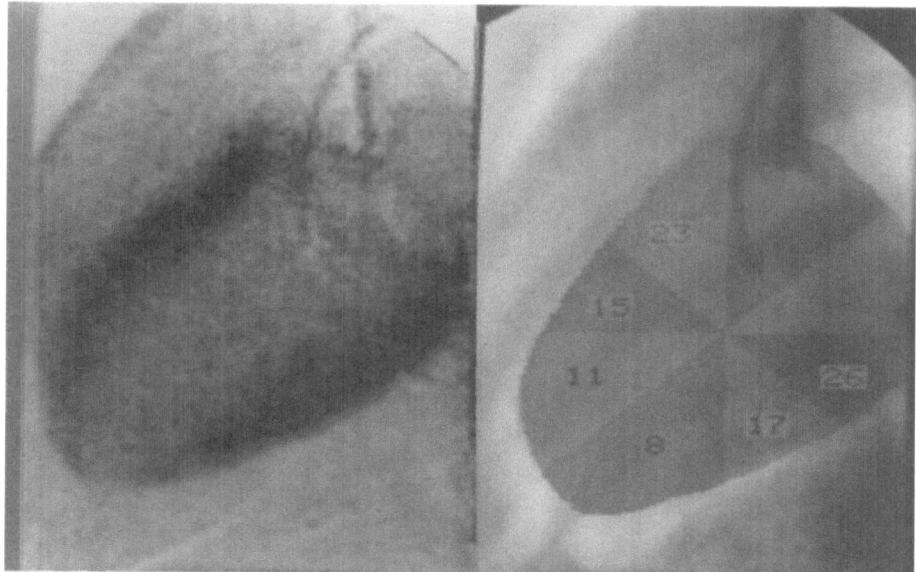

Fig. 4. Computer-processed images of the normal heart in lateral roentgen projection. Distribution of the contrast medium is quantitatively determined by integral density measurements within each of the six segments as depicted in the right picture. The percent numbers indicate average values of the mass of contrast medium for each region. There is a fairly symmetrical distribution of contrast medium as related to the anterior and posterior wall of the left ventricle

objectively study abnormal myocardial opacification, a densitometric analysis program was implemented in our system. After having manually outlined the external contours of the left ventricle, the long axis was used as a symmetry line for four segments at each side in order to establish integral absorption values that were indicative for the mass of contrast material accumulated in the different projection areas (Fig. 4). By that means an estimation of abnormal regional perfusion (percent of total perfusion) was obtained in the infarction study (Fig. 5).

If this method is going to be applied as a diagnostic procedure, perfusion studies in individual cases will be dependent upon comparison with regional perfusion data in normals. The reproducibility of such measurements and the pattern of normal values (mean value, standard deviation) is presently studied for the lateral X-ray projection of the heart.

Ventricular Wall Imaging

Myocardial images were combined with left ventricular cavity images for contour detection of the inner and outer borders of the left ventricular wall in biplane projections. Optimal opacification of the myocardium was obtained if

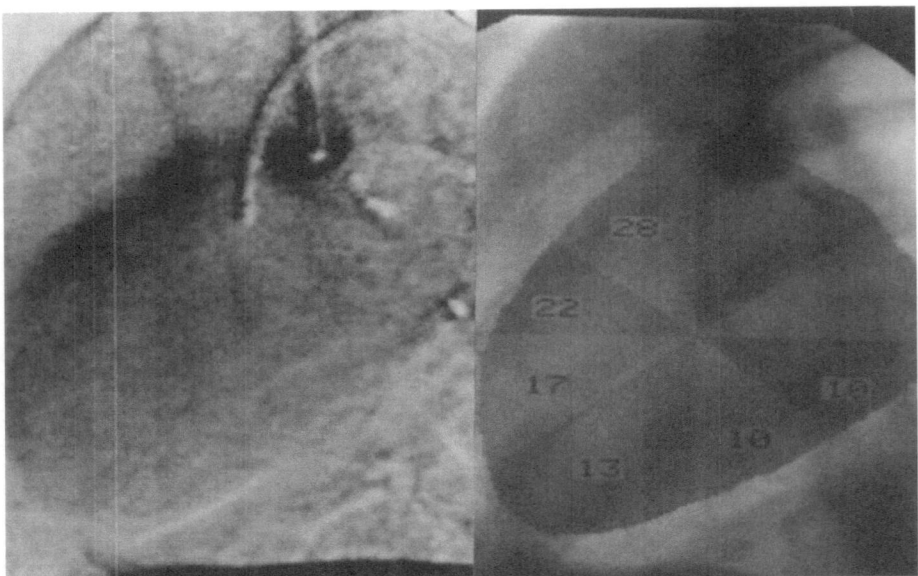

Fig. 5. Radiopaque distribution analysis after complete embolization of the circumflex artery (same pig as Fig. 4). The percent values of regional perfusion indicate significantly reduced perfusion at the posterior wall segments. Postmortem studies revealed an infarction size of 50%

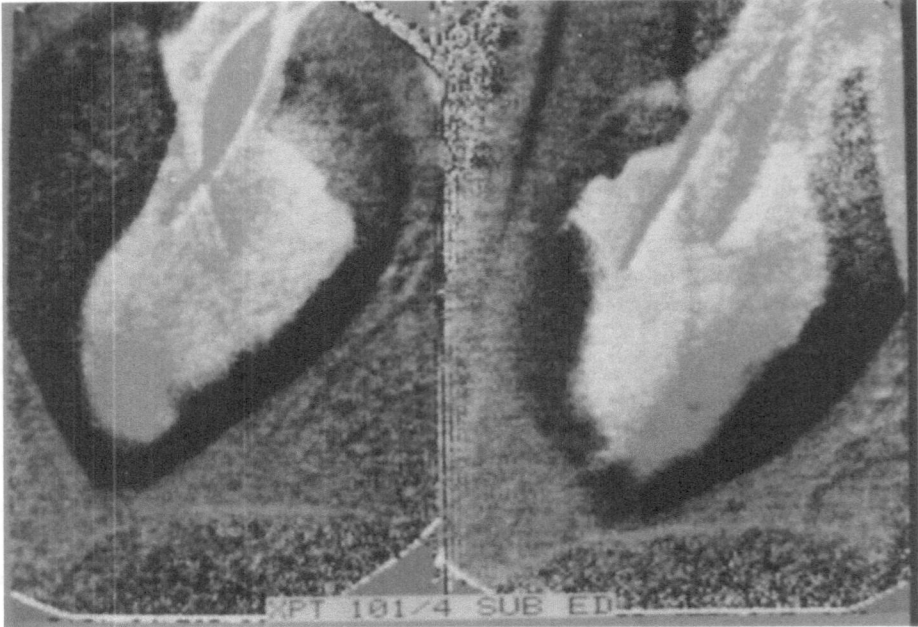

Fig. 6. Composed image from the myocardial and cavity perfusion phases of a pig in biplane projection (normal circulation). Superimposition of images provides detection of the inner and outer contours of the left ventricular wall

1 ml/kg body weight was injected within 1 s into the left ventricle. An example of such composed end-diastolic images is presented in Fig. 6. The cavity appears bright while the extending area of the perfused myocardium shows up in dark gray, indicating opacification of the myocardial wall. Density and mass information are lost in the central parts (cavity area) of the myocardium, and perfusion abnormalities in this processing technique can be judged only from the external ring (myocardial wall), which certainly is a limiting factor in small infarctions. On the other hand, it provides the unique feature to calculate left ventricular volumes and also to approximate the extent of myocardial infarction. According to angiocardiographic methods of dimensional volume determination of the heart chambers, two volume calculations were performed in each study, namely, left ventricular cavity volume (inner contours), and total left ventricular volume (outer contours). As a difference of these two values, left ventricular myocardial volume was obtained. In a control study (13 animals) an excellent correlation was found by comparing these data with postmortem muscle mass measurements (Radtke 1981; Radtke et al. 1981b). Angiographic data calculated from the end-diastolic cardiac phases revealed a correlation of $r = 0.89$, whereas end-systolic data correlated even better with $r = 0.94$. Neither comparative study showed statistically significant differences.

Validation of this principle using dimensional measurements of muscle volumes was a constituent for another approach of infarction size measurements.

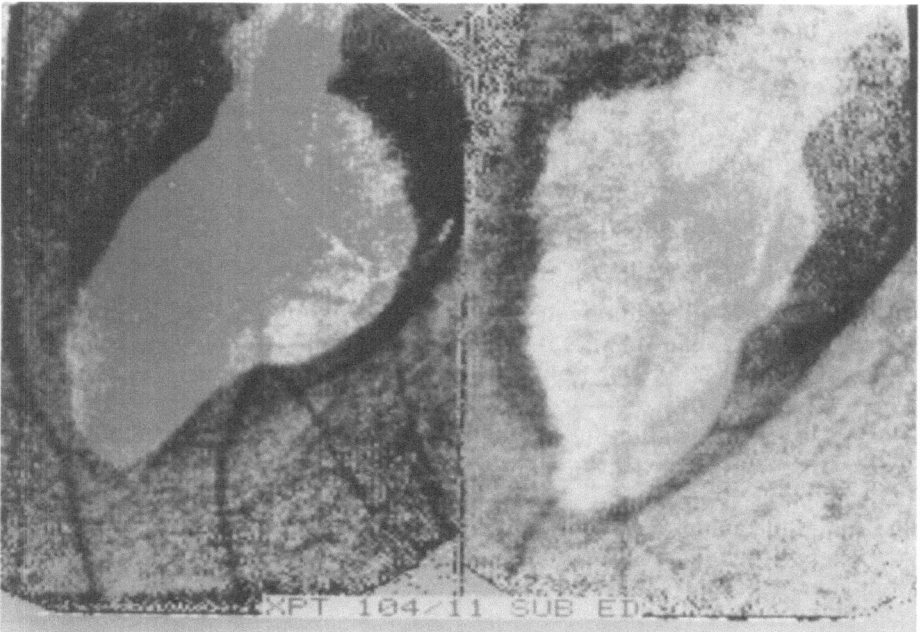

Fig. 7. Composed image for contour detection of the left ventricular wall in an infarction study (same pig as Fig. 6). Nonperfused myocardial wall can be recognized to a large extent at the apex in the left picture

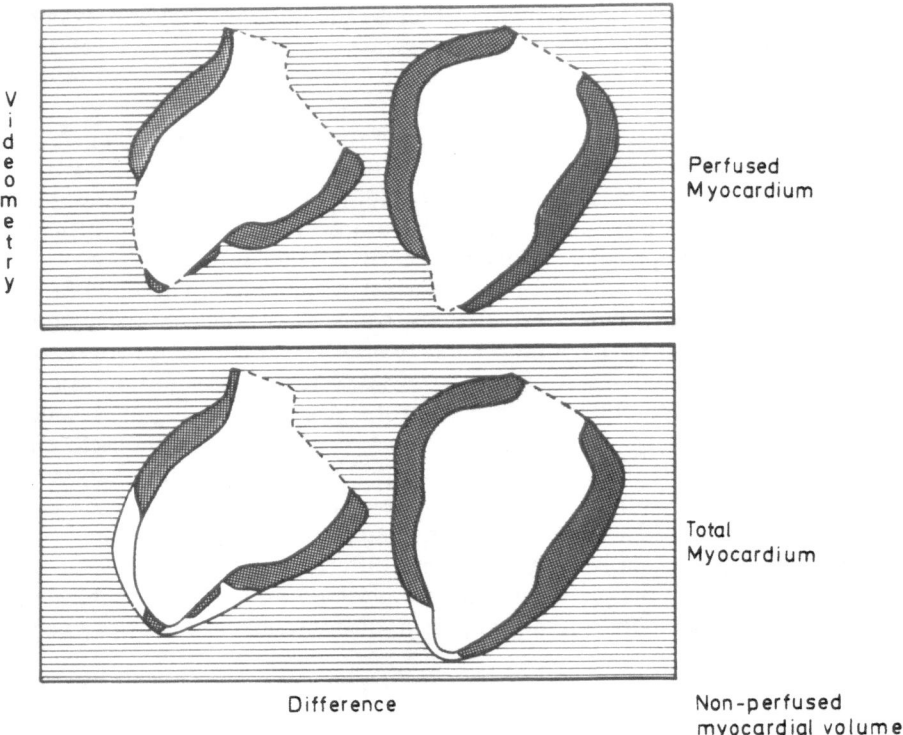

Fig. 8. Illustration of the two outlining procedures for myocardial volume determination using videometry (Heintzen et al. 1971). Calculation of the perfused myocardium is based on the actual contours of the opacified wall (*upper panel*). At nonperfused regions the external contour is identical to the cavity border. Calculation of the total myocardium implies estimation of the external borders by assuming a certain wall thickness derived from the perfused wall regions (*lower panel, white wall segments*)

In a first step of calculation, the total myocardial volume was determined by assuming mostly uniform wall thickness at the total circumference of the ventricular wall which provided external contour information even at those sites where myocardial opacification was extremely poor or not visible (Fig. 7). In the second step of calculation the volume was calculated from the actually visible outer contours, thereby excluding the nonperfused myocardial regions (Fig. 8). On this basis, nonperfused muscle volume (infarction) was determined as a fraction of the assumed total volume from end-diastolic images. The correlation coefficient was found to be $r = 0.80$ when angiocardiographic measurements were compared with the postmortem data.

Comment

In the near future, digital processing of angiocardiograms will become clinically feasible for the enhancement of angiographic contrast in a variety of diagnostic procedures. As indicated in this experimental study, it provides quantitative evaluation of parenchymal perfusion abnormalities which may be similarly applied to other organs such as the brain and kidneys. With regard to cardiac studies, visualization of the myocardial wall may also become useful for the assessment of ventricular wall dynamics. Regional systolic wall thickening can be analyzed in order to study the contractile behavior of the heart.

Acknowledgements. The authors would like to thank Ms W. Twißelmann and Mrs. U. Bürsch, Mr. G. Gonschior, and Mr. L. Meissner for their skilled technical assistance and preparation of the manuscript.

References

Brennecke R, Brown TK, Bürsch JH, Heintzen PH (1976) Digital processing of videoangiographic image series using a minicomputer. Proc Computer Cardiology, IEEE Computer Society, Long Beach, pp 255–260

Brennecke R, Brown TK, Bürsch JH, Heintzen PH (1977) Computerized video-image preprocessing with applications to cardio-angiographic roentgen-image series. In: Nagel HH (ed) Digitale Bildverarbeitung. Springer, Berlin Heidelberg New York, pp 244–262

Brennecke R, Brown TK, Bürsch JH, Heintzen PH (1978) A digital system for roentgen video image processing. In: Heintzen PH, Bürsch JH (eds) Roentgen-Video-Techniques. Thieme, Stuttgart, pp 150–157

Heintzen PH, Malerczyk V, Pilarczyk J, Scheel KW (1971) On-line processing of the video-image for left ventricular volume determination. Comput Biomed Res 4:474–485

Heintzen PH, Brennecke R, Bürsch JH (1978) Computerized ECG-gated angiocardiography. Excerpta Medica, Amsterdam, pp 1124–1126

Radtke W (1981) Die angiokardiographische Bestimmung des linksventrikulären Myokardvolumens mit Hilfe der digitalen Bildverarbeitung. Inauguraldissertation, Universität Kiel

Radtke W, Bürsch JH, Brennecke R, Hahne HJ, Meissner L, Heintzen PH (1981a) Visualization of the left ventricular wall by digital angiocardiography. Eur Heart J 2:135

Radtke W, Bürsch JH, Brennecke R, Hahne HJ, Heintzen PH (1981b) Bestimmung der linksventrikulären Muskelmasse mittels digitaler Angiokardiographie. Z Kardiol 70:302

Smith HC, Robb RA, Ritman EL (1978) Roentgen videodensitometric assessment of myocardial blood flow: clinical applications. In: Heintzen PH, Bürsch JH (eds) Roentgen-Video-Techniques. Thieme, Stuttgart, pp 39–48

Assessment of Regional Coronary Blood Velocity and Flow Using Roentgen Densitometry: Clinical Experience

R. SIMON, I. AMENDE, and P. R. LICHTLEN

Medizinische Hochschule Hannover, Department of Cardiology, Karl-Wiechert-Allee, D – 3000 Hanover, FRG

Introduction

Conventional analysis of coronary angiograms provides information regarding the morphology and anatomical abnormalities of the coronary arteries. Application of roentgen densitometric techniques may in addition offer an objective quantitation of coronary function, namely, the delivery of blood to the dependent regions of the myocardium (Rutishauser et al. 1970; Smith et al. 1973).

When we started to use densitometry in patients during clinical catheterization, we felt that the procedure in the laboratory should be as simple and short as possible, for the benefit and comfort of the patient and the investigator.

We therefore thought that the procedure should mimic the technique of routine angiography, since this would allow us to insert densitometric measurements between diagnostic angiograms without unnecessary delay. It would further allow the use of standard equipment for coronary angiography as well as for densitometry. Since videodensitometry has been shown to fulfill these requirements (Smith et al. 1978), we have chosen this method for application during patient investigation.

Methods

Our technique is similar to that described by Smith and coworkers (1973, 1978). For densitometric assessment, a projection is chosen that displays the vessel under study as parallel to the input screen of the intensifier as possible. As an example, Fig. 1 shows a bypass graft to the left anterior descending artery (LAD) in a right anterior oblique projection. A motor-driven, crescent-shaped copper filter that is mounted in the housing of the X-ray tube, is adjusted to the border of the heart in order to obtain a homogeneous background. The patient is asked to hold his breath and a rapid bolus injection of 2–3 cc of contrast material (Urografin 76%) is performed at the coronary ostium under fluoroscopy. This scene, which takes about 15 s, is stored on videotape for later densitometric evaluation. Concomitantly, biplane cineangiograms of the vessel are taken in the same projection for morphometric measurements of vessel dimensions. A grid of small metal spheres attached to the intensifier input screen enables compensation for image distortion as well as the detection of

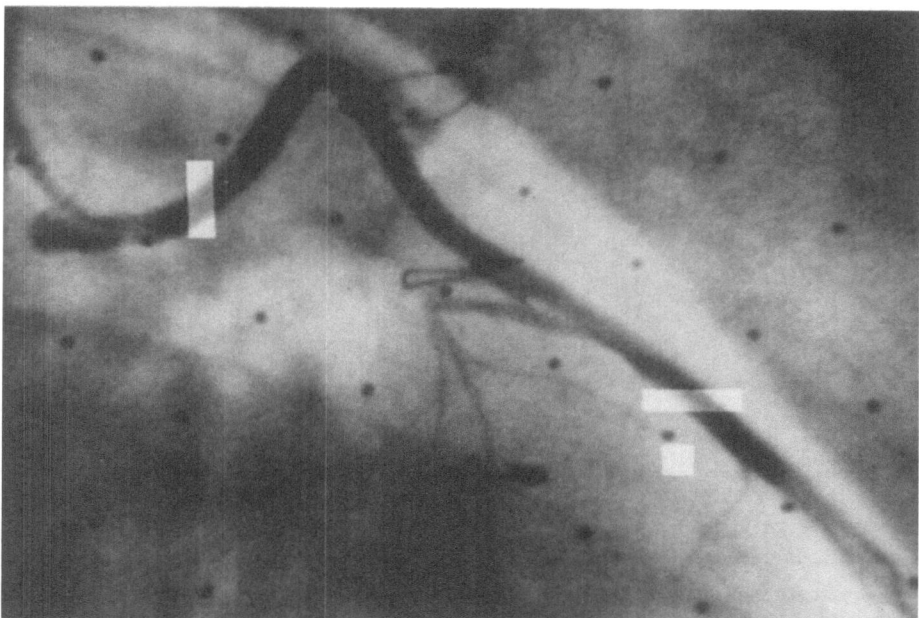

Fig. 1. Aortocoronary venous bypass graft to a left anterior descending artery in RAO projection, superimposed by densitometric measuring windows and calibration grid

corresponding sites in both cine and video images (see Fig. 1). When the tape is replayed, two densitometric sampling fields, so-called "windows," are placed over up- and downstream parts of the vessel, shown as white rectangles. A third window is positioned adjacent to the vessel over the myocardium. It drives special circuitry that will automatically compensate for the accumulation of contrast in the superimposed muscle (Simon et al. 1979).

By means of a two-channel videodensitometer that provides high fidelity logarithmic conversion of the video signal (Brennecke et al. 1978; Simon et al. 1979), contrast dilution curves are registered at the site of the proximal and distal window (Figs. 2 and 3). The original densograms (upper curve in Fig. 2) are superimposed by uniform undulations that occur in synchrony with the heart cycle, due to the cyclic alterations in thickness and blood contents of the structures superimposing the vessel. These undulations have to be subtracted to obtain the contrast-specific signal. Since this has to be done in a dynamic beat-by-beat manner, computer assistance is to be recommended. The lower curve in Fig. 2 shows the same densogram after computer processing for background compensation. The control cycle that has been subtracted from the entire curve is a mean of several beats before contrast injection; it is shown in the upper right corner.

The correction is carried out for the proximal and distal densograms and the travelling time of the bolus is calculated as the difference between mean transit times of both curves (Fig. 3). Since we use hand injections, we cannot neglect a possible influence of the time course of the injection on the shape of the curve.

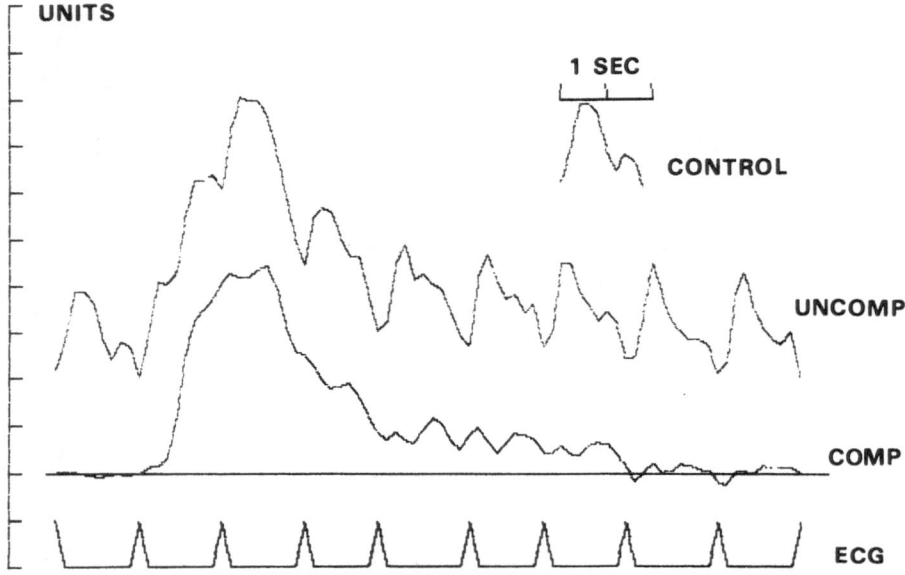

Fig. 2. Densogram from proximal window in Fig. 1. *Upper curve:* original densogram (*uncomp*). *Lower curve:* computer-processed densogram (*comp*) after beat-to-beat subtraction of a mean cycle derived from several beats before contrast injection (*control*). *Bottom:* computer-stored QRS complex of the ECG used for compensation of mean cycle length to actual cycle length

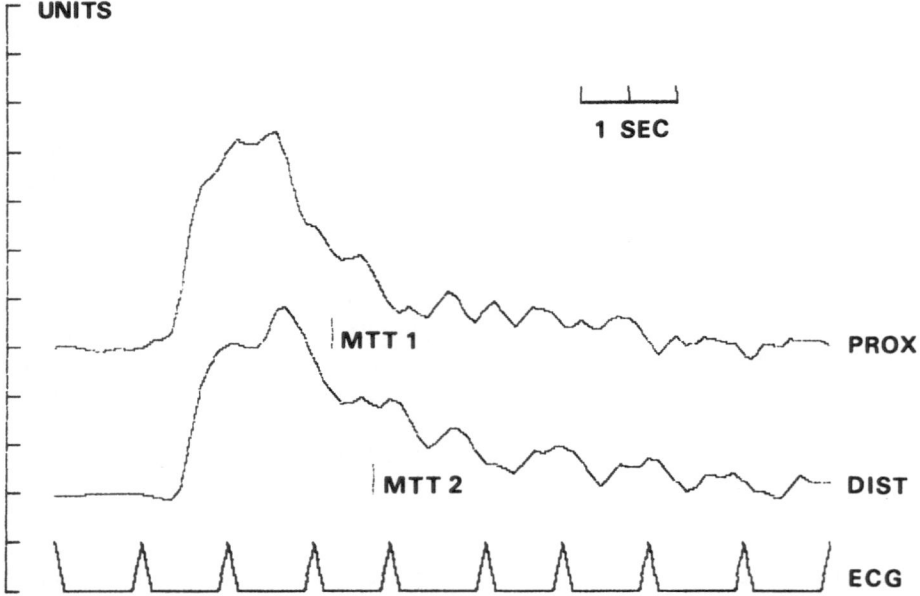

Fig. 3. Computer-processed densograms from the patient in Fig. 1. *Flags* indicate mean transit times of the proximal (*prox*) and the distal (*dist*) densogram

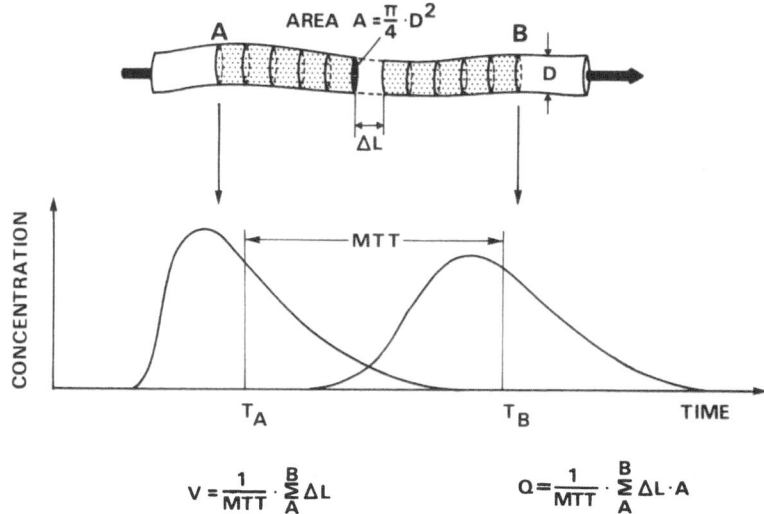

$$V = \frac{1}{MTT} \cdot \sum_{A}^{B} \Delta L \qquad\qquad Q = \frac{1}{MTT} \cdot \sum_{A}^{B} \Delta L \cdot A$$

Fig. 4. Principles of the assessment of mean blood velocity and flow in single vessels by densitometry: T_A, T_B, mean transit times of the proximal and distal curve; V, mean blood velocity; Q, mean blood flow.

We therefore use as many points of the curve as possible and apply the classical concept of Zierler (1962), where transit time T for each densogram is derived as:

$$T = \frac{\int t \cdot c\,(t) \cdot \mathrm{d}t}{\int c\,(t) \cdot \mathrm{d}t}$$

where $c\,(t)$ is the amplitude of the densogram at time t.

From travelling time and vessel dimensions obtained from cineangiograms, blood velocity and flow through the vessel under study can be calculated according to the principles outlined in Fig. 4. Between the windows, the vessel is divided into equidistant segments. For each segment the true spatial length and the volume is calculated by reconstruction from the orthogonal biplane cineangiograms. Total length is given by the sum of segmental length, total volume between the windows is obtained as the sum of segmental volumes. Mean blood velocity is derived by dividing length by travelling time, and mean flow is obtained by dividing volume by travelling time.

Previous validation of this method has demonstrated an excellent correlation with simultaneous electromagnetic flowmetry in animal experiments (Smith et al. 1973). For patients, sufficient reproducibility was proven by replicate determinations of bolus travelling time in our laboratory (Fig. 5).

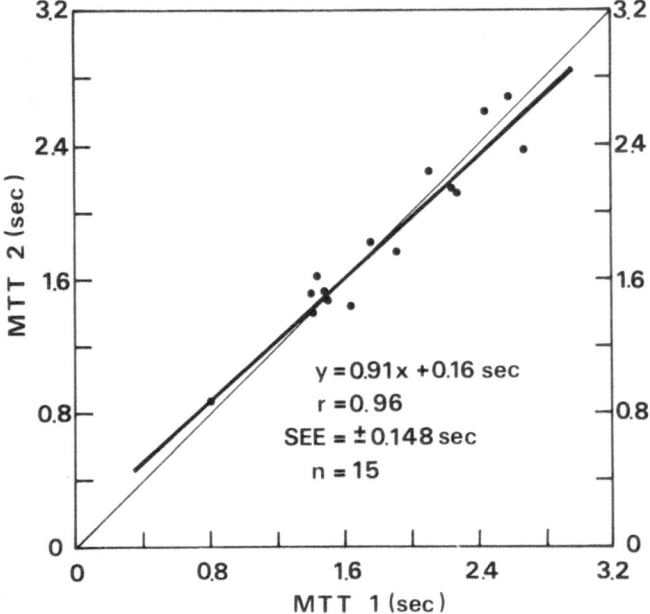

Fig. 5. Replicate determinations of bolus travelling time in 15 native LAD. Since the spatial distance between windows was kept constant between measurements, reproducibility also refers to velocity measurements. *MTT 1,* control measurement; *MTT 2,* repeated assessment 2 min later

Results

Bypass Grafts

We have used this method that is especially suited for unbranched vessels, to assess bypass graft hemodynamics in more than 40 patients in the postoperative state. Figure 6 presents hemodynamics of 36 nonobstructed aorto-to-coronary venous bypass grafts under resting conditions. Large variations were observed for velocity as well as for flow values, velocity ranging from 3 to 32 cm/s and flow from 15 to 160 ml/min. There were no differences for different graft locations. Velocity was also not related to graft dimensions. For flow, a tendency to decrease with a decrease in graft size was observed, if the luminal diameter of the graft was below 3 mm. Beyond this value, however, flow did not show any relation to graft size. These data suggest that bypass grafts beyond 3 mm simply serve as conductive tubing without significant effects on graft flow, whereas smaller veins may influence graft function to a certain extent.

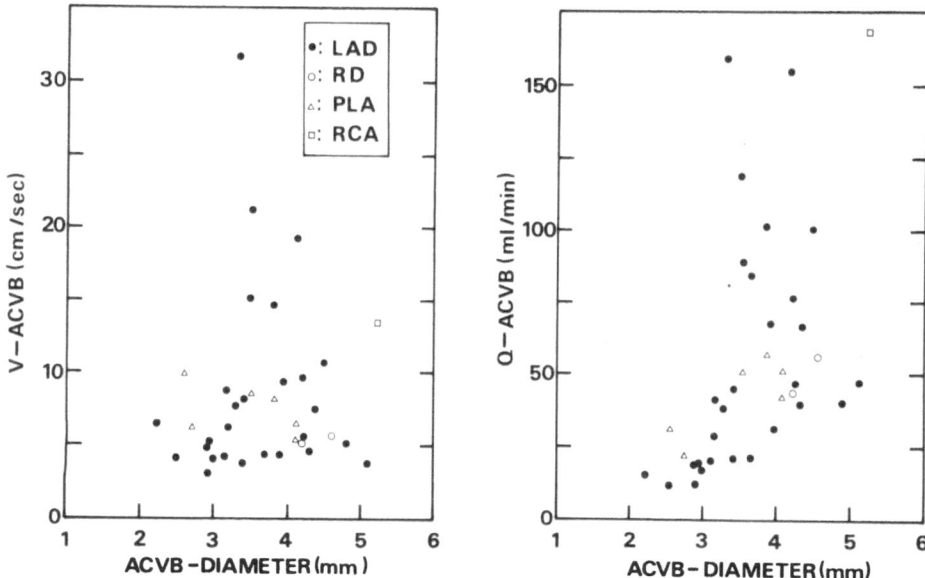

Fig. 6. Mean blood velocity and flow with relation to average graft diameter in 36 nonobstructed venous bypass grafts. Different symbols refer to grafts to the LAD, to diagonal branches (*RD*), to marginal branches of the left circumflex artery (*PLA*), or the right coronary artery (*RCA*)

Native Coronary Arteries

We also attempted to assess regional hemodynamics in native coronary arteries. Blood velocity in a given segment of an artery can be derived following the principles described above. Figure 7 presents the results of densitometric measurements of mean blood velocity in 33 native coronary arteries in patients. Blood velocity ranged from 2 to 22 cm/s, the average being about 7 cm/s. There was no correlation between blood velocity and vessel diameter in this group. Note also that velocity did not depend on the presence or absence of obstructions.

It is obvious that blood flow cannot be calculated according to the principles outlined in Fig. 4, since flow through the side branches would be neglected. This problem could be easily circumvented if one could assume that blood velocity is a constant in all segments of the epicardial arteries. Then, measured velocity in any segment multiplied by the cross section of the artery at its proximal take-off, should result in total influx to the vessel. Our experience so far suggests, however, that the simplifying assumption of a constant velocity does not hold true for the human coronary arteries. In Fig. 8, measured velocity is displayed with relation to the spatial distance of the measuring windows on the LAD in 27 patients. In all cases, the proximal window was positioned at the take-off of the LAD from the left main coronary. As can be seen, measured velocity decreases

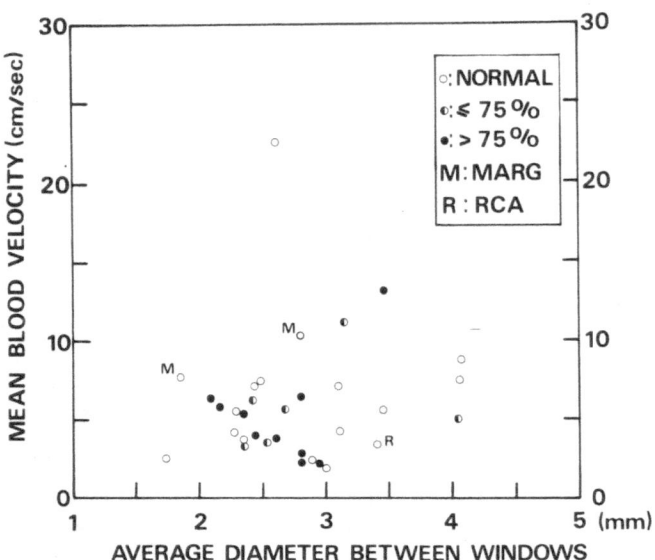

Fig. 7. Mean blood velocity with relation to average vessel diameter between measuring windows in 33 native coronary arteries. *Open circles:* nonobstructed vessels; *halfclosed circles:* arteries obstructed ≤ 75% in diameter; *closed circles:* obstructions > 75% of vessel diameter. Symbols refer to native LAD ($n = 30$), if not marked as R (right coronary artery, $n = 1$) or M (marginal branch of left circumflex artery, $n = 2$)

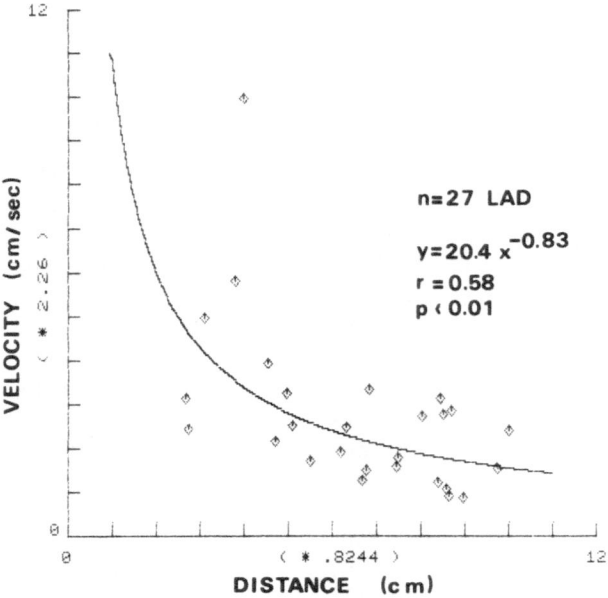

Fig. 8. Blood velocities in the native LAD in 27 patients with regard to the (spatial) distance of the measuring windows on the vessel. Proximal window in all cases at the take-off of the LAD from the main left coronary artery. *Abscissa:* window distance in multiples of 0.824 cm. *Ordinate:* velocity in multiples of 2.26 cm/s

significantly with an increasing distance on the vessel. This is not unexpected, since we know that in branching arteries, the total vascular cross section including the stem and the side branches increases after each branching. Since total outflow of the system equals influx, velocity must decrease after branching. Our densitometric method obtains a weighted average of velocities within a given arterial segment that does not represent the actual velocity in the proximal part of the artery. This means that to date there is no simple densitometric technique that can assess blood flow through branched coronary arteries in patients.

We may, however, take estimated flow as an equivalent of flow in order to assess *changes* in regional blood flow, for example, after interventions. To test this hypothesis, in 10 patients coronary flow was altered by the systemic application of nitroglycerin, nifedipine, or dipydamole. Changes in blood flow were assessed in a single LAD bypass in four patients, and in the native LAD in six patients without coronary disease.

Simultaneously, the continuous thermodilution technique (Ganz et al. 1971) was used to measure blood flow in the great cardiac vein that has been reported to refer closely to LAD blood flow (Pepine et al. 1978). As demonstrated by Fig. 9, a sufficient correlation between both measurements was obtained to indicate that changes in blood flow induced by interventions can be estimated by this simple technique, even in branched native arteries such as the LAD.

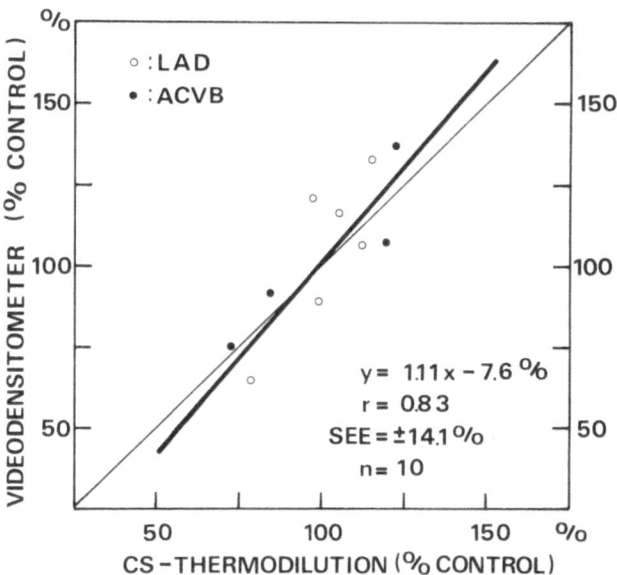

Fig. 9. Comparison of the simultaneous assessments of flow changes using videodensitometry and thermodilution, both expressed in percentage of the control values. *Symbols* refer to densitometric measurements on native left anterior descending arteries (*LAD*) or bypass grafts to the *LAD (ACVB)*

Comment

We conclude that videodensitometry offers an objective quantitation of regional coronary function during clinical catheterization. In our experience, the method proved to be without hazards for the patient and simple for the investigator.

We regard it as advantageous that standard roentgen equipment and conventional radiopaque indicators and techniques are employed. This considerably facilitates implementation during routine coronary angiography. So far, blood velocity can be assessed in absolute terms in unbranched and branched vessels, whereas flow can only be measured in unbranched vessels such as bypass grafts. Nonetheless, relative flow *changes* are reflected correctly when assessed in branched parts of the arteries. Thus, the method has been used to assess the effects of drug application on the coronary circulation in our laboratory.

References

Brennecke R, Bürsch HJ, Heintzen PH (1978) Improvements in videodensitometric measurement techniques. In: Heintzen PH, Bürsch HJ (eds) Roentgen-video-techniques for dynamic studies of structure and function of the heart and circulation. Thieme, Stuttgart, pp 15–22

Ganz W, Tamura K, Marcus HS, Donoso R, Yoshida S, Swan HJC (1971) Measurement of coronary sinus blood flow by continuous thermodilution in man. Circulation 44:181–195

Pepine CJ, Mehta J, Webster WW Jr, Nicholas WW (1978) In vivo validation of a thermodilution method to determine regional left ventricular blood flow in patients with coronary disease. Circulation 58:795–802

Rutishauser W, Noseda G, Bussmann WD, Preter B (1970) Blood flow measurement through single coronary arteries by roentgen densitometry. Am J Roentgenol 109:21–24

Simon R, Ziegler K, Grimm J (1979) Videodensitometer mit automatischer Regelung des Videoeingangs. Biomed Tech 24:156–157

Smith HC, Sturm RE, Wood EH (1973) Videodensitometric system for measurement of vessel blood flow, particularly in the coronary arteries, in man. Am J Cardiol 32:144–150

Smith HC, Robb RA, Ritman EL (1978) Roentgen videodensitometric assessment of myocardial blood flow: clinical applications. In: Heintzen PH, Bürsch HJ (eds) Roentgen-video-techniques for dynamic studies of structure and function of the heart and circulation. Thieme, Stuttgart, pp 39–48

Zierler KL (1962) Theoretical basis of indicator dilution methods for measuring flow and volume. Circ Res 3:393–407

Videodensitometric Measurement of Coronary Flow

K. L. Neuhaus, G. Sauer, H. Krause, and U. Tebbe

Department of Internal Medicine, Division of Cardiology, University of Göttingen, Robert-Koch-Straße 40, D-3400 Göttingen, FRG

Introduction

The first attempts to measure coronary artery flow velocities using densitometry were done nearly 15 years ago (Rutishauser et al. 1967, 1970a, 1970b; Smith et al. 1971). Methodological improvements have been reported by Pannek et al. (1978) and Fermor et al. (1979). Using the method described below, phasic flow velocity in native human coronary arteries can be obtained during routine coronary angiography.

Methods and Material

Three to five bolus injections of 0.8–2.0 ml contrast medium at a rate of 3 or 4 ml/s were given during routine coronary angiography (biplane cineangiography, 100 frames/s). The transit time of the contrast medium was measured from the leading slopes of densograms (50% increase, Bürsch et al. 1979), taken from two sites of the coronary artery (Fig. 1). The method has been described in detail by Krause et al. (1980).

In 54 of the first 81 patients to whom contrast bolus injections were given, a quantitative evaluation of systolic and diastolic coronary flow velocities was obtained. Ten of these patients were normal (no coronary or valvular heart disease), ten patients were investigated 3 weeks after an acute myocardial infarction and early recanalisation of the infarct-related artery by intracoronary or intravenous streptokinase. Another eight patients with a history of angina pectoris but not coronary artery disease showed a significantly reduced flow velocity and were taken as a separate "slow flow" group.

Results

The mean flow velocity of the normal patients was 16.2 ± 1.5 cm/s in the left anterior descending (LAD) and 16.4 ± 2.0 cm/s in the right coronary artery (RCA). During systole, flow velocity was significantly lower than during early and late diastole (Fig. 2).

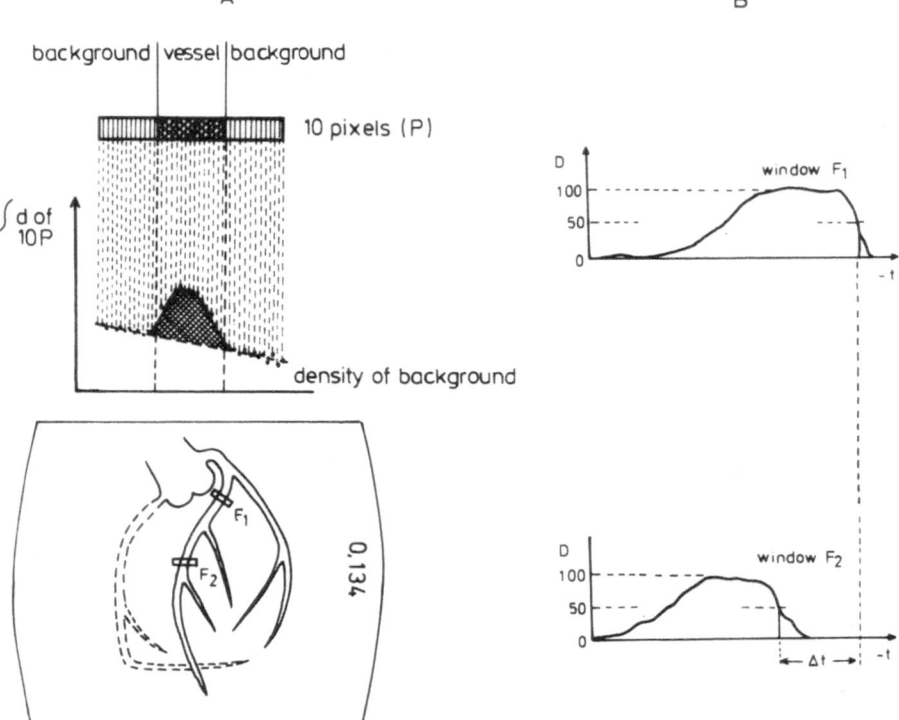

Fig. 1. *Lower left:* coronary arterial tree. F_1 and F_2, densitometric windows positioned over the left anterior descending coronary artery. *Upper left:* principle of densitometric measurement. *Cross-hatched areas,* contrast density of the vessel. For background correction density is measured on both sites of the vessel, too. *Right:* redrawn densograms taken from both windows (read from right to left). Δt is measured from the 50% increase of the leading slopes

The highest flow velocities were measured during early diastole (RCA, 22.3 ± 3.0 cm/s; LAD, 25.0 ± 2.4 cm/s). Three weeks after early recanalisation of infarct-related coronary arteries, mean flow velocity in these vessels on the average was almost normal (16.3 ± 0.7 cm/s; Fig. 3). There was a significant reduction of the amplitude of the velocity pattern. The difference between systolic and early diastolic flow was 14.0 ± 1.6 cm/s in normal vessels and 10.3 ± 1.9 cm/s in recanalised infarct-related vessels (Fig. 3).

In the "slow flow" group only mean flow velocity is quoted (Fig. 4). It was 5.8 ± 1.0 cm/s in the RCA and 7.4 ± 1.1 cm/s in the LCA, which is a statistically significant reduction in comparison with normal.

Discussion

According to our present experience, videodensitometric measurements of coronary flow velocity can be made in native human coronary arteries in about two-thirds of patients; this proportion has been improved to more than 80% in

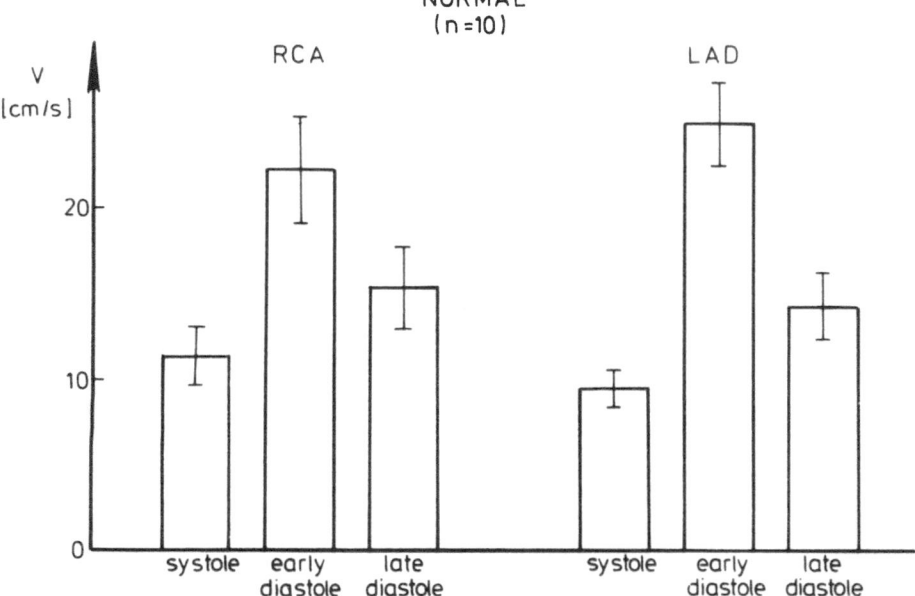

Fig. 2. Mean values and SEM of systolic and diastolic flow velocities in the right (*RCA*) and left anterior descending (*LAD*) coronary artery

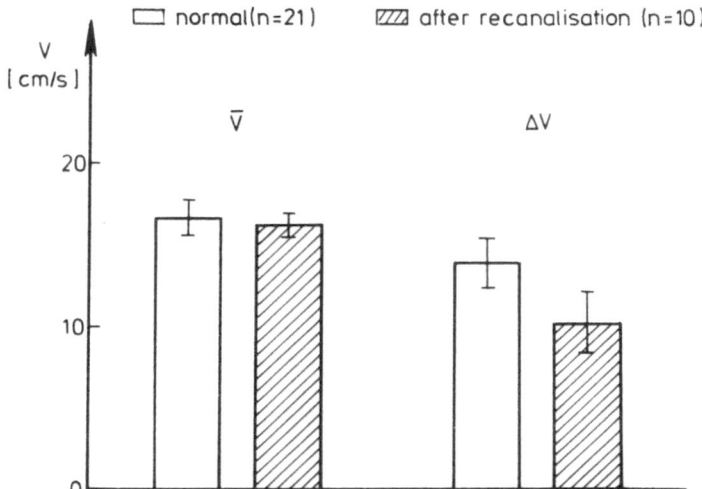

Fig. 3. Mean values and SEM of coronary flow velocities in normal and infarct-related coronary arteries 3 weeks after early recanalisation. $\overline{V}$, mean flow velocity; ΔV, difference of systolic and early diastolic flow velocity. ΔV is significantly reduced in the recanalised coronary arteries

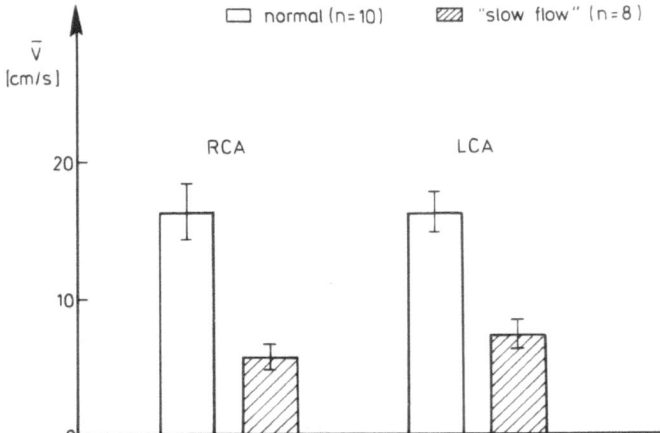

Fig. 4. Mean values and SEM of mean coronary flow velocities in normals and in the "slow flow" group

the last 40 patients. The reproducibility of the method as assessed from independent velocity determinations by two observers showed no systematic deviation. Interobserver variation was found to be 20% ± 8%, mainly due to inaccurate determinations of coronary artery segment length. This problem has been largely reduced by a computer-assisted segment length determination using a light-pen drawing of the coronary arteries in both planes of coronary arteriograms (which in addition reduces the time for evaluation by about two-thirds).

The coronary flow velocities in normal patients agree well with comparable measurements by other authors (Pannek et al. 1978). Estimates of coronary blood flow from known figures by independent methods and myocardial oxygen demand are in the same order of magnitude (105–135 ml/min for the left ventricle), as the flow can be calculated from our flow velocity measurements and coronary artery diameters. Flow velocity patterns during the cardiac cycle accurately reflect the flow patterns, which have been measured using electromagnetic flowmetry both in the experimental animal and in man (Hackbarth et al. 1980) (Fig. 5).

The reduced amplitude of phasic flow velocity in recanalised infarct-related vessels can be explained either by a high-grade residual stenosis or by a diminished systolic-diastolic difference of coronary artery resistance due to a lack or at least a decrease of contractile function in the myocardium supplied by these vessels. Mean flow, however, is about normal – indicating the minor importance of the residual coronary artery stenoses.

The "slow flow" phenomenon which has been observed in eight patients with a history of angina pectoris, but no coronary artery stenosis, is not yet understood. The striking reduction of flow velocity to an average of less than 50% of the so-called normal patients flow velocity is at present thought to be a dysregu-

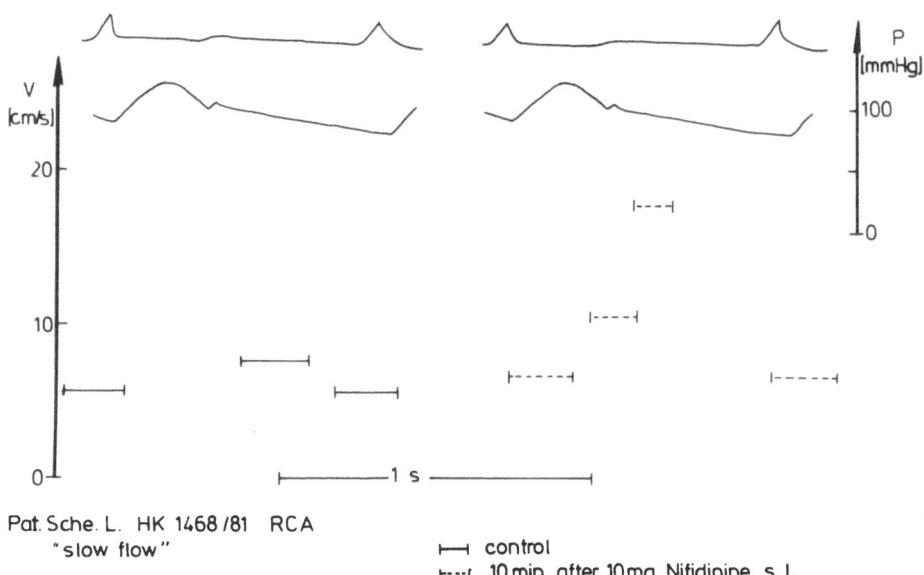

Pat. Sche. L. HK 1468/81 RCA
"slow flow"

⊢—⊣ control
⊢---⊣ 10 min after 10 mg Nifidipine s.l.

Fig. 5. Coronary flow velocity in a patient with "slow flow" phenomenon. *Left:* control values; the *horizontal bars* indicate flow velocities during the cardiac cycle. *Right:* after nifedipine flow velocities are nearly normal

lation of coronary artery resistance on the arteriolar level. Some of these patients complained about anginal symptoms at the time of velocity measurement, others did not. Only one patient had a transient ST segment depression at that time. In one of these patients nifedipine was given sublingually, resulting in a normalisation of the "slow flow" (Fig. 5).

Further intervention studies and simultaneous analyses of myocardial metabolism such as arterovenous oxygen and lactate differences will help to bring further insight into this problem.

References

Bürsch JH, Hahne HJ, Brennecke A, Hetzer R, Heintzen PH (1979) Funktionsangiogramme als Ergebnis der densitometrischen Analyse digitalisierter Röntgenbildserien. Biomed Tech 24 [Suppl] :189–190

Fermor U, Huber H, Neuhaus KL, Schmiel FK, Spiller P (1979) Measurement of flow velocity in the model circulation by videodensitometry. Methodological investigations. Basic Res Cardiol 73:361–377

Hackbarth W, Birks W, Pölitz B, Körfer R, Schmiel FK, Spiller P (1980) Vergleich videodensitometrischer und elektromagnetischer Flußmessung in aortocoronaren Bypassgefäßen. Fortschr Geb Röntgenstr Nuklearmed 132:554–560

Krause H, Neuhaus KL, Sauer G, Schröder R (1980) Videodensitometrische Messung der Flußgeschwindigkeit in Koronararterien. Biomed Tech 25:253–255

Pannek H, Neuhaus KL, Schmiel FK, Spiller P (1978) Röntgenvideodensitometrische Flußmessungen in aortokoronaren Bypass-Gefäßen. Z Kardiol 67:787–796

Rutishauser W, Simon H, Stucky J, Wellauer G (1967) Evaluation of roentgen-cine-
densitometry for flow measurements in models and in the intact circulation. Circulation
36:951

Rutishauser W, Bussmann WD, Noseda G, Meier W, Wellauer J (1970a) Blood flow measurement through single coronary arteries by roentgen videodensitometry. Part I. Am J
Roentgenol Radium Ther Nucl Med 109:12–20

Rutishauser W, Noseda G, Bussmann WD, Preter B (1970b) Blood flow measurement
through single coronary arteries by roentgen densitometry. Part II. Am J Roentgenol
Radium Ther Nucl Med 109:21–24

Smith HC, Frye RL, Donald DE, Davis GD, Pluth JR, Wood EH (1971) Roentgen videodensitometric measure of coronary flow. Mayo Clin Proc 46:800–806

Densitometric Measurement of Phasic Blood Flow in the Coronary Artery System

F. K. Schmiel, M. Block, J. Jehle, B. Pölitz, and P. Spiller

Medizinische Klinik und Poliklinik B, University of Düsseldorf, Moorenstr. 5, D-4000 Düsseldorf, FRG

Since the principle of densitometric flow measurement has already been described by Neuhaus et al. and Simon et al. (this volume), I want to focus here on three methodological problems arising from the application of densitometry on flow measurements in coronary arteries. These are that:
1. The flow rates in coronary arteries are altered by the injection of contrast medium.
2. The motion of the coronary arteries throughout the cardiac cycle is superimposed on the propagation of the contrast medium.
3. The length of the densitometric measurement section is restricted by the ramifications of the coronary arteries.

In order to study the effect of contrast medium on coronary blood flow, we intraoperatively performed electromagnetic flow measurements in aortocoronary bypass grafts and cineangiography simultaneously during revascularization [5]. Figure 1 shows a typical example of a flow recording during and immediately after the injection of contrast medium.

The contrast medium (amidotricoate) was injected as a bolus of 1.5 ml by an ECG-triggered power injector (flow rate, 5 ml/s). The time of injection is indicated by the square pulse with the higher amplitude. Compared with the cycle before the injection, there is a slight increase in flow of about 5% during the first cycle after the injection, due to the increased perfusion pressure. This period is followed by a decrease of flow caused by the high viscosity of the contrast medium. Five seconds after the injection there is a marked increase, which amounts in some cases to more than 100%. About 30 s later the flow reaches its initial value.

If the transit time of the contrast medium is measured from the two densograms using the lines of gravity, the flow measurement is performed just during that interval, where the flow has markedly increased. This problem can be avoided if the flow velocities are determined from the leading slopes of the densograms instead of from the lines of gravity. By this procedure the measurement is usually finished at least 200 ms after the onset of the injection [3]. As can be seen from our electromagnetic flow measurements, during this period almost no changes of flow induced by the injection can be observed [2]. Additionally, this method has the advantage that the measured flow rates can be attached to a definite time interval of the cardiac cycle. Therefore, this can be used as a sampling technique.

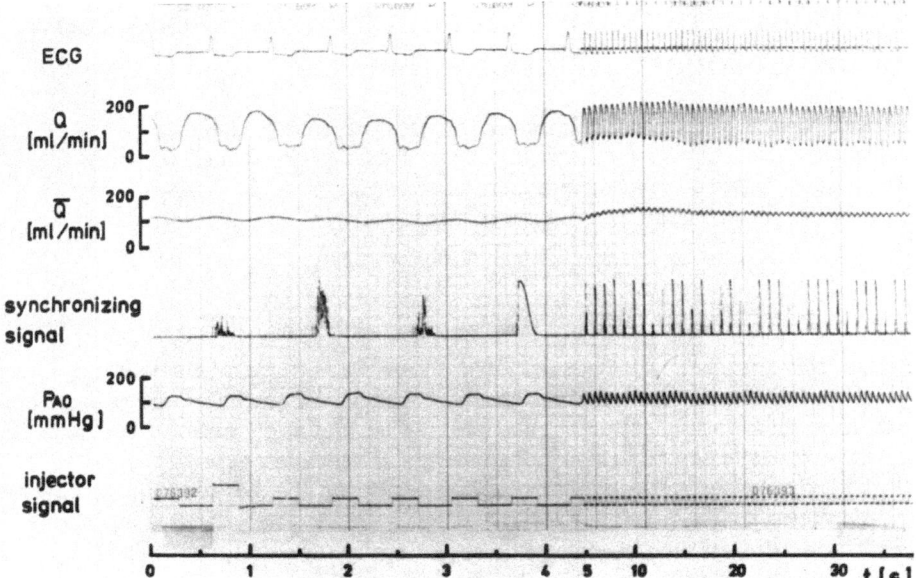

Fig. 1. Recording of the electromagnetically measured graft flow during and immediately after the injection of contrast medium. *From top to bottom:* ECG, instantaneous flow Q, mean flow $\overline{Q}$, synchronizing signal, aortic pressure *PAO*, injector signal (the pulse with the higher amplitude indicates the time of the injection)

The second problem, the motion of the coronary arteries, becomes evident in Fig. 2. If the densitometric measurement windows are held in a fixed position, the vessel motions induce a deformation of the densograms, especially if the artery moves parallel to the vessel axes. In this example the densograms with exclusively horizontal positioning of the windows (lower part) and with a two-dimensional positioning of the windows (upper part) were recorded. The latter method takes both transverse and parallel motion of the vessel into consideration. The transit times determined from the resulting densograms are 110 ms and 180 ms, respectively. To avoid this artifact, control of the position of the windows transverse and parallel to the vessel axes is imperative. As the problem of an automatic two-dimensional control of the window position has not yet been solved, for flow measurements in coronary arteries we use a photodensitometric system with manually positioned windows [4].

The problem of the short measurement section caused by the ramifications of the coronary arteries becomes especially relevant in high-flow velocitites. The two densitometric windows define a fixed length of the measurement segments. The flow velocity is calculated by dividing this length by the measured transit time. Consequently, the relative error of the velocity depends upon the relative error of the time measurement. As the resolution in time of the method is restricted by the cine frame rate on 10 ms, the relative error increases with a decreasing transit time.

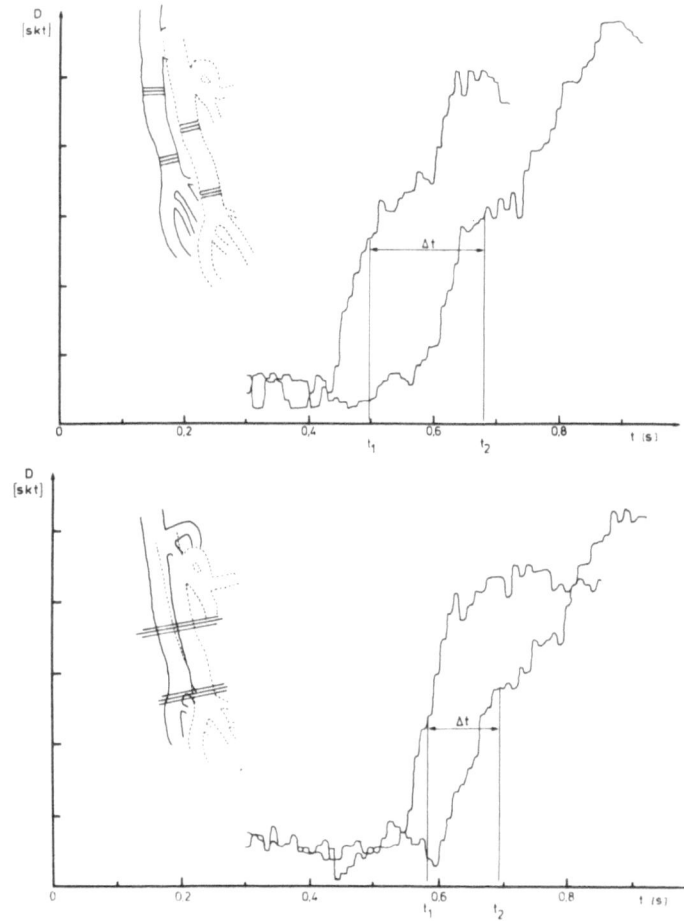

Fig. 2. Densograms resulting from two different position control modes. *Upper panel:* position of the measurement windows is controlled according to the motion of the coronary artery parallel and transverse to the vessel axes. Resulting transit time, 180 ms. *Lower panel:* position of the measurement windows is controlled exclusively transverse to the vessel axes. The densograms are artificially altered by the superimposed vessel motion. The corresponding transit time is shortened to 110 ms

These relationships are explained schematically in Fig. 3. Let us assume a fixed length of 100 m and a transit time of 10 s with an error of ±0.1 s (upper part). The resulting velocity amounts to 10 m/s with a relative error of ±1%. If the measurement distance is reduced from 100 m to 2 m, the transit time will be only 0.2 s, i.e., the resulting relative error will increase to 50%, although the absolute error is the same (middle part). This is just the situation that corresponds to the short measurement segments of the coronary arteries combined with high flow rates.

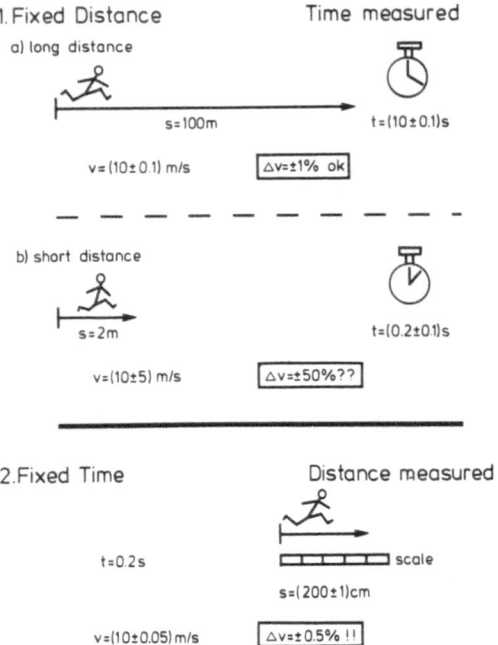

Fig. 3. Relative errors of flow velocities resulting from different measurement principles. *Panel 1:* transit time (resolution ± 0.1 s) is measured for a fixed distance. *a* Long distance, resulting error of calculated velocity ± 1%. *b* Short distance, resulting error of calculated velocity ± 50%. *Panel 2:* displacement (resolution ± 1 cm) is measured for a fixed time interval (same distance and velocities as *1b*). Resulting error of calculated velocity, ± 0.5%

One possible solution of this problem is depicted in the lower part of Fig. 3. If the measurement principle is turned upside down by taking a fixed time interval and measuring the covered displacement – let us assume 0.2 s and 2 m, respectively – the relative error of the velocity depends upon the error in length measurement. This way, the relative error is reduced from 50% to only 0.5%, if the error in length measurement amounts to ±1 cm. This modified principle can be applied on flow measurements using a digital image subtraction system, which will be described later on.

Another possibility to avoid the problem results from our findings in branching vessels [1]. Using photodensitometry, we determined the flow velocities in different segments of the same artery distal and proximal to a ramification (Fig. 4). The velocities measured are plotted on the abscissa and ordinate, respectively. As can be seen from this slide, these velocities are nearly the same in both segments. This agrees with the assumption that the total cross section of the epicardial coronary arteries does not essentially change proximal and distal to ramifications. It is therefore not necessary to worry about branchings lying between the two densitometric windows. It should, however, be considered as a restriction that these results apply only in unstenosed branches.

Finally, our digital image-processing system will be described, by which the displacement of the front of the contrast medium from frame to frame can be measured. As mentioned previously, the flow velocity can be calculated by dividing the measured displacement through the fixed time interval defined by the two corresponding cine frames. The main task of this system is to locate the

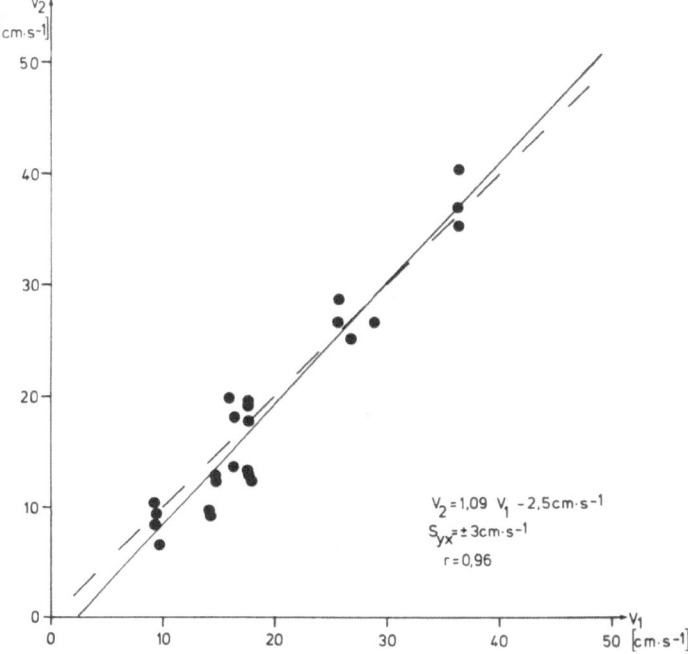

Fig. 4. Flow velocities V_1, V_2 in different unstenosed segments of the same coronary artery (branching vessels or proximal and distal to ramifications). The flow velocities remain almost unchanged

position of the front on each separate frame. Assuming that the only difference between two consecutive frames is a distal displacement of the front, the front can be visualized by subtracting these two consecutive frames. The brightness of the resulting difference image becomes zero in all parts where the two frames are identical, i.e., the difference image shows structures only in those regions where the front of the contrast medium has moved foreward.

The hardware (Fig. 5) of our system is similar to that used by Prof. Heintzen's group (Brennecke and Heintzen, this volume). The cine frame is scanned by a video camera, the output of which is digitized with a rate of 10 MHz and 8-bit resolution (i.e., 256 gray levels). As the transfer rate of our computer (PDP 11/10) is only 1 MHz, the scanned image is buffered as a matrix in a fast semiconductor memory (RAM, 128 kB). From here the frames are transferred via a DMA-interface (DR-11B) into the computer, where the difference images are calculated. After restoring this information in the buffer memory, the difference images can be displayed via a digital-to-analog converter on a TV monitor.

The performance of the system is demonstrated on Fig. 6. The upper panels show two consecutive single frames of a cineangiogram of the left coronary artery at the early filling with contrast medium. From these two frames the difference image is calculated (lower left panel). The positions of the front of

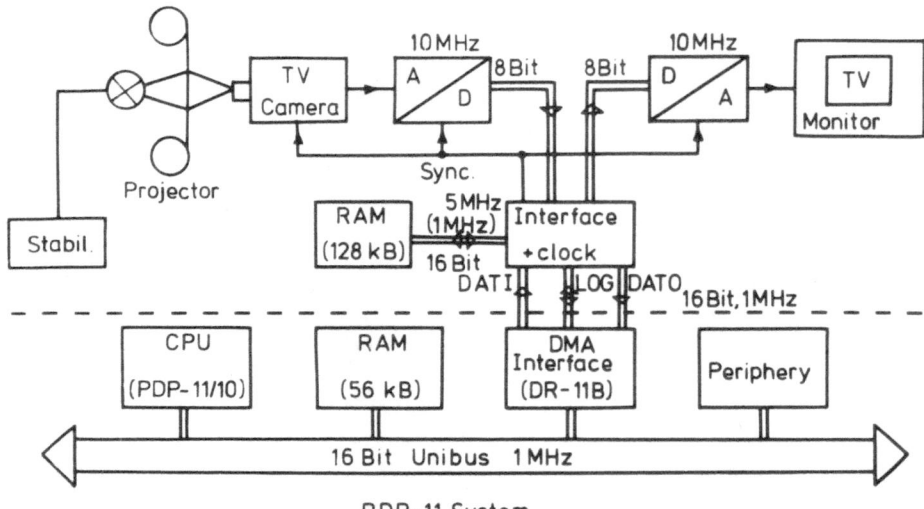

Fig. 5. Digital image processing system. The cine frames are scanned by a video camera and digitized with a rate of 10 MHz. As the transfer rate of the computer system is only 1 MHz, the digitized image is buffered as a matrix in a fast semiconductor memory (RAM, 128 kB). The difference images are calculated by the computer and restored in the buffer memory (RAM, 128 kB), the contents of which can be displayed on a TV monitor

the contrast material in the left anterior descending and circumflex artery are indicated by the triangular structures. The structures over the vessel are caused by inhomogenous mixing of the contrast medium. The grainy structure of the total background is due to a nonuniform distribution of silver in the film emulsion. The quality of the image can be improved by digital filtering and smoothing (lower right panel).

Flow velocities cannot be determined from only one difference image. For this purpose a series of images is necessary (Fig. 7). The propagation of the front can be tracked from frame to frame (indicated by the cross-hair marks). The velocity of the front can be quantified by plotting the position vs time. An example of the resulting displacement-time diagram is shown in Fig. 8. The diagram consists of two phases, each being linear, i.e., the flow velocity during each phase remains constant. In all biphasic displacement-time curves we have found the flow velocity of the first phase to be higher than that of the second one. From this we infer that the first phase is caused artificially by the pressure increase due to the injection of the contrast medium. The velocity during the second phase in this example equals 15 cm/s. Regarding the abscissa of this diagram, it can be seen that the propagation of the front can only be traced correctly for about 100 ms. The slope of the plot corresponds to the velocity of the front. As this period is relatively short with respect to a heart cycle, this method must be used as a sampling technique. This is done by ECG-triggered bolus injections covering different phases of a cardiac cycle.

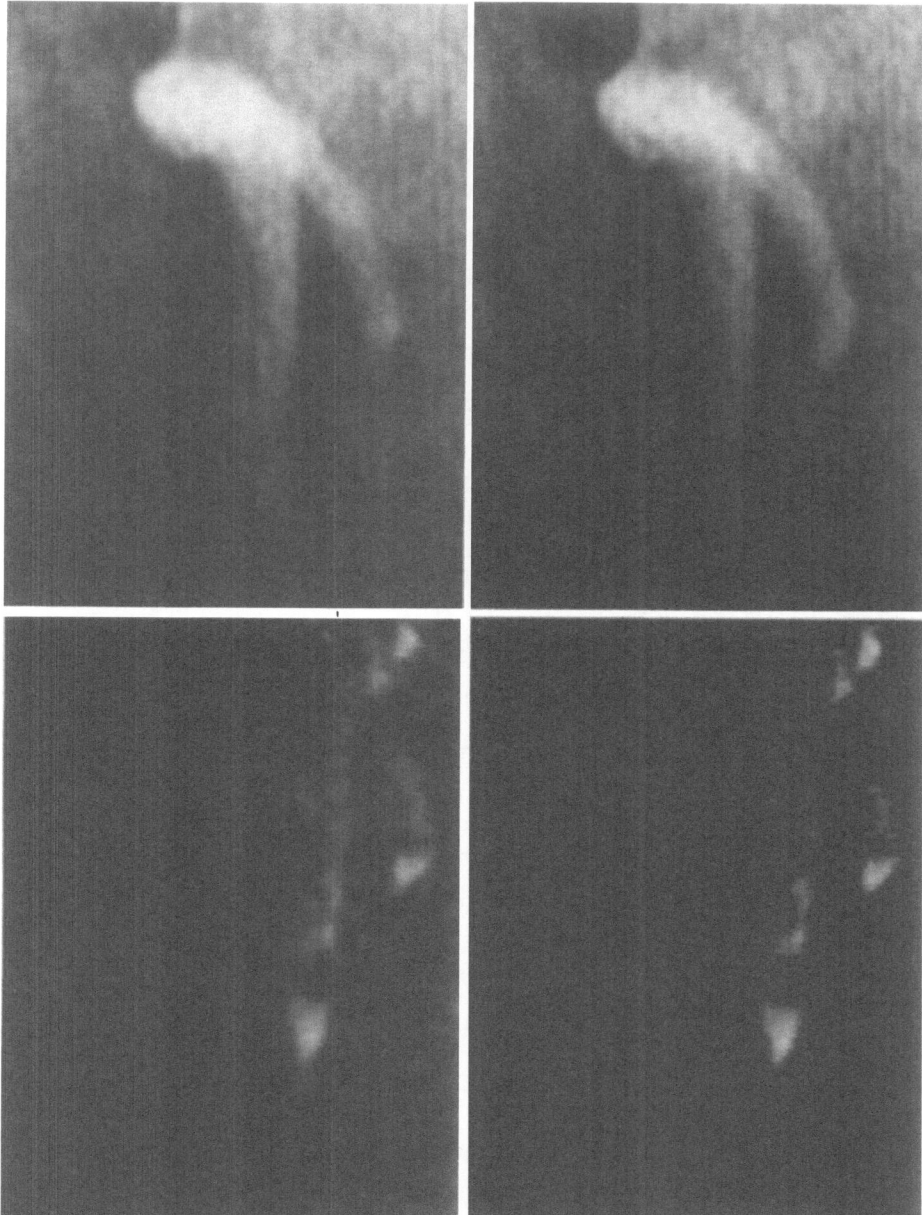

Fig. 6. Two consecutive single frames of the left coronary artery (*upper left* and *right*). The inhomogeneous background structures of the corresponding difference image (*lower left*) can be removed by digital filtering (*lower right*). The positions of the front of the contrast medium are visualized by the triangular structures

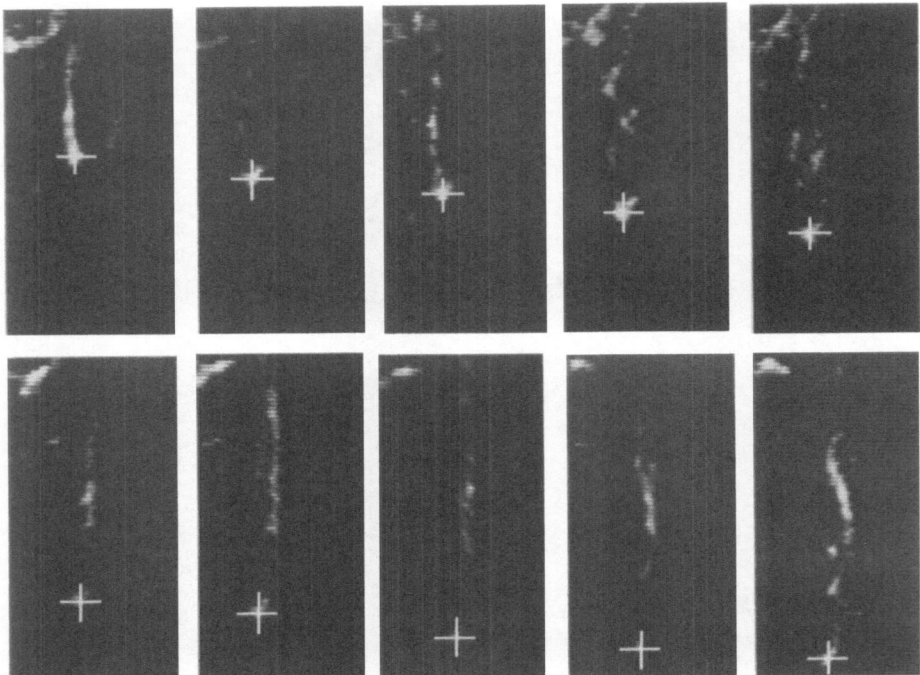

Fig. 7. Ten consecutive difference images of the passage of the contrast medium through the left coronary artery. The position of the front is indicated by the *cross-hair marks*

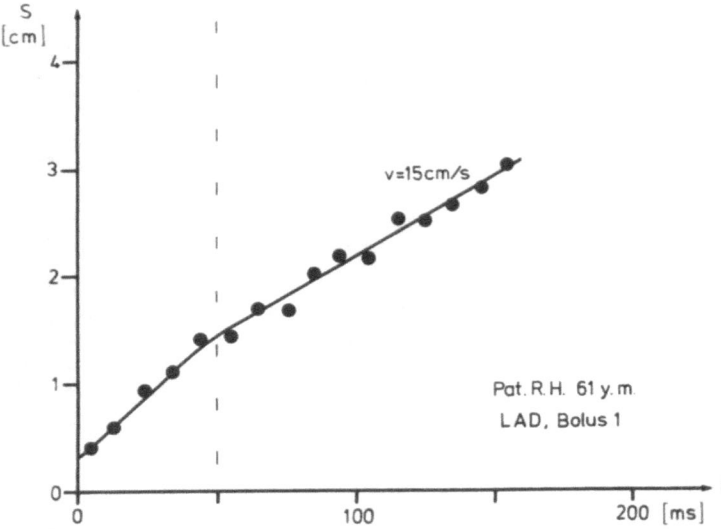

Fig. 8. Displacement-time diagram resulting from a series of difference images. The displacement (*ordinate*) is plotted vs time (*abscissa*). The velocity is determined from the slope. The steeper slope during the first 50 ms is caused by the increased perfusion pressure due to injection

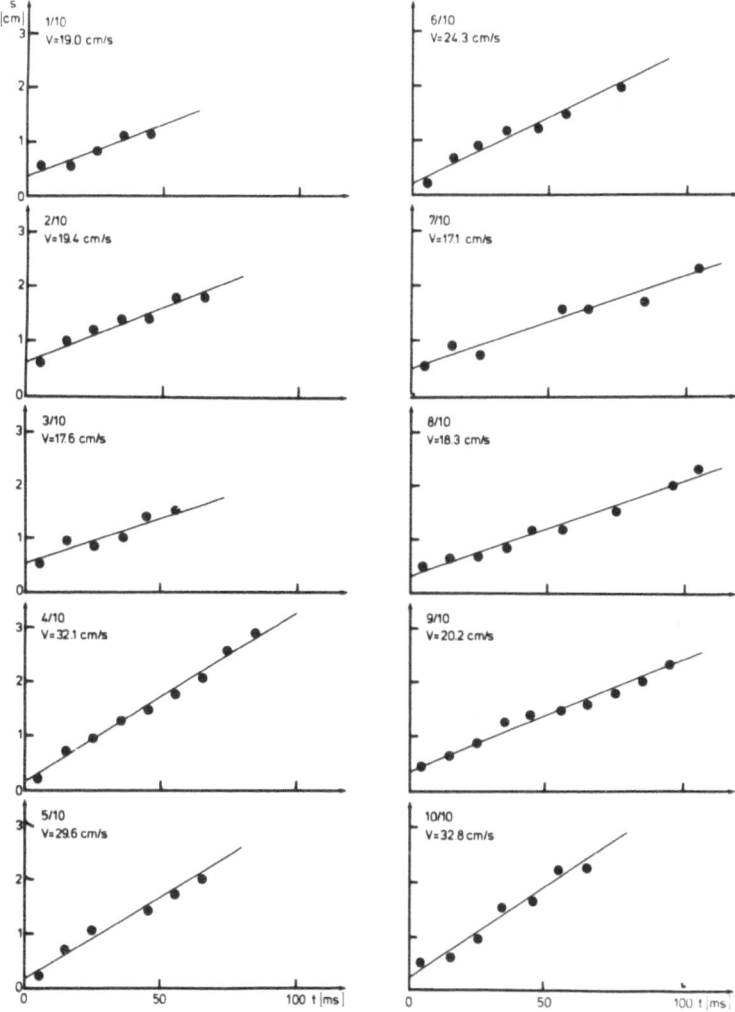

Fig. 9. Displacement-time diagrams and corresponding flow velocities determined from ten bolus injections into the right coronary artery. The measurements cover different phases of a cardiac cycle (sampling technique)

As an example, Fig. 9 demonstrates the displacement-time functions of a right coronary artery, where 10 boli of contrast medium had been injected. From the resulting velocities the flow curve can be reconstructed (Fig. 10). The ordinate depicts the velocity, the abscissa the corresponding time interval. The reconstructed flow curve (indicated by the dashed line) shows the typical pulsatile flow, as known from electromagnetic measurements.

In summarizing the advantages of digital densitometry for flow measurements in coronary arteries, it can be stated that:

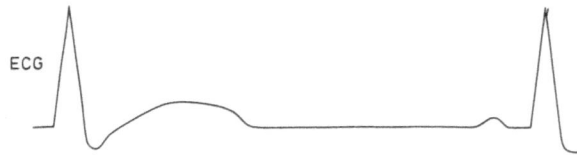

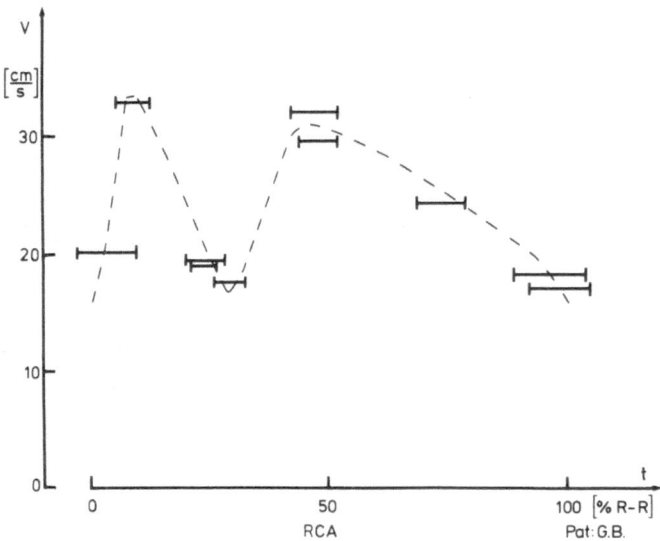

Fig. 10. Flow curve of the right coronary artery (*dashed line*) reconstructed from the ten bolus injections (Fig. 9). The *horizontal bars* depict the flow velocity (*ordinate*) and the time interval (*abscissa*) during which the flow was measured. The *abscissa* is calibrated in percentages of the R-R interval of the patient's ECG (*upper part*)

1. Instead of time measurement, digital densitometry allows the measurement of displacement of contrast medium. The velocities are determined from plots and not from a single measurement as in videodensitometry. This is combined with higher accuracy, especially in high flow rates.
2. Superimposed vessel motions are visualized in the difference image and can easily be taken into account. We plan to automate this procedure using a program for pattern recognition.

References

1. Block M, Jehle J, Pölitz B, Schmiel FK, Spiller P (1982) Bestimmung der phasischen Flußgeschwindigkeiten im Koronargefäßsystem mit einem einfachen, fotodensitometrischen Verfahren. Fortschr Rontgenstr 136:283–290

2. Hackbarth W, Bircks W, Pölitz B, Körfer R, Schmiel FK, Spiller P (1980) Vergleich videodensitometrischer und elektromagnetischer Flußmessungen in aortokoronaren Bypassgefäßen. Fortschr Rontgenstr 132:554–560
3. Pannek H, Neuhaus KL, Schmiel FK, Spiller P (1978) Röntgenvideodensitometrische Flußmessungen in aortokoronaren Bypass-Gefäßen. Z Kardiol 67:787–796
4. Pölitz B, Block M, Jehle J, Schmiel FK, Spiller P (1980) Bestimmung der systolischen und diastolischen Flußgeschwindigkeit im Koronargefäßsystem mit einem einfachen, photo-densitometrischen Verfahren. Biomed Tech 25:365–367
5. Schmiel FK, Hackbarth W, Körfer R, Pölitz B, Spiller PW, Bircks W (1979) Flow measurements and simultaneously performed angiography of aorto-coronary bypass grafts during bypass surgery. Thorac Cardiovasc Surg 27:386–389

Subject Index